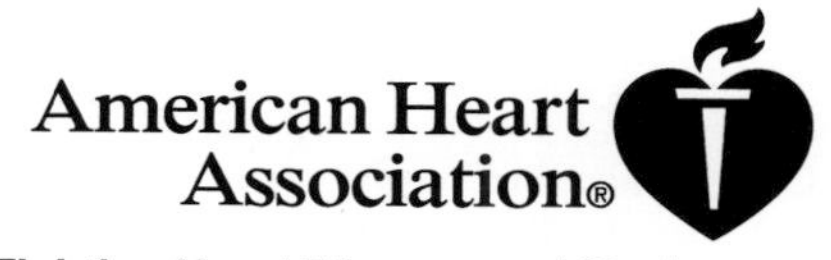

Fighting Heart Disease and Stroke

Monograph Series

HEART FAILURE: *PROVIDING OPTIMAL CARE*

Previously published in the American Heart Association Monograph Series:

Cardiovascular Applications of Magnetic Resonance
Edited by Gerald M. Pohost, MD

Cardiovascular Response to Exercise
Edited by Gerald F. Fletcher, MD

Congestive Heart Failure: Current Clinical Issues
Edited by Gemma T. Kennedy, RN, PhD and Michael H. Crawford, MD

Atrial Arrhythmias: State of the Art
Edited by John P. DiMarco, MD, PhD and Eric N. Prystowsky, MD

Invasive Cardiology: Current Diagnostic and Therapeutic Issues
Edited by George W. Vetrovec, MD and Blase Carabello, MD

Syndromes of Atherosclerosis: Correlations of Clinical Imaging and Pathology
Edited by Valentin Fuster, MD, PhD

Pathophysiology of Tachycardia-Induced Heart Failure
Edited by Francis G. Spinale, MS, MD, PhD

Exercise and Heart Failure
Edited by Gary J. Balady, MD and Ileana L. Piña, MD

Sudden Cardiac Death: Past, Present, and Future
Edited by Sandra B. Dunbar, RN, DSN, Kenneth A. Ellenbogen, MD, and Andrew E. Epstein, MD

Hormonal, Metabolic, and Cellular Influences on Cardiovascular Disease in Women
Edited by Trudy M. Forte, PhD

Discontinuous Conduction in the Heart
Edited by Peter M. Spooner, PhD, Ronald W. Joyner, MD, PhD, and José Jalife, MD

Frontiers in Cerebrovascular Disease: Mechanisms, Diagnosis, and Treatment
Edited by James T. Robertson, MD and Thaddeus S. Nowak, Jr., PhD

Current and Future Applications of Magnetic Resonance in Cardiovascular Disease
Edited by Charles B. Higgins, MD, Joanne S. Ingwall, PhD, and Gerald M. Pohost, MD

Pulmonary Edema
Edited by E. Kenneth Weir, MD and John T. Reeves, MD

The Vulnerable Atherosclerotic Plaque: Understanding, Identification, and Modification
Edited by Valentin Fuster, MD, PhD

Obesity: Impact on Cardiovascular Disease
Edited by Gerald F. Fletcher, MD, Scott M. Grundy, MD, PhD, and Laura L. Hayman, PhD, RN, FAAN

The Fetal and Neonatal Pulmonary Circulations
Edited by E. Kenneth Weir, MD, Stephen L. Archer, MD, and John T. Reeves, MD

Ventricular Fibrillation: A Pediatric Problem
Edited by Linda Quan, MD and Wayne H. Franklin, MD

Markers in Cardiology: Current and Future Clinical Applications
Edited by Jesse E. Adams III, MD, Fred S. Apple, PhD, Allan S. Jaffe, MD, and Alan H.B. Wu, PhD

Compliance in Healthcare and Research
Edited by Lora E. Burke, PhD, MPH, RN and Ira S. Ockene, MD

Cerebrovascular Disease: Momentum at the End of the Second Millennium
Edited by Dennis W. Choi, MD, PhD, Ralph G. Dacey, Jr., MD, Chung Y. Hsu, MD, PhD, and William J. Powers, MD

Assessing and Modifying the Vulnerable Atherosclerotic Plaque
Edited by Valentin Fuster, MD, PhD and William Insull, Jr., MD

Interactions of Blood and the Pulmonary Circulation
Edited by E. Kenneth Weir, MD, Helen L. Reeve, PhD, and John T. Reeves, MD

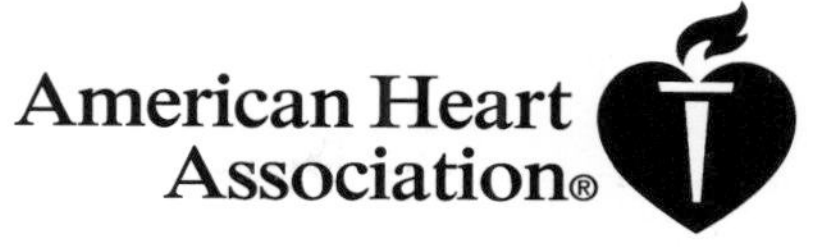

Monograph Series

Heart Failure:
Providing Optimal Care

Edited by

Mariell Jessup, MD, FACC, FAHA
Associate Professor of Medicine
Medical Director
Heart Failure/Transplantation Program
Division of Cardiovascular Medicine
Hospital of the University of Pennsylvania
Philadelphia, Pennsylvania

and

Kathleen M. McCauley, PhD, RN, CS, FAAN, FAHA
Associate Professor of Cardiovascular Nursing
Cardiovascular Clinical Specialist
University of Pennsylvania
School of Nursing
Philadelphia, Pennsylvania

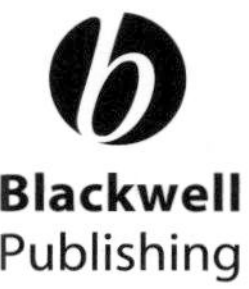

Futura, An imprint of Blackwell Publishing

Blackwell Publishing, Inc./Futura Division, 3 West Main Street, Elmsford, New York 10523, USA
Blackwell Publishing, Inc., 350 Main Street, Malden, Massachusetts 02148-5020, USA
Blackwell Publishing Ltd, 9600 Garsington Road, Oxford OX4 2DQ
Blackwell Science Asia Pty Ltd, 550 Swanston Street, Carlton, Victoria 3053, Australia

02 03 04 05 5 4 3 2 1

ISBN: 1-4051-0375-2

Library of Congress Cataloging-in-Publication Data

Heart failure: providing optimal care/edited by Mariell Jessup and Kathleen M. McCauley.
p.; cm.
Includes bibliographical references and index.
ISBN 1-4051-0375-2
1. Heart failure.
[DNLM: 1. Heart Failure, Congestive—therapy. 2. Heart Failure, Congestive—prevention & control. WG 370 H43654 2004] I. Jessup, Mariell L. II. McCauley, Kathleen M., 1949–

RC685.C53H446 2004
616.1'29—dc21 2003014050

A catalogue record for this title is available from the British Library

Acquisitions: Steven Korn
Production: Julie Elliott
Typesetter: SNP Best-set Typesetter Ltd., Hong Kong
Printed and bound by MPG Books Ltd, Bodmin, Cornwall, UK

For further information on Blackwell Publishing, visit our website:
www.futuraco.com

Preface

As the science of medicine has grown, so too have the number of options for disease specific interventions, therapies and treatments. This expansion of *the state of science* has left the practitioner with an equally bewildering *state of the practice* to understand and from which to prescribe. All too often it is one matter to produce a guideline and a very different one to follow it and implement it in the individual patient. The successful management of the patient with heart failure involves the utilization of a growing number of sophisticated diagnostic tests and a complex array of medicines, pacing devices, and surgical approaches. Patients with apparently identical systolic dysfunction may be dissimilar with respect to functional status, mitral valve competency, degree of ischemia, or pulmonary hypertension, all of which will determine therapy and/or prognosis.

It is our goal that this monograph will help bridge the chasm between science and practice for the busy clinician confronted with a patient suffering from heart failure symptoms. Specifically, we selected contributors who could address evidenced-based practice across the range of patient acuity and clinical care settings. These authors interpret basic research and apply the results to the real world of practice. We are very grateful, indeed, for the efforts of our contributors and we hope that you will find this monograph helpful in your day to day management of the patient with heart failure.

We are, likewise, indebted to the Council on Cardiovascular Nursing from the American Heart Association in proposing this partnership with Futura Publishing so that this, and future disease management monographs, could be developed.

Mariell Jessup, MD, FACC, FAHA
Kathleen McCauley, PhD, RN, CS, FAAN, FAHA

Contributors

Michael A. Acker, MD Associate Professor of Surgery, Division of Cardiothoracic Surgery, Department of Surgery, University of Pennsylvania School of Medicine, Philadelphia, PA

Nancy M. Albert, MSN, RN, CCNS, CCRN, CNA Manager, Heart Failure Disease Management Program, George M. and Linda H. Kaufman Center for Heart Failure, The Cleveland Clinic Foundation, Cleveland, OH

David W. Baker, MD, MPH Associate Professor of Medicine, Center for Health Care Research and Policy, Case Western Reserve University at MetroHealth Medical Center, Cleveland, OH

Suzette Cardin, RN, DNSc, FAAN Adjunct Assistant Professor, UCLA School of Nursing, Los Angeles, CA

Arthur M. Feldman, MD, PhD Magee Professor and Chair, Department of Medicine, Jefferson Medical College, Philadelphia PA

John M. Fontaine, MD Associate Professor of Medicine, MCP Hahnemann University; Director of Arrhythmia Services, Medical College of Pennsylvania Hospital, Philadelphia, PA

Anna Gawlinski, RN, DNSc, CS, ACNP Director, Evidence-based Practice Initiative, Associate Adjunct Professor, University of California, Los Angeles, Medical Center and School of Nursing, Los Angeles, CA

Lee R. Goldberg, MD, MPH, FACC Assistant Professor of Medicine, Division of Cardiovascular Medicine, Heart Failure/Transplant Program, Hospital of the University of Pennsylvania, Philadelphia, PA

Mariell Jessup, MD, FACC, FAHA Associate Professor of Medicine, Medical Director, Heart Failure/Transplantation Program, Division of Cardiovascular Medicine, Hospital of the University of Pennsylvania, Philadelphia, PA

Kathleen M. McCauley, PhD, RN, CS, FAAN, FAHA Associate Professor of Cardiovascular Nursing, Cardiovascular Clinical Specialist, University of Pennsylvania School of Nursing, Philadelphia, PA

Salpy V. Pamboukian, MD, FACC Rush Presbyterian St. Luke's Medical Center, Rush Heart Failure and Cardiac Transplant Program, Chicago, IL

Sara Paul, RN, MSN, FNP Director, Heart Function Clinic, Hickory Cardiology Associates, Hickory, NC

David Rabin, MD, FACC North Shore Cardiovascular Associates, Salem, MA

Virginia Schneider, RN The Cardiovascular Institute of the UPMC Health System, Pittsburgh, PA

Ozlem Soran, MD The Cardiovascular Institute of the UPMC Health System, Pittsburgh, PA

Lynne Warner Stevenson, MD Associate Professor of Medicine, Harvard Medical School, Director, Heart Failure and Cardiomyopathy Program, Brigham and Women's Hospital, Boston, MA

James B. Young, MD Kaufman Center for Heart Failure, Department of Cardiovascular Medicine, Cleveland Clinic Foundation, Cleveland, OH

David Zeltsman, MD The Glover Clinic, Thoracic and Cardiovascular Surgery; Delaware County Memorial Hospital, Drexel Hill PA; Mercy Fitzgerald Hospital, Darby, PA

Contents

Chapter 1

Heart Failure as a National Health Problem: the Burden of Heart Failure

Arthur M. Feldman, MD, PhD,
Virginia Schneider, RN, and Ozlem Soran, MD

The Burden of Heart Failure

Heart failure is a disease of epidemic proportions in the U.S., but only recently have health-care organizations, governmental agencies, and the general public begun to recognize this disease as a major cause of human suffering and a contributor to increased health-care cost. The term *heart failure* does not describe a single "disease," but rather a constellation of signs and symptoms, including shortness of breath, overwhelming fatigue, and edema. These symptoms can be caused by a variety of specific cardiovascular diseases, including dilated cardiomyopathies, restrictive and constrictive myopathies, hypertrophic cardiomyopathies, and valvular heart disease; however, dilated cardiomyopathies and systolic dysfunction predominate as a cause of heart failure in the U.S. Although physicians recognize the significance of the diagnosis of heart failure, the term *heart failure* has always been confusing for patients, as it implies that the heart has "failed" or stopped, rather than the fact that heart failure represents a progressive, though usually lethal, disease. Indeed, heart failure has frequently been confused with a "heart attack" or with sudden death. As the U.S. population ages and clinicians have become increasingly adept at ameliorating the immediate consequences of acute coronary syndromes, the population of patients with heart failure has increased steadily and has been associated with a dramatic increase in health-care costs. Thus, the impact of heart failure in

From: Jessup M, McCauley KM (eds). *Heart Failure: Providing Optimal Care.* Elmsford, NY: Futura, an imprint of Blackwell Publishing; ©2003.

patients in both the U.S. and around the world continues to rise. In this first chapter, we will review our current understanding of:

- The incidence of heart failure
- Its associated morbidity and mortality
- The influence of gender, race and socioeconomic status on the demographics of heart failure
- The effects of heart failure on health-care costs
- How new therapeutic interventions might alter the demographics of heart failure in the future

The Incidence of Heart Failure

Seminal studies assessing the incidence of heart failure have come from the ongoing Framingham Heart Study. Begun in 1949, the Framingham study enrolled men and women between the ages of 30 and 62 and followed them throughout their lives. The initial Framingham report on the incidence and natural history of heart failure, by McKee and colleagues in 1971,[1] was one of the first reports to alert clinicians to the overwhelming burden of heart failure in a representative community population. Although the absolute number of individuals with heart failure was relatively small (142 cases), the initial observations were largely confirmed over time as the data were reanalyzed, with an increasing number of the over 5000 participants in the study being found to have the disease. Evaluation in the 1980s found that the annual age-adjusted incidence of heart failure in persons greater than or equal to 45 years of age was 7.2 cases/1000 in men and 4.7 cases/1000 in women.[2] In addition, the age-adjusted prevalence of overt heart failure was 24/1000 in men and 25/1000 in women. The Framingham studies have also shown a marked relationship between incidence of heart failure and age. Heart failure was found to affect nearly 1% of subjects in their 50s and rose progressively with age, affecting nearly 10% of people in their 80s.[3] The annual incidence also increased with age: the diagnosis was made in 0.2% of individuals between the ages of 45 and 54 and 4.0% of men aged 85 to 94 years. Indeed, the incidence of heart failure nearly doubled with each increasing decade of age,[3] with the lifetime risk of developing heart failure estimated at being 20% for men and women.[4] Similar epidemiologic data from the Rochester Epidemiology Project, which identified persons with a new diagnosis of congestive heart beginning in 1982 in Rochester, Minnesota, found similar results—underscoring the importance of heart failure in community populations.[5] Furthermore, the epidemiology of heart failure in the United States does not differ substantially from that in Europe (Table 1).[6] Unfortunately, despite improvements in the treat-

Table 1

Incidence* of Congestive Heart Failure: Comparison of the Framingham, Massachusetts, and Swedish Cohorts with the Population of Rochester, Minnesota. (Reproduced with permission from Rodeheffer et al.[5])

	Framingham†		Rochester	
Age (yr)	Men	Women	Men	Women
45–54	200	100	80	0
55–64	400	300	402	128
65–74	800	500	1319	724

	Swedish men born in 1913‡	Rochester (men)
50–54	150	86
55–60	430	402
61–67	1020	1618

*Rates per 100,000 person-years.

† Data based on 34 years of follow-up experience.[3]

‡ Data based on 17 years of follow-up experience.[95]

ments for ischemic heart disease and hypertension, the incidence of heart failure did not decline appreciably during progressive follow-up,[7,8] a finding that might be attributable to the aging of the population and/or improved techniques for preserving ischemic myocardium.[9]

Both systolic and diastolic dysfunction can result in the clinical syndrome of heart failure. However, early population or community-based studies were not able to differentiate adequately between systolic and diastolic dysfunction. More recently, using echocardiography, investigators assessed the proportions of individuals with impaired left ventricular systolic dysfunction (defined as an ejection fraction less than 50%) versus those with normal left ventricular function in a subgroup of the Framingham Heart Study cohort.[10] Subjects with heart failure were compared with age- and gender-matched control subjects. Of the patients with heart failure, 51% had normal systolic function. Similar results were obtained in a comparable community-based study assessing all incident cases of heart failure in Olmsted County, Minnesota, in 1991.[11] In the Framingham Study, the group with normal left ventricular function had a higher proportion of women (65%), whereas the group with diminished systolic function had a larger proportion of men (75%). Interestingly, the risk of death in the two populations was similar (adjusted hazard ratio with normal ejection fraction 4.06; with decreased ejection fraction 4.31). Since hypertension is a major cause of both hypertrophy and eventual systolic dysfunction, it is not surprising that in over 5000 subjects from the original Framingham Heart Study and the Framingham Offspring Study, the most common risk factor for the development of heart failure was hypertension.[12] Additional risk factors among hypertensive subjects included a myocardial infarction, diabetes, left ventricular hypertrophy, and valvular heart disease.

In all assessments of the epidemiology of heart failure, investigators include patients who have been diagnosed by their physicians as having heart failure. This diagnosis is usually based on symptoms at the time of presentation to an outpatient office or in-patient facility. Using these criteria, current estimates suggest that there are over 5 million patients in the United States who carry the diagnosis of heart failure. However, these evaluations may grossly underestimate the total population of patients with left ventricular dysfunction, as many patients have left ventricular dysfunction and remain asymptomatic. Recently, investigators performed echocardiograms on the first-degree, asymptomatic relatives of patients with nonischemic dilated cardiomyopathy. These studies revealed that 29% of the patients who were studied demonstrated abnormalities on their echocardiograms. Additional support for the presence of a large number of patients with asymptomatic left ventricular dysfunction in the U.S. comes from a study measuring echocardiographic parameters in a population of patients without heart failure or a history of a myocardial infarction.[13] In 4744 subjects, 5.2% of men and 1.9% of women had diminished fractional shortening on their baseline studies. Furthermore, 74 of 4744 subjects developed heart failure during up to 11 years of follow-up. While these studies are highly suggestive of a large number of asymptomatic individuals, it should be noted that echocardiographic diagnostic criteria for classification of the heart failure phenotype need to be developed and standardized.[14,15]

Heart Failure and Survival

A pathognomonic feature of heart failure is that patients have an absolutely abysmal prognosis. Indeed, the Framingham study found that the probability of death within 4 years of the first diagnosis of heart failure was 52% in men and 34% in women, regardless of the underlying cause of the disease. These statistics did not change substantially over time, as later studies assessing survival in 652 members of the Framing-

Table 2

Survival after Congestive Heart Failure as Estimated by Kaplan–Meier Methods. (Adapted from Ho and colleagues[7])

	Survival rates			
	1 year	2 years	5 years	10 years
Men	0.57	0.46	0.25	0.11
Women	0.64	0.56	0.38	0.21

ham Heart Study who developed heart failure between 1948 and 1988 demonstrated a median survival after the onset of heart failure of 1.7 years in men and 3.2 years in women.[2] Overall 1-year and 5-year mortality rates were 43% and 75% in men and 36% and 62% in women, respectively (Table 2). Mortality increased with advancing age in both sexes; however, the prognosis did not appear to change over the 40 years of observation. These data have been substantiated by a number of different studies. Franciosa and colleagues[16] found that the overall mortality rate was 34% at 1 year, 59% at 2 years, and 76% at 3 years in a population of 182 patients with symptomatic heart failure. In the Olmsted County studies, two incident cohorts were followed—one first identified in 1981 and the second in 1991.[8] The 1-year mortality was 28% and 23% in the two groups, respectively. More recently, Cowie and colleagues identified 220 new cases of heart failure from a population of 151,000 individuals who had undergone echocardiography during 1995 and 1996. The 6- and 12-month mortality rates were 30% and 38%, respectively.[17]

Similar studies have also been performed in Europe. In a group of unselected patients with heart failure in Scotland, a country in which all hospitalizations and deaths are captured in a single database, 66,547 patients were studied over a period of 10 years from 1986 to 1995.[18] When measuring case fatality rates, median survival rates were 1.47 years in men and 1.39 years in women. Unlike studies in Olmsted County, in which survival did not differ in a community population between 1981 and 1991,[8] case fatality rates in Scotland decreased statistically, albeit modestly (18% in men and 15% in women) during the study period. These results are also in conflict with recent studies in the U.S. suggesting that the overall mortality for heart failure does not appear to have changed over the past two decades in community populations.[19] The apparent benefit in Scotland might be due to the fact that the database came from hospital admissions, the patients were older than other studies, including Framingham, the study population more adequately represented the gender mix of the population than do most clinical trials, or there may have been better compliance with recommended medical therapies by either physicians or patients. Alternatively, because the database lacks extensive clinical information which could more definitively identify the characteristics of the population, the relationship between the results of the database study and the real world might be skewed.[20] Regardless of this, the MacIntyre study[18] points out our need to assiduously assess the changing population dynamics of heart failure.

A large number of variables have been identified that can accurately predict prognosis in patients with heart failure. By multivariate analysis, a key predictor of a poor outcome is the presence of ischemic heart disease as an etiologic factor.[21,22] Mortality is also improved in patients whose care is provided in a major teaching hospital compared with a minor teaching or nonteaching hospital.[23] Hemodynamic indices, including left ventricular filling pressure,[16] have variably been reported to predict prognosis, while other factors have also been independently associated with prognosis, including New York Heart Association functional class, the presence of a third heart sound, cardiac output, mean arterial pressure, and pulmonary artery diastolic pressure.[24] However, the most commonly used predictive tool in patients being evaluated for cardiac transplantation is the peak Vo_2.[25,26] Interestingly, the presence of biopsy-proven myocarditis did not appear to increase the 5-year prognosis in comparison with patients having idiopathic dilated cardiomyopathy.[27] Future predictors of prognosis will likely include markers of a patient's genotype, as recent studies have suggested that the presence of maladaptive polymorphisms can accurately predict outcome in patients with heart failure awaiting cardiac transplantation.[28,29]

Heart Failure Hospitalizations

Heart failure is associated with a substantial morbidity as well as an abysmal prognosis. Although "morbidity" is difficult to define, it has conveniently been defined as hospitalization for worsening heart failure. Indeed, this would appear to be a reasonable definition of morbidity, since patients are most likely to seek medical attention when their symptoms have worsened. Objective data regarding hospitalization for heart failure can be obtained from the National Hospital Discharge Survey.[30] When assessing data for the years 1985 through 1995, Haldeman and colleagues reported that the number of hospitalizations increased from 577,000 to 871,000 for a first-listed diagnosis and from 1.7 to 2.6 million for any diagnosis of heart failure.[30] Almost 78% of the men and 85% of the women who were hospitalized with heart failure were 65 years of age or older—a finding that was not surprising, in light of the fact that heart failure is the most common principal diagnosis for patients of this age group who are hospitalized in the U.S.[9] Indeed, it has been projected that over 1,000,000 patients will be hospitalized for heart failure in 2001. With the population increasingly aging (the number of adults over the age of 65 is expected to double by the year 2030),[31] the overwhelming burden of heart failure will naturally increase. However, aggressive efforts to control the cost of care for patients with congestive heart failure with disease management programs may show long-term benefit on hospital admission rates. For example, in Oregon, a region in which aggressive attempts have been made to decrease hospitalization rates, the number of hospital admissions between 1991 and 1995 remained relatively stable. The age- and sex-standardized admission rates among people aged 65 years or older were 13.9/1000 in 1991 and 12.9/1000 in 1995.[32] Furthermore, the average length of stay was decreased from 5.01 to 3.95 days during that same period, and the in-hospital mortality rate decreased from 6.9% to 4.7%. Another recent study at a single academic medical center demonstrated a significant decrease in adjusted length of stay between 1986 and 1996, with an accompanying decrease in in-hospital mortality.[33] However, the use of cardiac procedures and overall costs increased during that time period. In addition, it is important to point out that while admissions have increased, so have readmissions. Indeed, a recent study by Vinson and colleagues[34] demonstrated that 47% of elderly patients discharged from the hospital with the diagnosis of heart failure were readmitted within 3 months of the initial discharge. Both medical care and social support (e.g., education) appear to be important factors in contributing to readmission rates.[35] In a retrospective study of over 42,000 patients, hospital readmission was most common in black people, in patients with Medicare and Medicaid insurance, patients with more comorbid illnesses, and in those in whom telemetry monitoring was used during the index hospitalization.[36] However, recent studies suggest that measurement of plasma levels of B-natriuretic peptide (BNP) may provide a sensitive measure of the risk of rehospitalization in patients with heart failure.[37]

Gender and Race in the Demographics of Heart Failure

Although heart failure affects all genders and races, studies over the past three decades have demonstrated profound differences in the demographics of heart failure in men and women (Fig. 1). In the Framingham Study, for every 5-year age group from 30 to 62 years of age, the incidence of heart failure was greater in men than in women.[1] This difference was thought to be due to the fact that coronary artery disease, a major cause of

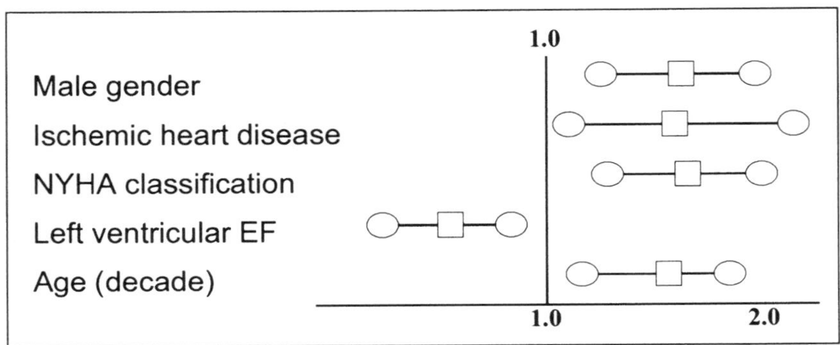

Figure 1. Predictors of relative risk of death in patients with heart failure using the Cox Proportional Hazard model. (Adapted from Adams et al. [45].)

heart failure in both men and women, was far more common in men.[1,22] Reevaluation of the Framingham database in the 1980s demonstrated similar findings when assessing the age-adjusted incidence of heart failure among persons greater than 45 years of age; however, the age-adjusted prevalence of overt heart failure was not different between genders.[7] Similarly, the National Health and Nutrition Examination Survey demonstrated similar prevalence of heart failure in men and women when evaluating over 23,000 noninstitutionalized persons between the ages of 1 and 74.[38]

However, the Framingham Study also demonstrated for the first time that the probability of survival was significantly better in women (42%) than in men (62%). This gender-related difference in survival was also identified in subsequent analysis of the Framingham study group[7] and the National Health and Nutrition Examination Survey I (NHANES-I) study,[38] but not in the smaller European *Épidémiologie de l'Insuffisance Cardiaque Avancée en Lorraine* (EPICAL) study.[6] As in EPICAL, women did not fare better than men in the Studies of Left Ventricular Dysfunction (SOLVD) trial, a study in which all patients had reduced left ventricular ejection fractions, thus precluding the confounding problem of heart failure secondary to diastolic dysfunction.[39] It has been suggested that the disparities in these different studies might be attributable to a failure to identify underlying pathologies (e.g., obesity or pulmonary disease),[40,41] a higher incidence of inaccurate diagnosis in women,[9] or a higher incidence of diabetes in women.[42,43] Investigators have also proposed that the lower incidence of coronary disease is an etiologic factor in heart failure in women, which could result in improved survival in this group. This hypothesis was supported by studies by Bart and colleagues, who found that in a population of over 3700 patients with ejection fractions of less than or equal to 40%, survival was substantially better in patients with nonischemic heart disease than in those with heart failure secondary to ischemic heart disease.[22] Similarly, the SOLVD databases demonstrated a higher number of women than men with heart failure secondary to coronary disease. However, several studies questioned this hypothesis. First, while the incidence of myocardial infarction is lower in women than in men, women who do suffer a myocardial infarction are more likely to develop heart failure.[44] Furthermore, women are more likely to develop heart failure after coronary artery bypass grafting in comparison with men.[45]

In order to clarify the disparity between the different epidemiologic studies that have appeared in the literature, Adams and colleagues observed the natural history of heart failure in a prospective and long-term study using the University of North Carolina (UNC) Heart Failure Database.[46] In over 500 patients with heart failure who were followed for between one and 10 years, they found that women were significantly less likely to die than men. Furthermore, a significant association was found between female gender and better survival. Consistent with the hypothesis of Bart and colleagues,[22] the improved survival was seen only in women who had nonischemic heart failure, and not in women in whom heart failure was due to ischemic heart disease. Etiology was scrupulously documented by angiographic, autopsy, and clinical data, and in the majority of patients the diagnosis was made by angiography. In contrast to earlier epidemiologic studies, patients were included in the UNC database only if they had documentation of systolic dysfunction within 6 months of study entry. Thus, this database provides one of the most compelling arguments that gender and outcome are tightly coupled in patients with heart failure.

If mortality were in fact worse in men than in women, we would expect that hospitalizations for heart failure would also be more common in men than in women. Indeed, studies in the UK,[15] Sweden,[47] The Netherlands,[48] and the U.S.[49,50] have all demonstrated higher hospital admission and discharge rates for men in younger age groups. However, this difference diminishes in older age categories.[22] Furthermore, the possibility of a sex bias in referring patients—and especially women with heart failure—to hospitals cannot be excluded.

Important information regarding the epidemiology of cardiovascular disease can often be gleaned from assessing the data obtained from large multicenter randomized clinical trials. Unfortunately, such information is difficult, if not impossible, to obtain from the many large studies of patients with heart failure, due to a marked under-representation of women. Indeed, the percentage of women in the major heart failure clinical trials that have been carried out over the past two decades has for the most part been less than 25%.[51–57] While these studies were not powered to assess differences in treatment effects between men and women, post-hoc analysis of the Cardiac Insufficiency Bisoprolol Study-II (CIBIS-II) demonstrated that the probability of death in women with heart failure was reduced by 36% in comparison with that in men when there was adjustment for baseline differences.[58] While beta-blocker therapy appeared to be more effective in women than in men, the effect was not significant in multivariate analysis.

In only a small number of studies have investigators specifically addressed the possibility that gender (and/or sex hormone therapy) has an impact on survival. Liao and coworkers[59] demonstrated when assessing a group of African-American patients without evidence of coronary artery disease that left ventricular hypertrophy had a greater impact on survival in women in comparison with men. By contrast, Adams, et al.[60] reported data from the Flolan International Randomized Survival Trial (FIRST) study. Among patients with nonischemic etiology of heart failure, the relative risk of death for men was significantly greater than that for women. By contrast, the relative risk of death for men versus women with heart failure secondary to ischemic heart disease was not different. More recently, Reis and colleagues[61] assessed whether there was an association between estrogen use and survival in 1134 women enrolled in the studies of vesnarinone in the therapy of patients with heart failure. All-cause 12-month mortality was 15% among the 237 women who received hormone replacement, whereas mortality was 27.1% among the 897 women who did not receive estrogen. Furthermore, regression analysis demonstrated that estrogen use was independently associated with improved survival, as were advanced age, low ejection fraction, Caucasian race and abnormal serum electrolyte levels. These markedly positive results were not influenced by whether or not women had ischemic or nonischemic disease. Taken together, the large number of studies suggesting that women with heart failure—and in particular those with disease that was not attributable to coronary artery disease, have improved survival—suggests that female gender provides a benefit in terms of heart muscle function. However, whether or not women profit from the same medical therapy as men remains to be established.

While studies are increasingly assessing the demographic differences amongst males and females with heart failure, a paucity of information is available regarding differences between incidence and outcomes amongst different racial groups. This lack of knowledge is due at least in part to the fact that minority groups have been largely underrepresented in populations studied in large community databases such as the Framingham Heart studies. In addition, studies using hospital-based and payer-based databases have yielded conflicting results. In a recent study prospectively evaluating the incidence of heart failure in a long-term health-care facility caring for an older population, there was no difference between the incidence of heart failure in African-Americans, Hispanics, and Caucasians.[62] Information can also be gleaned-from assessing deaths attributed to heart failure. In 1995, deaths attributable to heart failure were highest for black men (8.8/100,000) in comparison with black women (7.1/100,000), white men (6.7/100,000), and white women (5.4/100,000).[63–65] Similarly, data from the National Health and Nutrition Examination Survey III, carried out between 1988 and 1991, demonstrated that approximately 2.8% of non-Hispanic adult white men and 2.2% of women had heart failure, while approximately 3.2% of non-Hispanic black men and 2.8% of women have the disease.[66] Similarly, recent studies suggest that black adults may be twice as likely as white adults younger than 60 years of age to have a first hospitalization for heart failure.[50,67] Conflicting data were seen when assessing national Medicare hospital claims records for 1984 through 1986 and Medicare enrollment records from 1986 through 1992.[68] Only 16% of white men survived 6 years after their first hospitalization for heart failure, while survival was 19% in black men, 25% in black women, and 23% in white women. In addition, white men had a 10% greater mortality than did black men after adjustment for age.

Unfortunately, many of the studies assessing the burden of heart failure in minority populations have inherent limitations: they do not separate systolic from diastolic dysfunction, they do not account for concomitant disease, they do not assess potential differences in treatment algorithms, and the populations are often biased by age or method of data/patient recruitment. For example, race and gender influence care process and hospital-based case outcomes for patients hospitalized with heart failure.[69] Furthermore, blacks hospitalized for heart failure are less likely to receive care from a cardiologist,[70] an intervention that has been shown to substantially affect both cost and outcome in patients hospitalized for heart failure.[71] In addition, in adjusted analysis of data from Medicare beneficiaries hospitalized for congestive heart failure between 1991 and 1992 in three large states, black patients with heart failure received a lower quality of care than other patients, as assessed by both explicit process criteria and implicit review.[72]

In many instances, demographic and epidemiologic data have been obtained from large-scale clinical trials assessing the efficacy of new therapeutic agents for the treatment of heart failure. Unfortunately, black patients have been under-represented in many of these studies, resulting in conflicting information. For example, the percentage of black patients in Veterans Administration Heart Failure Trials (V-HeFT) I and II[73,74] was 27%, in SOLVD[75,76] it was 12%, and in a group of other large clinical studies it was substantially lower because of the inclusion of large numbers of European centers.[54,73,77–79] In a recent matched-cohort analysis of data from the SOLVD trial, the angiotensin-converting enzyme inhibitor enalapril proved beneficial in reducing the risk of heart failure hospitalization in white patients, but not in similar black patients.[80] Similar data were seen in analysis of the Beta-Blocker Evaluation of Survival trial, which randomized patients with heart failure to treatment with the beta-blocker bucindolol or a placebo.[81] However, the beta-blocker carvedilol appeared to benefit both black and nonblack patients with heart failure, although the number of events was quite small.[82] These differences may be attributable to genetic differences between different racial populations;[29] however, it is imperative that large and prospective studies be carried out to better understand both the demographics of heart failure in minority populations as well as racial differences in response to therapeutic interventions.

The Economic Burden of Heart Failure

Although heart failure exerts an enormous burden on patients and their families, the disease also has an enormous impact on the cost of health care. Indeed, according to Health Care Financing Administration (HCFA) data from 1991, the cost of hospitalizations for patients in the U.S. with heart failure was over twofold greater than that for the combined costs for treatment of the five most common diagnosis-related groups for cancer, and higher than either of the most common drug-related groups used to define patients discharged after a myocardial infarction.[79] Although it is clear that the "cost" of heart failure is enormous, it has been difficult to definitively assess the exact dollar burden. A frequently cited aggregate cost for the care of patients hospitalized with heart failure is $8 billion.[83,84] However, this figure likely underestimates the hospital cost and does not include outpatient costs. The most in-depth assessment of the cost of heart failure was first reported in 1994. The authors reported that hospital charges for heart failure management were approximately $10,000 per discharge (mean length of stay of 6.3 to 7.7 days) and that almost 75% of the costs associated with these hospitalizations occurred within the first 48 hours.[79] In addition, with hospital readmissions averaging between 15% and 30% at 90 days,[53,85] they estimated that the total expenditure in 1991 for heart failure hospitalizations was nearly $23 billion. However, a more recent study reported an even higher per-patient hospital cost.[86] Thus, despite advances in heart failure care, the total cost for heart failure management in 1999 was estimated by O'Connell to be $56 billion.[86]

The enormous cost of care for patients with heart failure in the U.S. is also seen in other areas of the world. For example, fully-loaded costs for care of heart failure in Sweden are approximately 2000–2600 million kronor, or nearly 2% of the Swedish health-care budget.[87] Hospitalization accounts for between 65% and 75% of those costs. Similarly, studies in Europe have demonstrated that heart failure encompasses a similar percentage of the total health-care budget as in the U.S. (U.S., 1.5%; France, 1.9%; UK, 1.2%; Netherlands, 1.0%).[88] In addition, the cost of care for patients with heart failure increased between twofold and fourfold in patients with New York Heart Association class III symptoms in comparison with patients having class I and II symptoms, and in France, the cost of care for patients with class IV symptoms was twice that of patients with class III disease. Interestingly, European trials suggested that the cost of outpatient therapy might exceed that of in-patient care.

The enormous burden of health-care costs has led economists to study the cost-effectiveness of new technologies. This analysis assesses the relative benefits of new therapies by analyzing the relationship between the extra benefits produced and the associated cost.[84] Economists also assess the ability of new therapies to minimize costs by effecting changes at a lower cost. The ultimate goal of any new therapy, from an economic perspective, is to lower costs while at the same time improving outcomes. Several recent initiatives have met at least some of these economic thresholds. For example, a recent study demonstrated that the use of a multidisciplinary, home-based intervention consisting of home visits by a cardiac nurse after discharge decreased the rate of unplanned readmissions and associated health-care costs while at the same time prolonging event-free and total survival.[89] In a similar study in which patients in northern California were enrolled in a patient home-monitoring program that included patient education and notification of physicians when changes were noted in weight, vital signs, or symptoms, the intervention significantly decreased medical claims by approximately $1000 per year, whereas claims in the control group doubled over the same time period.[90] However, salutary effects of home health care were not seen in a small population of patients with severe symptoms, many of whom required inotropic therapy.[91] The use of newer pharmacologic therapies for the treatment of patients with heart failure have also been shown to be cost-effective.[92,93] Indeed, the cost per life-year gained is substantially less than that of other cardiovascular interventions. However, improved longevity has its own inherent costs, and complex models are thus needed to explore the relationships between clinical data and economic consequences in heart-failure populations.[93]

The Future of Heart Failure Demographics

It is clear from various community-based studies, reviews of Medicare databases, and assessment of health-care costs that heart failure is a disease that is not only of epidemic proportions, but one that will be associated with an increasing burden as the current populations in industrialized societies age. The morbidity and mortality associated with heart failure are greater than those associated with most other human diseases, and the cost of care for patients with heart failure is nearly twofold greater than that of all common cancers combined. However, we face continued challenges to better understand and more accurately document the burden of heart failure. New technologies, including left ventricular assist devices and implantable artificial hearts, will require careful assessment to identify those patients in whom such expensive therapy will be most warranted. Furthermore, the use of novel molecular genetic techniques to develop unique but costly recombinant proteins and monoclonal antibodies will further tax the already overburdened finances that support care—particularly in the elderly population. In addition, novel interventional technology, including resynchronization therapy, may nearly double the cost of outpatient care. Thus, difficult questions will need to be raised as to which endpoints must be met to warrant the expense of these new therapies. Our ability to answer these questions will depend on improved methods of accurately monitoring heart failure demographics, including survival, hospitalizations, and disease costs.

In addition, it will become increasingly important to learn which patients benefit from certain therapies. The increasing understanding of the relationships between pharmacologic therapies and patient genotype, as well as more assiduous attempts to relate therapeutic success to patient phenotype, may help not only to improve morbidity and mortality but also to lower costs. The development of techniques to identify single-nucleotide polymorphisms may help to identify subsets of patients who respond to specific drug therapies, rather than treating entire populations to see benefit in a few. While it is easy to assume that the burden of heart failure is widely recognized, to do so would be shortsighted. This is most evident from a recent study by Gross and colleagues, which compared disease-specific funding in 1996 by the National Institutes of Health (NIH) with data on measures of the burden of 29 human diseases.[94] While the data suggested a relationship between disease burden and NIH funding, heart failure was not included in the data analysis. In fact, if it had been included in the analysis, it would have been the outlier in an otherwise linear relationship. Thus, even in 2001, we must continue to insure that governmental agencies, private endowments, hospital administrators, and patients and their families understand the "burden" of heart failure both in the U.S. and around the world.

Acknowledgments. The author would like to thank Tracey Barry for preparation of this manuscript. This work was supported in part by National Institutes of Health grant NIH RO1 (HL60032-01).

References

1. McKee PA, Castelli WP, McNamara PM, et al. The natural history of congestive heart failure: the Framingham Study. *N Engl J Med* 1971;285:1441–1446.
2. Ho KL, Anderson KM, Kannel WB, et al. Survival after the onset of congestive heart failure in Framingham heart study subjects. *Circulation* 1993;88:107–115.
3. Kannel WB, Belanger AL. Epidemiology of heart failure. *Am Heart J* 1991;121: 951–957.
4. Lloyd-Jones DM. The risk of congestive heart failure: sobering lessons from the Framingham Heart Study. *Curr Cardiol Rep* 2001;3:184–190.
5. Rodeheffer RJ, Jacobsen SJ, Gersh BJ, et al. The incidence and prevalence of congestive heart failure in Rochester, Minnesota. *Mayo Clin Proc* 1993;68: 1143–1150.
6. Zannad F, Briancon S, Juilliere Y, et al. Incidence, clinical and etiologic features, and outcomes of advanced chronic heart failure: the EPICAL Study. *J Am Coll Cardiol* 1999;33:734–742.
7. Ho KK, Pinsky JL, Kannel WB, et al. The epidemiology of heart failure: the Framingham Study. *J Am Coll Cardiol* 1993;22:6A–13A.
8. Senni M, Tribouilloy CM, Rodeheffer RJ, et al. Trends in incidence and survival in a 10-year period. *Arch Intern Med* 1999;159:29–34.
9. Rich MW. Epidemiology, pathophysiology, and etiology of congestive heart failure in older adults. *J Am Geriatr Soc* 1997;45:968–974.
10. Vasan RS, Larson MG, Benjamin EJ, et al. Congestive heart failure in subjects with normal versus reduced left ventricular ejection fraction. *J Am Coll Cardiol* 1999;33:1948–1955.
11. Senni M, Tribouilloy CM, Rodeheffer RJ, et al. Congestive heart failure in the community: A study of all incident cases in Olmsted County, Minnesota, in 1991. *Circulation* 1998;98:2282–2289.
12. Levy D, Larson MG, Vasan RS, et al. The progression from hypertension to congestive heart failure. *JAMA* 1996;275:1557–1562.
13. Vasan RS, Larson MG, Benjamin EJ, et al. Left ventricular dilatation and the risk of congestive heart failure in people without myocardial infarction. *N Engl J Med* 1997;336:1350–1356.
14. Hershberger RE, Ni H, Crispell KA. Familial dilated cardiomyopathy: echocardiographic diagnostic criteria for classification of family members as affected. *J Card Fail* 1999;5:203–212.
15. Vasan RS, Levy D. Defining diastolic heart failure: A call for standardized diagnostic criteria. *Circulation* 2000;101:2118–2121.
16. Franciosa JA, Wilen M, Ziesche S, et al. Survival in men with severe chronic left ventricular failure due to either coronary heart disease or idiopathic dilated cardiomyopathy. *Am J Cardiol* 1983;51:831–836.
17. Cowie MR, Wood DA, Coats AJS, et al. Survival of patients with a new diagnosis of heart failure: a population based study. *Heart* 2000;83:505–510.
18. MacIntyre K, Capewell S, Stewart S, et al. Evidence of improving prognosis in heart failure: Trends in case fatality in 66,547 patients hospitalized between 1986 and 1995. *Circulation* 2000;102:1126–1131.
19. Khand A, Gemmel I, Clark AL, et al. Is the prognosis of heart failure improving? *J Am Coll Cardiol* 2000;36:2284–2286.
20. Konstam MA. Progress in heart failure management? Lessons from the real world. *Circulation* 2000;102:1076–1078.
21. Gradman A, Deedwania P, Cody RJ, et al. Predictors of total mortality and

sudden death in mild to moderate heart failure. *J Am Coll Cardiol* 1989;14:564–570.
22. Bart BA, Shaw LK, McCants CB, et al. Clinical determinants of mortality in patients with angiographically diagnosed ischemic or nonischemic cardiomyopathy. *J Am Coll Cardiol* 1997;30:1002–1008.
23. Rosenthal GE, Harper DL, Quinn LM, et al. Severity-adjusted mortality and length of stay in teaching and nonteaching hospitals. *JAMA* 1997;278:485–490.
24. Campana C, Gavazzi A, Berzuini C, et al. Predictors of prognosis in patients awaiting heart transplantation. *J Heart Lung Transplant* 1993;12:756–765.
25. Mudge GH, Goldstein S, Addonizio LJ, et al. Task Force 3: recipient guidelines/prioritization. *J Am Coll Cardiol* 1993;22:21–31.
26. Costanzo MR, Augustine S, Bourge R, et al. Selection and treatment of candidates for heart transplantation: a statement for health professionals from the Committee on Heart Failure and Cardiac Transplantation of the Council on Clinical Cardiology, American Heart Association. *Circulation* 1995;92:3593–3612.
27. Grogan M, Redfield MM, Bailey KR, et al. Long-term outcome of patients with biopsy-proved myocarditis: comparison with idiopathic dilated cardiomyopathy. *J Am Coll Cardiol* 1995;26:80–84.
28. Loh E, Rebbeck TR, Mahoney PD, et al. Common variant in the *AMPD1* gene predicts improved clinical outcome in patients with heart failure. *Circulation* 1998;99:1422–1425.
29. Wood AJ. Racial differences in the response to drugs: Pointers to genetic differences. *N Engl J Med* 2001;344:1393–1395.
30. Haldeman GA, Croft JB, Giles WH, et al. Hospitalization of patients with heart failure: national hospital discharge survey, 1985 to 1995. *Am Heart J* 1999;137:352–360.
31. Rice DP. Beneficiary profile: yesterday, today, and tomorrow. *Health Care Financ Rev* 1996;18:23–46.
32. Ni H, Nauman DJ, Hershberger RE. Analysis of trends in hospitalizations for heart failure. *J Card Fail* 1999;5:79–84.
33. Polanczyk CA, Rohde LE, Dec W, et al. Ten-year trends in hospital care for congestive heart failure. *Arch Intern Med* 2000;160:325–332.
34. Vinson JM, Rich MW, Sperry JC, Shah AS, McNamara T. Early readmission of elderly patients with congestive heart failure. *J Am Geriatr Soc* 1990;38:1290–5.
35. Chin MH, Goldman L. Correlates of early hospital readmission or death in patients with congestive heart failure. *Am J Cardiol* 1997;79:1640–1644.
36. Philbin EF, DiSalvo T. Prediction of hospital readmission for heart failure: development of a simple risk score based on administrative data. *J Am Coll Cardiol* 1999;33:1560–1566.
37. Maisel A, Koon J, Krishnaswamy P, et al. Utility of B-natriuretic peptide as a rapid, point-of-care test for screening patients undergoing echocardiography to determine left ventricular dysfunction. *Am Heart J* 2001;141:367–374.
38. Schocken DD, Arrieta MI, Leaverton PE, et al. Prevalence and mortality rate of congestive heart failure in the United States. *J Am Coll Cardiol* 1992;20:301–306.
39. Bourassa M, Gurne O, Bangdiwala SI, et al. Natural history and current practices in heart failure. *J Am Coll Cardiol* 1993;22(suppl):14A–19A.
40. Wheeldon NM, MacDonald TM, Flucker CJ, et al. Echocardiography in chronic heart failure in the community. *Q J Med* 1993;86:17–22.

41. Remes J, Miettinen H, Reunanen A, et al. Validity of clinical diagnosis of heart failure in primary health care. *Eur Heart J* 1991;12:315–321.
42. Olivetti G, Giordano G, Corradi D, et al. Gender differences and aging: effects on the human heart. *J Am Coll Cardiol* 1995;26:1068–1079.
43. Grohe C, Kahlert S, Lobbert K, et al. Cardiac myocytes and fibroblasts contain functional estrogen receptors. *FEBS Lett* 1997;416:107–112.
44. Vaccarino V, Parsons L, Every NR, et al. Sex-based differences in early mortality after myocardial infarction. *N Engl J Med* 1999;341:217–232.
45. Hoffman RM, Psaty BM, Kronmal RA. Modifiable risk factors for incident heart failure in the Coronary Artery Surgery Study. *Arch Intern Med* 1994;154:417–423.
46. Adams KF, Dunlap S, Sueta CA, et al. Relation between gender, etiology and survival in patients with symptomatic heart failure. *J Am Coll Cardiol* 1996;28: 1781–1788.
47. Andersson B, Waagstein F. Spectrum and outcome of congestive heart failure in a hospitalized population. *Am Heart J* 1993;126:632–640.
48. Reitsma JB, Mosterd A, De Craen AJM, et al. Increase in hospital admission rates for heart failure in the Netherlands 1980–1993. *Heart* 1996;76:388–392.
49. Gillium RF. Heart failure in the United States 1970–1985. *Am Heart J* 1987;113: 1043–1045.
50. Ghali JK, Cooper R, Ford E. Trends in rates for heart failure in the United States 1973–1986: evidence for increasing population prevalence. *Arch Intern Med* 1990;150:769–773.
51. Pitt B, Poole-Wilson PA, Segal R, et al. Effect of losartan compared with captopril on mortality in patients with symptomatic heart failure: randomised trial—the Losartan Heart Failure Survival Study, ELITE II. Lancet 2000;355: 1582–1587.
52. Pitt B, Zannad F, Remme WJ, et al. The effect of spironolactone on morbidity and mortality in patients with severe heart failure. Randomized Aldactone Evaluation Study Investigators. *N Engl J Med* 1999;341:709–717.
53. Lechat P, Escolano S, Golmard JL, et al. Prognostic value of bisoprolol-induced hemodynamic effects in heart failure during the Cardiac Insufficiency Bisoprolol Study (CIBIS). *Circulation* 1997;96:2197–2205.
54. MERIT-HF Study Group. Effect of metoprolol CR/XL in chronic heart failure: metoprolol CR/XL randomised intervention trial in congestive heart failure (MERIT-HF). *Lancet* 1999;353:2001–2007.
55. Heart Outcomes Prevention Evaluation Study Investigators. Effects of an angiotensin-converting enzyme inhibitor, ramipril, on cardiovascular events in high-risk patients. *N Engl J Med* 2000;342:145–153.
56. PROVED Investigative Group. Randomized study affecting the effect of digoxin withdrawal in patients with mild to moderate chronic congestive heart failure: results of the PROVED trial. *J Am Coll Cardiol* 1993;22:955–962.
57. Digitalis Investigation Group. The effect of digoxin on mortality and morbidity in patients with heart failure. *N Engl J Med* 1997;336:525–533.
58. Simon T, Mary-Krause M, Funck-Brentano C, et al. Sex differences in the prognosis of congestive heart failure results from the Cardiac Insufficiency Bisoprolol Study (CIBIS II). *Circulation* 2001;103:375–380.
59. Liao Y, Cooper RS, Mensah GA, et al. Left ventricular hypertrophy has a greater impact on survival in women than in men. *Circulation* 1995;92:805–810.
60. Adams KF, Sueta CA, Gheorghiade M, et al. Gender differences in survival in advanced heart failure: Insights from the FIRST study. *Circulation* 1999;99: 1816–1821.

61. Reis SE, Holubkov R, Young JB, et al. Estrogen is associated with improved survival in women with congestive heart failure: analysis of the vesnarinone studies. *J Am Coll Cardiol* 2000;36:529–533.
62. Gilbert EM, Sandoval A, Larrabee P, et al. Lisinopril lowers cardiac adrenergic drive and increases P-receptor density in the failing human heart. *Circulation* 1993;88:472–480.
63. Goldberg RJ. Assessing the population burden from heart failure. *Arch Intern Med* 1999;159:15–17.
64. American Heart Association. *Heart and Stroke Statistical Update, 1998*. Dallas, TX: American Heart Association, 1998.
65. National Institutes of Health/National Heart, Lung and Blood Institute. *Morbidity and Mortality Chartbook on Cardiovascular, Lung, and Blood Diseases, 1990–1994*. Bethesda, MD: U.S. Department of Health and Human Services, 1994.
66. *Phase I, National Health and Nutrition Examination Survey III (NHANES III)*. Bethesda, MD: National Center for Health Statistics/American Heart Association, 1995.
67. Alexander M, Grumbach K, Selby J, et al. Hospitalization for congestive heart failure: explaining racial differences. *JAMA* 1995;274:1037–1042.
68. Croft JB, Giles WH, Pollard RA, et al. Heart failure survival among older adults in the United States: A poor prognosis for an emerging epidemic in the Medicare population. *Arch Intern Med* 1999;159:5205–510.
69. Philbin EF, DiSalvo T. Influence of race and gender on care process, resource use, and hospital-based outcomes in congestive heart failure. *Am J Cardiol* 1998;82:76–81.
70. Auerbach AD, Hamel MB, Califf RM, et al. Patient characteristics associated with care by a cardiologist among adults hospitalized with severe congestive heart failure. *J Am Coll Cardiol* 2000;36:2119–2125.
71. Reis SE, Holubkov R, McNamara DM, et al. Treatment of hospitalized patients with congestive heart failure: specialty-related disparities in practice patterns and outcomes. *J Am Coll Cardiol* 1997;30:733–738.
72. Ayanian JZ, Weissman JS, Chasan-Taber S, et al. Quality of care by race and gender for congestive heart failure and pneumonia. *Med Care* 1999;37:1260–1269.
73. Cohn JN, Johnson G, Ziesche S, et al. A comparison of enalapril with hydralazine isosorbide dinitrate in the treatment of chronic congestive heart failure. *N Engl J Med* 1991;325:303–310.
74. Cohn JN, Archibald DG, Ziesche S, et al. Effect of vasodilator therapy on mortality in chronic congestive heart failure. *N Engl J Med* 1986;314:1547–1552.
75. SOLVD Investigators. Effect of enalapril on survival in patients with reduced left ventricular ejection fractions and congestive heart failure. *N Engl J Med* 1991;325:293–302.
76. SOLVD Investigators. Effect of enalapril on mortality and the development of heart failure in asymptomatic patients with reduced left ventricular ejection fractions. *N Engl J Med* 1992;327:685–691.
77. CONSENSUS Trial Study Group. Effects of enalapril on mortality in severe congestive heart failure. *N Engl J Med* 1987;316:1429–1435.
78. Packer M, Bristow MR, Cohn JN, et al. The effect of carvedilol on morbidity and mortality in patients with chronic heart failure. *N Engl J Med* 1996;334:1349–1355.
79. CIBIS-II Investigators and Committee. The Cardiac Insufficiency Bisoprolol Study II (CIBIS-II): a randomised trial. *Lancet* 1999;353:9–13.

80. Exner DV, Dries DL, Domanski MJ, et al. Lesser response to angiotensin converting enzyme inhibitor therapy in black as compared with white patients with left ventricular dysfunction. *N Engl J Med* 2001;344:1351–1357.
81. Eichhorn EJ, Domanski MJ, Krause- Steinrauf MS, et al. A trial of the beta blocker bucindolol in patients with advanced chronic heart failure. *N Engl J Med* 2001;344:1659–1667.
82. Yancy C, Fowler M, Colucci WS, et al. Race and the response to adrenergic blockade with carvedilol in patients with chronic heart failure. *N Engl J Med* 2001;344:1358–1365.
83. Krumholz HM, Chen Y, Wang Y, et al. Predictors of readmission among elderly survivors of admission with heart failure. *Am Heart J* 2000;139:72–77.
84. Mark DB. Economics of treating heart failure. *Am J Cardiol* 1997;80:33H–38H.
85. Swedberg K, Bristow MR, Cohn JN, et al. Effects of sustained-release moxonidine, an imidazoline agonist, on plasma norepinephrine in patients with chronic heart failure. *Circulation* 2002;105:1797–1803.
86. O'Connell JB. The economic burden of heart failure. *Clin Cardiol* 2000; 23(suppl 3):III6–10.
87. Ryden-Bergsten T, Andersson F. The health care costs of heart failure in Sweden. *J Intern Med* 1999;246:275–284.
88. Malek M. Health economics of heart failure. *Heart* 1999;82(suppl 4):IV11–13.
89. Stewart S, Marley JE, Horowitz JD. Effects of a multidisciplinary, home-based intervention on unplanned readmissions and survival among patients with chronic congestive heart failure: a randomized controlled study. *Lancet* 1999;354:1077–1083.
90. Heidenreich PA, Ruggerio CM, Massie BM. Effect of a home monitoring system on hospitalization and resource use for patients with heart failure. *Am Heart J* 1999;138:633–640.
91. Wilson JR, Smith JS, Dahle KL, et al. Impact of home health care on health care costs and hospitalization frequency in patients with heart failure. *Am J Cardiol* 1999;83:615–617.
92. Szucs TD. Pharmacoeconomics of angiotensin-converting enzyme inhibitors in heart failure. *Am J Hypertens* 1997;10:272S–279S.
93. Cleland JGF. Health economic consequences of the pharmacological treatment of heart failure. *Eur Heart J* 1998;19:P32–P39.
94. Gross CP, Anderson GF, Powe NR. The relation between funding by the national institutes of health and the burden of disease. *N Engl J Med* 1999;340: 1881–1887.
95. Eriksson H, Svardsudd K, Larsson B, et al. Risk factors for heart failure in the general population: The study of men born in 1913. *Eur Heart J* 1989;10:647–656.

Chapter 2

Heart Failure Guidelines and Disease Management

David W. Baker, MD, MPH

Numerous studies have shown that the quality of health care in the United States is suboptimal.[1] Patients are often not prescribed medications or given treatments that could improve their survival and quality of life. Conversely, many people undergo procedures or diagnostic tests that have not been shown to be beneficial. These issues are most problematic for patients with chronic diseases, as described in detail by a recent report from the Institute of Medicine.[2]

The care for patients with heart failure typifies these inadequacies, with perceived and documented problems of late and incorrect diagnosis, inadequate evaluation of patients with overt heart failure, and management errors.[3–8] For example, Jencks and coworkers recently reported that approximately one-third of Medicare patients hospitalized in the United States with a principal diagnosis of heart failure did not have their left ventricular ejection fraction (LVEF) documented.[5] Moreover, of those who did, one-third of patients with LVEF $<40\%$ were not prescribed an angiotensin-converting enzyme (ACE) inhibitor. In many states, performance was much worse than this. The available evidence suggests that care for outpatients with heart failure may be even poorer.[9]

These widespread deficiencies in quality of care and unexplained variations in use of health-care services led the Agency for Health Care Policy and Research (now the Agency for Health Care Research and Quality) and other public and private organizations to explore clinical practice guidelines as a way to improve care.[10] Since the early 1990s, numerous groups, including physician subspecialty organizations, have jumped on the guideline bandwagon. What are clinical practice guidelines? The Institute of Medicine defines clinical practice guidelines as

From: Jessup M, McCauley KM (eds). *Heart Failure: Providing Optimal Care.* Elmsford, NY: Futura, an imprint of Blackwell Publishing; ©2003.

"systematically developed statements to assist practitioner and patient decisions about appropriate health care for specific clinical circumstances." Although guidelines have the *potential* to improve care by providing information on best practices to health-care providers and patients, there is little evidence that guidelines have improved quality of care or outcomes. This is not surprising, since most experts agree that continuing medical education programs are not effective in changing physician practice.[11] So, guidelines may be necessary but not sufficient for changing physician behavior. Formal dissemination and implementation plans are needed to achieve greater awareness of recommendations and increased adoption of these recommendations into practice. Disease management programs usually incorporate guideline recommendation into their practice plans. In this manner, disease management may result in rapid adoption of guideline recommendations and improvements in quality of care. This paper describes the steps necessary to develop guidelines[12–14] and speed dissemination of awareness and adoption of guideline recommendations.[15]

Developing Clinical Practice Guidelines

Rigorous methods are necessary to ensure that a guideline is valid, credible, clear, and clinically appropriate. Several publications are available that fully describe proper methodology for guideline development.[13,14,16] Only a brief overview is provided here.

The Institute of Medicine has outlined eight key attributes of clinical practice guidelines (Table 1). First and foremost, the guideline recommendations must be *valid*: if practitioners adopt the recommendations, patients would live longer and feel better. This is also referred to as a *process–outcome link*. The validity of guidelines is most certain when recommendations are based on systematic literature reviews of all randomized controlled trials of a therapy, with careful attention to the quality of

Table 1

Eight Attributes of Good Practice Guidelines

- Validity of recommendations
- Reproducibility of recommendations
- Recommendations are clinically applicable
- Recommendations are flexible
- Recommendations are clear and concise
- Developed by multidisciplinary process
- Scheduled review and update as needed
- Documentation of procedures and methods

the clinical trial.[17] Uncontrolled studies can be used as evidence supporting a recommendation, but the guideline must clearly indicate that the level of evidence supporting the recommendation is weaker. If careful attention is given to ensure a thorough literature review and appropriate rating of the quality of clinical trials, guideline recommendations should be *reliable and reproducible*.

What defines a beneficial treatment? The goal of the guideline development process is to identify those diagnostic tests and therapies that make patients live longer and/or feel better. Assessing whether a therapy reduces mortality for patients with heart failure is the easy part. Measuring changes in health-related quality of life is more challenging. Currently, there is no clearly valid surrogate for health-related quality of life. The Agency for Health Care Policy and Research (AHCPR) heart failure panel explicitly stated that it would not make recommendations to use a therapy if the only evidence supporting its effectiveness was improvement in exercise time, maximum oxygen uptake, ejection fraction, or other tests.[18] Changes in these measures have only modest correlation with patients' symptoms. The 6-minute walk appears to be the test that best captures patients' symptoms, but the correlation is still only modest.[12] Thus, health-related quality of life is best assessed by direct patient self-report, and guidelines should base recommendations on studies that have used one of several validated measures of health-related quality of life as their outcome.[3]

Even if a definite process–outcome link can be established from two or more multicenter randomized trials, a recommendation based upon these data often comes with the caveat that patients with heart failure in clinical trials are frequently quite different from those in the general population.[19] Specifically, patients in clinical trials tend to be younger, white, male, and have fewer comorbidities. Thus, guideline panels must often use potentially biased data sources (observational studies and expert opinion) to decide the limits, if any, of the patient population to which their recommendation should apply (*clinical applicability*). For example, are the benefits of ACE inhibitor or beta-blockers proven for patients age 80 and above (who form a significant proportion of the population with heart failure)? It is essential that guideline panels indicate when they extend the generalizability of their recommendations beyond the eligibility criteria used in clinical trials. Otherwise, guidelines risk writing in stone a recommendation that may not be valid for some patients. By identifying the limits of our knowledge and the frontiers of our ignorance, guideline committees can point to where future clinical trials or high quality observational studies are needed.

What has been given far less attention by guidelines is whether the benefits reported in a clinical trial will be achieved equally in general practice. Clinical trials establish the *efficacy* of a therapy (i.e., whether it improves outcomes in an idealized setting). However, the *effectiveness* (i.e., the outcomes achieved in the real world) may be far less if therapies are used in a different manner than in the clinical trials (i.e., little or no patient education about medications, less stringent follow-up) or if they are applied to patients that would have been excluded from trials. There are even examples in which apparently beneficial therapies appeared harmful in general practice.[20] Thus, guidelines must go beyond merely saying *what* therapies are recommended and they must make clear recommendations about *how* to put these recommendations into practice to achieve optimal outcomes (*clarity*).

Each of these steps in guideline development poses unique challenges. However, the most difficult task in guideline development usually begins when leaving "evidence-based medicine" and entering the world of "expert opinion." For example, there was heated debate over which patients should undergo cardiac catheterization during the development of the Agency for Health Care Policy and Research heart failure guideline in 1992, and that debate has continued in more recent guideline panels. No studies on the benefits of cardiac catheterization were found in the literature to help guide the expert panel's decision. Making recommendations when there is no clear consensus among experts threatens the validity and reproducibility of the guideline development process. If there are no data to guide a decision and no consensus among experts, a guideline's recommendation on a topic becomes highly dependent upon random or systematic bias in how panelists were selected. Are the opinions of the guideline panel representative of the overall population of heart failure experts? Previous studies have shown that if there is a consensus among experts that a therapy is beneficial (despite an absence of data from controlled trials), future clinical trials are likely to bear out the experts' beliefs.[21] However, we have no analogous data supporting the validity of "majority opinions." If there is no consensus, it is probably better to simply state this, rather than make a recommendation that may not be valid.

My belief that guidelines should avoid making recommendations when both data and consensus of opinion are lacking is also based on pragmatism. Such recommendations will probably do little to change practice patterns, because in the absence of strong supporting evidence, a recommendation may lack credibility among the providers. Moreover, in the absence of a clear process–outcome link, a recommendation should not be used as a measure of quality.[22] There is an old saying that not everything that is important can be measured, and not everything that can be measured is important. Nevertheless, managed care organizations, state peer-review organizations, and the Health Care Financing Administration cannot target a recommendation for quality improvement efforts unless compliance with that recommendation can be measured. Thus, the inability to translate a recommendation into a quality measure further decreases the impetus to change. For these reasons, guideline development may be more efficient and effective by concentrating on areas where there is strong evidence or overwhelming expert opinion in favor of a recommendation.

The issue of whether a guideline should make recommendations in the absence of data begs another more fundamental question. What is the purpose of the guideline? Is it a compendium of best practices (based on data and the majority opinion of experts)? Or is it a quality improvement tool? Most guidelines to date appear to have been written from the former perspective. For example, the first American College of Cardiology/American Heart Association (ACC/AHA) guideline attempted to cover the entire spectrum of heart failure and contained approximately 100 separate recommendations.[23] It is simply not possible to simultaneously target 100 issues for quality improvement efforts. If the second perspective is adopted with a goal of identifying key targets to improve care and health outcomes, then it would be preferable to produce a document with fewer recommendations based on the strongest available data. From this latter perspective, recommendations based on weak consensus only serve to clutter a guideline and detract from the main quality improvement goals.

Have Guidelines Been Effective?

To date, there have been four published guidelines for heart failure. The AHCPR guideline was published in 1994[18] and the ACC/AHA guideline was published shortly after that, in 1995.[23] More recently, the ACTION-HF guideline was published in 1999,[24] and the Heart Failure Society of America (HFSA) guideline was released in 2000.[25] Has care changed? All four guidelines have recommended ACE inhibitors for patients with heart failure and systolic dysfunction (e.g., LVEF ≤0.40). Two large studies have assessed whether ACE inhibitors were prescribed for Medicare patients discharged with a principal diagnosis of heart failure and documented low ejection fraction. The Large State Peer Review Organization found that among patients hospitalized in 1993 and 1994, approximately 70% of patients received ACE inhibitors at discharge.[4] Jencks and colleagues reassessed states' performance in 1997–99 and found that little had changed.[26] A direct comparison of these two studies (Fig. 1) suggests that ACE inhibitor use may have actually decreased slightly. The difficulties in increasing use of ACE inhibitors raises even more serious concerns about whether we can get physicians to increase use of beta-blockers, which were viewed until recently as contraindicated in heart failure with systolic dysfunction.

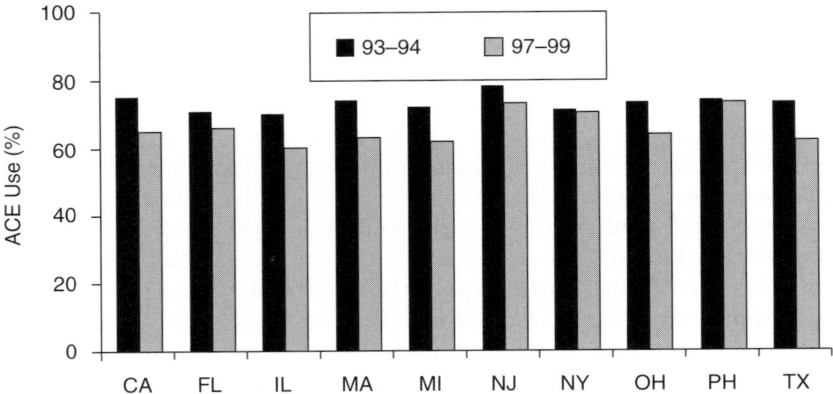

Figure 1. Proportion of Medicare patients hospitalized with heart failure who were discharged on an angiotensin-converting enzyme (ACE) inhibitor in 1993–94 and 1997–99 in ten large states.

Why haven't guidelines worked? Have the guidelines met the Institute of Medicine (IOM) criteria for high quality (Table 1)? From the perspective of validity, reproducibility, and clinical applicability and flexibility, the guidelines appear to have met the mark. All reviewed published literature and made key recommendations based on published clinical trials. The similarity of the recommendations is a testament to their reproducibility. All dealt with common problematic situations, such as what to do with patients who could not tolerate an ACE inhibitor or had comorbid renal insufficiency, making them relevant to the broad population of patients with heart failure and flexible enough to accommodate frequently encountered challenges.

However, on other counts they do not fare quite as well. Although most have made some attempt to make the guideline development panels multidisciplinary (i.e., to include primary-care physicians, nurses, cardiothoracic surgeons, and patients), only the AHCPR guideline really achieved this goal. In fact, creating a functioning multidisciplinary group is problematic, because of the differing levels of expertise and areas of interest of the groups named above. Nevertheless, broader involvement of other disciplines may be helpful for dissemination of a guideline and adoption of its recommendations. Specifically, primary-care physicians' lack of awareness of guideline recommendations may be ameliorated by increasing their involvement in the process and involving primary-care organizations more actively in the dissemination process. So, multidisciplinary development of guidelines, in one way or another, remains a worthy goal.

In addition, "concise" is certainly not an adjective that most people would use to describe the AHCPR or the ACC/AHA guidelines, each of which issued dozens of recommendations on everything from the initial physical examination to the use of cardiac catheterization. This gets back to the question posed previously about defining the goal of guideline development. If what is desired is a clear, concise statement regarding "best practices" for the use of key diagnostic tests and therapies, the AHCPR and ACC/AHA guidelines missed the mark. The HFSA guidelines come far closer to this goal, and have begun to look more like the "position papers" issued by the American College of Physicians and published in *Annals of Internal Medicine*. It may be that a concise guideline is an oxymoron: calling something a guideline compels the developers to be comprehensive and abandon attempts to focus on key targets. The "position paper" may be a fruitful alternative to explore.

In summary, developers of published heart failure guidelines have put in a solid performance when measured against the yardstick laid down by the Institute of Medicine for how guidelines should be developed. Nevertheless, published guidelines appear to have had minimal impact on quality of care. This suggests that we may be operating under a fundamentally wrong assumption that "better" guidelines (as per the IOM criteria) will be more effective at promoting improvements in quality of care. We need to look more closely at how change occurs, and why it sometimes does not occur, to understand how we can improve guidelines and increase their effectiveness.

Accelerating Change: Lessons From Technology Diffusion Studies

In 1601, an English sea captain found that citrus fruits reduced scurvy deaths from 40% to nearly zero.[27] Almost 150 years later, James Lind, a British navy physician, found that giving scurvy victims citrus fruits could cure the disease. Nevertheless, it was not until 1795 that the British navy instituted routine provision of citrus fruits on all ships. But perhaps the most incredible part of the story is that it took another 70 years before the British merchant marine adopted a similar policy! There are two morals to this story. First, just because something is a good idea (or better than a previous one) does not mean that it will be accepted. Second, even if a practice is accepted in one group (e.g., the British navy or American cardiologists), it does not mean it will be rapidly adopted by another group (e.g., the British merchant marine or American primary-care physicians).

Technology diffusion models[15] suggest the rate of adoption of a new technology is affected by:

Table 2

Characteristics Affecting the Rate of Adoption of Beta-blockers and Spironolactone

	Beta-blockers	Spironolactone
Supporting evidence*	A	B
Mortality rate reduction	1/3	1/3
Complexity of use	Difficult	Easy
Compatible with previous beliefs	No	Yes
Can try on limited basis	Difficult	Easy
Observable effect	Yes	No

* American College of Cardiology/American Heart Association criteria for rating evidence.

- The perceived advantage of a new technology
- The complexity of learning its use
- Its compatibility with previously held attitudes and beliefs
- The ability to try the technology on a limited basis
- Whether beneficial effects are observable

Awareness of a new technology is not enough if there are barriers to its adoption. Thus, there may be a lag time of several years between awareness and actual use (the "knowledge–attitude–practice gap"), or it may never be adopted at all.

It is instructive to view two new heart failure therapies from this perspective: beta-blockers and spironolactone (Table 2). Both have been shown to reduce mortality rates by approximately one-third in one or more randomized controlled trials.[28–33] But there are important differences. Use of beta-blockers is substantially more complex, requiring careful assessment of fluid status prior to initiation, counseling regarding side effects and what to do if weight increases or edema develops; and the dose must be steadily increased over a period of weeks to months to reach the target doses used in controlled trials. By comparison, spironolactone initiation is far easier, and titration may not be needed for many patients. More importantly, the use of beta-blockers in patients with heart failure and systolic dysfunction was anathema until recently, so the rapid shift in status from "contraindicated" to "indicated" creates substantial cognitive dissonance for physicians who are unaware of the long literature suggesting that high catecholamine levels may be injurious.[34] By comparison, the use of spironolactone is completely coherent with the prevailing and widely emphasized view that blockade of the renin–angiotensin system is beneficial for patients with heart failure. The sole advantage of beta-blockers that could lead to more rapid adoption is that the beneficial effects may be readily apparent (improved exercise tolerance, increase in left ventricular ejection fraction), whereas spironolactone appears to reduce mortality, but does not affect symptoms or physical functioning. Which will be adopted more rapidly? Spironolactone is the odds-on favorite, because of its perceived simplicity and compatibility with previous beliefs.

If guidelines are going to overcome the barriers to beta-blocker use, they will need to do far more than make sweeping statements about the efficacy of these agents. For example, guidelines could provide:

- A set of questions to determine whether a patient is an appropriate candidate for beta-blocker initiation (e.g., questions to exclude patients with New York Heart Association (NYHA) class IV symptoms or evidence of uncontrolled volume overload)
- Essential points for educating patients about the therapy, along with actual patient education materials and weight monitoring sheets that could be downloaded from the Internet
- A dose initiation and titration schedule, with some flexibility to account for patients' functional class and LVEF.

These materials could be kept in physicians' offices, in their pocket, or even on a hand-held computer.

It remains unclear whether including information such as this would help overcome some physicians' fears of starting beta-blockers. However, it would certainly decrease the complexity of learning the new technology and increase the ability to try it out on a limited basis without having to reinvent the wheel for their own practice. Downloading documents would even allow physicians to customize messages for their own practice, further increasing the flexibility of the guideline.

Guidelines may also need to directly confront the myths and misconceptions that pose barriers to change. Primary-care physicians appear to be overly concerned about initiating an ACE inhibitor for patients with low blood pressure (i.e., 100/70* mmHg) or mild renal insufficiency (serum creatinine 2.0 mg/dL).[35] Similarly, for patients with heart failure and comorbid atrial fibrillation, they overestimate the risk of major bleeding and the adverse effects on quality of life if a patient is prescribed warfarin.[35] Thus, guidelines need to address these issues head on. The AHCPR guideline attempted to do this.[18] For example, the section on ACE inhibitors states (page 55):

> *Side-effects of ACE inhibitors, particularly decreases in blood pressure and increases in serum creatinine and potassium, have been emphasized in many*

studies. These concerns may have made some physicians reluctant to use ACE inhibitors. However, the average changes in blood pressure and serum chemistries in the SOLVD trial were actually quite small, with systolic blood pressure decreasing an average of 5 mmHg, diastolic blood pressure decreasing 4 mmHg, creatinine increasing 0.1 mg/dL, and potassium increasing 0.2 mEq/L. Only 2.2% of those eligible had hypotension when enalapril was initiated.

However, simply providing this information is probably not enough to overcome many physicians' fears. It may be useful for guidelines to develop Internet-based programs where physicians can attempt to manage this type of difficult case and receive Council on Medical Education (CME) credits for going through the program.

So, guidelines may be a useful way to synthesize a complex body of knowledge about the use of a diagnostic test or treatment into a digestible "package" for clinicians. However, a palatable message is not enough. The technology diffusion literature suggests that the rate of change also depends upon individual characteristics of the adopter, the adopter's social network, the messenger, and incentives to change.[15] Some clinicians may be inherently resistant to adopting new technology. Others may not be influenced by expert cardiologists opinions and look to see what their "peers" are doing. Finally, many primary-care physicians may be ready and willing to change, but need some support structure to remind them of best practices for the vast number of conditions they must treat. For these physicians, more intensive measures are probably needed to achieve behavior change, and disease management programs may be a helpful tool.

The Promise of Disease Management for Improving Quality of Care

In contrast to the glacial rate of change in quality of care in the general population of patients with heart failure, disease management programs have shown the potential to rapidly improve compliance with guideline recommendations and, more importantly, improve patients' outcomes. What is disease management? Definitions vary, but the essence is "a comprehensive integrated system for managing patients . . . by using best practices, clinical practice improvement information technology, and other resources and tools to reduce overall costs and improve measurable outcomes in the quality of care."[36] However, the application of this concept is even more variable than the definitions: if you've seen one disease management program, you've seen one disease management program. There are three broad types that are most widely used:

- Hospital-based programs, which generally use a multidisciplinary team for evaluation and treatment
- The heart failure clinic
- The community case-management model, which follows patients across the entire continuum of care and heavily emphasizes home visits

Each of these will be briefly described below and published examples presented. For a more complete discussion, I refer the reader to the excellent book edited by Moser and Riegel.[37]

Hospital-Based Programs

The prototype for hospital-based disease management for heart failure was the study conducted by Rich and colleagues.[38] Patients hospitalized with heart failure were seen by a nurse-directed multidisciplinary team consisting of the heart failure nurse and a geriatric cardiologist, a dietician, and a social worker. The cardiologist adjusted medications as needed, including eliminating unnecessary medications. The dietician reviewed low-salt diet and other dietary requirements as indicated, and the nurse instructed the patient and family members about self-management principles. The nurse also conducted follow-up telephone calls after discharge. The intervention dramatically reduced the overall readmission rate, mostly due to a reduction in readmissions for heart failure exacerbations (Fig. 2). Medication compliance also improved. This in-patient model was used in a simplified form by Costantini and coworkers in a firm trial.[39] A faculty cardiologist and a nurse care manager reviewed each patient's chart and made guideline-based recommendations. Another group of patients received usual care. The rate of ACE inhibitor use prior to the intervention was 60%. After the start of the intervention period, ACE inhibitor use in the usual care group rose slightly to 75%. But ACE inhibitor use rose to 95% in the care-managed group, an increase more than double the expected temporal trend.

We have used a similar model in our Heart Failure Disease Management Program at MetroHealth. Prior to establishing the program, we identified five targets for quality improvement (Table 3). These were selected because a process–outcome link was believed to exist, and a baseline chart review suggested significant room for improvement. This is an example of the "less is more" philosophy that change is more likely to occur if quality improvement projects concentrate on only a few goals at a time. Once these goals are met, new ones can be established. We then hired a "heart failure nurse," who was assigned the key role of seeing all patients admitted with a heart failure exacerbation. Upon first seeing the

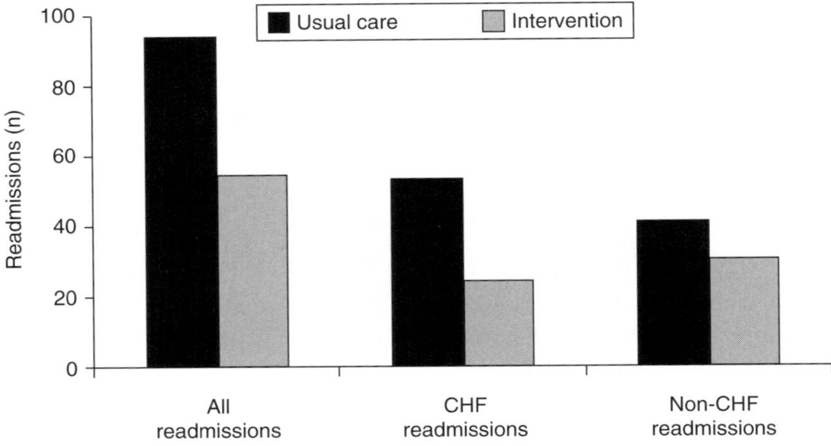

Figure 2. Number of readmissions within 90 days of discharge with usual care (black) and with a nurse-directed multidisciplinary disease management program (gray).

Table 3

Challenges in Quality of Care for Key Indicators before and after Initiation of a Disease Management Program at MetroHealth Medical Center

	Before (%)	After (%)
• Documentation of LVEF	77	95
• On ACE inhibitor (low LVEF)	85	98
• Prescribed at target dose	35	81
• On digoxin (low LVEF)	72	92
• On warfarin (atrial fibrillation)	41	100

ACE, angiotensin-converting enzyme; LVEF, left ventricular ejection fraction (low LVEF is ≤40%).

patient, she reviews compliance with the quality-of-care goals and contacts physicians if a patient has not had an echocardiogram or is not receiving an indicated medication. In addition, she conducts a readmission risk assessment (including inability to pay for medications, dementia, depression, low literacy, etc.), educates patients about their disease and self-management skills (including giving patients a free scale if they are unable to afford one), and provides a case-management function to try to reduce readmission risks. Several months after the program began, we repeated our chart review. Quality of care had improved for all measures

(Table 3). After this rapid improvement, we began to address other problematic areas, such as inadequate monitoring of daily weights and fluid balance and suboptimal diuretic dosing.

The Heart Failure Clinic

To expand the scope of disease management for heart failure, it is important to move beyond the hospital. Heart failure clinics care for patients discharged from the hospital and for patients with severe heart failure who require more intensive and more specialized outpatient care than is usually available in physicians' offices. Most rely on a multidisciplinary team to optimize medical therapy, educate patients about their condition and self-management (especially weight monitoring and the use of a flexible diuretic regimen), and provide long-term follow-up. Nurse practitioners and advance practice nurses play a prominent role in patients' care. Almost all clinics have used written guidelines or care paths. Because of this systematic approach, it is difficult for patients to "slip through the cracks" and not be prescribed indicated therapy.

Although almost all heart failure clinics have reported decreases in hospital admission rates, this should be interpreted cautiously, because only one study was a randomized trial.[40] Moreover, we have limited data on the degree to which heart failure clinics improve quality of care. Some of the reduction in hospitalizations is likely due to better patient education, and information on compliance with quality of care measures is sparse. Dahl and Penque reported higher rates of use of ACE inhibitors among patients who went through their clinic compared to historical controls,[41] and Fonarow and colleagues reported a doubling of the mean dose of ACE inhibitors for patients seen in their clinic.[42] Thus, heart failure clinics, like hospital-based programs, are very likely to improve quality of care. The more important issue is how to reach the large population of outpatients with heart failure that is not severe enough to require specialized care for the prevention of hospitalization. In our experience, many of the patients with milder heart failure are not receiving ACE inhibitors and beta-blockers. Although they may be at lower risk for hospitalization, they remain at risk for sudden death and progressive worsening of their cardiac function. Thus, it is important to find ways of extending the reach of heart failure clinics and other specialized outpatient programs such as community case management (see below).

Case-Management Models

Many patients with heart failure are elderly and have multiple comorbidities and social situations that put them at risk for adverse outcomes. For such individuals, having a case manager who follows them across the spectrum of care may be very helpful. The transition from hospital to home may be a particularly vulnerable period, so a home visit shortly after discharge may be helpful to reduce readmissions. Finally, education is likely to be more effective in a relaxed, familiar setting than at the time of discharge from the hospital. All of these factors have served as a rationale for community case management models of heart failure care.[43] Several studies have shown reductions in hospital admission for patients enrolled in a heart failure case management program. For example, in a randomized controlled trial, Stewart reported a 42% reduction in unplanned admissions.[44] Similarly, Naylor reported that patients randomized to a case management program had a readmission rate of 20.3%, compared to 37.1% for those under usual care.[45] These studies have not reported changes in compliance with guideline recommendations, but the reductions in readmissions suggest positive changes in processes of care.

Limitations of Disease Management

Although many think of their disease management programs as "population-based," they often deal with only a small segment of all patients with heart failure. Most are very selective as to which patients they enroll. Obviously, hospital-based programs only enroll patients who have been hospitalized. Heart failure clinics only care for patients who were referred to them, often for evaluation for transplant. Although case-management programs may have more of a population focus, they still generally have criteria for identifying patients, such as a past hospitalization or emergency department visit for a heart failure exacerbation. It is understandable that disease management programs would choose to concentrate efforts on patients with severe disease and high utilization. After all, the prime motivator for creating a disease management program is often to reduce costs (i.e., hospital admissions).

However, only a minority of patients with heart failure have had a recent hospitalization. For example, when we started our disease management program at MetroHealth in 1997, we conducted analyses to understand better the population of patients with heart failure cared for by our health system. We found that a total of 348 patients had been discharged one or more times in the previous year with a principal diagnosis of heart failure (International Classification of Disease-9 codes 402.11, 402.91, 425.xx, 428.0, 428.1, 428.9, 429.0, and 429.1). However, another 1975 had been given an outpatient diagnosis code (any of three positions) of heart failure. Thus, of the 2323 patients with heart failure as an active medical problem, 85% had not been hospitalized. However, during the subsequent year, a total of 8% of individuals with only an outpatient diagnosis of heart failure were hospitalized with a primary diagnosis of heart failure. This shows that the population of outpatients with heart failure is a reservoir for future hospitalizations. Because this group is less likely to have received subspecialty care, they may be less likely to be receiving indicated therapy such as ACE inhibitors and beta-blockers. Thus, disease management programs that do not attempt to improve quality of care for outpatients, particularly those cared for exclusively by primary-care physicians, miss an important opportunity to reduce morbidity, mortality, and hospitalizations.

It is unclear what type of disease management program will prove to be both acceptable and effective for patients who are cared for by office-based physicians, especially primary-care providers. These doctors would probably not be willing to refer their patients with mild to moderate disease to a heart failure clinic. They also may not be willing to work in a cooperative relationship with a case-manager employed by an insurance company, although one program has successfully accomplished this goal by actually having a nurse practitioner see patients with heart failure in physicians' offices. It should be a priority for future research to identify models of disease management that work for the large proportion of patients with mild to moderate symptoms who are cared for by office-based physicians.

New information technology may also help achieve this goal. At MetroHealth, we have a fully computerized medical records system. This has allowed us to create flags that identify patients with heart failure in the general medicine clinic who are not receiving an ACE inhibitor or a beta-blocker. When a physician sees such a patient, a note pops up on the screen to notify the clinician and asks the clinician to indicate why the patient is not on this medication; start the medication; or refer the patient to our heart failure clinic for possible initiation and titration of indicated medications. A controlled trial of computer reminders at Veterans' Administration outpatient clinics improved prescribing patterns, but this effect waned over time.[46] Thus, there is no panacea. The goal of rapidly changing physicians' care patterns to coincide with what experts consider to be optimal therapy remains elusive. We need to augment our research efforts to understand better how we can ensure that all patients with heart failure receive high-quality care.

References

1. Schuster MA, McGlynn EA, Brook RH. How good is the quality of health care in the United States? *Milbank Q* 1998;76:517–563.
2. Committee on Quality Health Care in America, Institute of Medicine. *Crossing the Quality Chasm: A New Health System for the 21st Century*. Washington, DC: National Academy Press, 2001.

3. Deaton C, Exner DV, Schron EB, Riegel B, Prevost S. Outcomes measurement in heart failure. In: Moser DK, Riegel B, eds. *Improving Outcomes in Heart Failure*. Gaithersburg, MD: Aspen, 2001:267–300.
4. The Large State Peer Review Organization Consortium. Heart failure treatment with angiotensin-converting enzyme inhibitors in hospitalized Medicare patients in 10 large states. *Arch Intern Med* 1997;157:1103–1108.
5. Jencks SF, Cuerdon T, Burwen DR, et al. Quality of medical care delivered to Medicare beneficiaries. *JAMA* 2000;284:1670–1676.
6. Chin MH, Wang JC, Zhang JX, Lang RM. Utilization and dosing of angiotensin converting enzyme inhibitors for heart failure: Effect of physician specialty and patient characteristics. *J Gen Intern Med* 1997;12:563–566.
7. Chin MH, Friedmann PD, Cassel CK, Lang RM. Differences in generalist and specialist physicians' knowledge and use of angiotensin-converting enzyme inhibitors for congestive heart failure. *J Gen Intern Med* 1997;12:523–530.
8. Krumholz HM, Wang Y, Parent EM, Mockalis J, Petrillo M, Radford MJ. Quality of care for elderly patients hospitalized with heart failure. *Arch Intern Med* 1997;157:2242–2247.
9. Stafford RS, Saglam D, Blumenthal D. National patterns of angiotensin-converting enzyme inhibitor use in congestive heart failure. *Arch Intern Med* 1997;157:2460–2464.
10. Field MJ, Lohr KN, Committee to Advise the Public Health Service on Clinical Practice Guidelines, Institute of Medicine, eds. *Clinical Practice Guidelines: Directions For A New Program*. Washington, DC: National Academy Press, 1990.
11. Davis D, O'Brien MAT, Freemantle N, Wolf FM, Mazmanian P, Taylor-Vaisey A. Impact of formal continuing medical education: Do conferences, workshops, rounds, and other traditional continuing education activities change physician behavior or health care outcomes? *JAMA* 1999;282:867–874.
12. Hadorn D, Baker D, Dracup K, Pitt B. Making judgements about treatment effectiveness based on health outcomes: Theoretical and practical issues. *Jt Comm J Qual Improv* 1994;20:547–554.
13. Hadorn DC, Baker DW. Development of the AHCPR-sponsored heart failure guideline: methodologic and procedural issues. *Jt Comm J Qual Improv* 1994; 20:539–547.
14. Field MJ, Lohr KN, Committee on Clinical Practice Guidelines, Division of Health Care Services, Institute of Medicine. *Guidelines for Clinical Practice: From Development to Use*. Washington, DC: National Academy Press, 1992.
15. Rogers EM. *Diffusion of Innovations*. New York: Free Press, 1995.
16. McCormick KA, Moore SR, Siegel RA, eds. *Methodology Perspectives: Clinical Practice Guideline Development*. Rockville, MD: U.S. Dept. of Health and Human Services, Public Health Service, Agency for Health Care Policy and Research, 1994. (AHCPR pub. no. 95–0009.)
17. Hadorn DC, Baker DW, Hodges JS, Hicks N. Rating the quality of evidence for clinical practice guidelines. *J Clin Epidemiol* 1996;49:749–754.
18. Konstam M, Dracup KA, Baker DW, et al. *Heart Failure: Evaluation and Care of Patients with Left-Ventricular Systolic Dysfunction*. Rockville, MD: Agency for Health Care Policy and Research, 1994. (Clinical Practice Guideline no. 11.)
19. Massie BM. Clinical trials in heart failure: can we expect the results to be replicated in general practice? *J Card Fail* 1998;4:243–247.
20. Katzan IL, Furlan AJ, Lloyd LE, et al. Use of tissue-type plasminogen activator for acute ischemic stroke: The Cleveland area experience. *JAMA* 2000;283: 1189–1191.

21. Shekelle PG, Chassin MR, Park RE. Assessing the predictive validity of the RAND/UCLA appropriateness method criteria for performing carotid endarterectomy. *Int J Technol Assess Health Care* 1998;14:707–727.
22. Krumholz HM, Baker DW, Ashton CM, et al. Evaluating quality of care for patients with heart failure. *Circulation* 2000;101:E122–E140
23. Anonymous. Guidelines for the evaluation and management of heart failure. Report of the American College of Cardiology/American Heart Association Task Force on Practice Guidelines (Committee on Evaluation and Management of Heart Failure). *Circulation* 1995;92:2764–2784.
24. Anonymous. Consensus recommendations for the management of chronic heart failure. On behalf of the membership of the advisory council to improve outcomes nationwide in heart failure. *Am J Cardiol* 1999;83:1A–38A.
25. Anonymous. Heart Failure Society of America (HFSA) practice guidelines. HFSA guidelines for management of patients with heart failure caused by left ventricular systolic dysfunction-pharmacological approaches. *J Card Fail* 1999;5:357–382.
26. Jencks SF, Cuerdon T, Burwen DR, et al. Quality of medical care delivered to Medicare beneficiaries: A profile at state and national levels. *JAMA* 2000;284: 1670–1676.
27. Mosteller F. Innovation and evaluation. *Science* 1981;211:881–886.
28. Hjalmarson A, Goldstein S, Fagerberg B, et al. Effects of controlled-release metoprolol on total mortality, hospitalizations, and well-being in patients with heart failure: the Metoprolol CR/XL Randomized Intervention Trial in Congestive Heart Failure (MERIT-HF). MERIT-HF Study Group. *JAMA* 2000;283:1295–1302.
29. Anonymous. Effect of metoprolol CR/XL in chronic heart failure: Metoprolol CR/XL Randomised Intervention Trial in Congestive Heart Failure (MERIT-HF). *Lancet* 1999;353:2001–2007.
30. Waagstein F, Bristow MR, Swedberg K, et al. Beneficial effects of metoprolol in idiopathic dilated cardiomyopathy. Metoprolol in Dilated Cardiomyopathy (MDC) Trial Study Group. *Lancet* 1993;342:1441–1446.
31. Packer M, Bristow MR, Cohn JN, et al. The effect of carvedilol on morbidity and mortality in patients with chronic heart failure. U.S. Carvedilol Heart Failure Study Group. *N Engl J Med* 1996;334:1349–1355.
32. Anonymous. The Cardiac Insufficiency Bisoprolol Study II (CIBIS-II):a randomized trial. *Lancet* 1999;353:9–13.
33. Pitt B, Zannad F, Remme WJ, et al. The effect of spironolactone on morbidity and mortality in patients with severe heart failure. Randomized Aldactone Evaluation Study Investigators. *N Engl J Med* 1999;341:709–717.
34. Francis GS, Cohn JN, Johnson G, Rector TS, Goldman S, Simon A. Plasma norepinephrine, plasma renin activity, and congestive heart failure: Relations to survival and the effects of therapy in V-HeFT II. The V-HeFT VA Cooperative Studies Group. *Circulation* 1993;87(suppl):VI40–148.
35. Baker DW, Hayes RP, Massie BM, Craig CA. Variations in family physicians' and cardiologists' care for patients with heart failure. *Am Heart J* 1999;138: 826–834.
36. Bernard S. Disease management: Pharmaceutical industry perspective. *Pharmacy Executive* 1995:48–50.
37. Riegel B, LePetri B. Heart failure disease management models. In: Moser DK, Riegel B, eds. *Improving Outcomes in Heart Failure*. Gaithersburg, MD: Aspen, 2001:267–281.
38. Rich MW, Beckham V, Wittenberg C, Leven CL, Freedland KE, Carney RM. A

multidisciplinary intervention to prevent the readmission of elderly patients with congestive heart failure. *N Engl J Med* 1995;333:1190–1195.

39. Costantini O, Huck K, Carlson MD, et al. Impact of a guideline-based disease management team on outcomes of hospitalized patients with congestive heart failure. *Arch Intern Med* 2001;161:177–182.
40. Fonarow GC, Creaser JW, Livingston N. The clinic model of heart failure care. In: Moser DK, Riegel B, eds. *Improving Outcomes in Heart Failure.* Gaithersburg, MD: Aspen, 2001:301–317.
41. Dahl J, Penque S. The effects of an advanced practice nurse-directed heart failure program. *Nurse Pract* 2000;25:61–8, 71.
42. Fonarow GC, Stevenson LW, Walden JA, et al. Impact of a comprehensive heart failure management program on hospital readmission and functional status of patients with advanced heart failure. *J Am Coll Cardiol* 1997;30:725–732.
43. Moser DK, Macko MJ, Hackett FK, Hutchins MR. *Community Case Management Models of Heart Failure Care.* In: Moser DK, Riegel B, eds. *Improving Outcomes in Heart Failure.* Gaithersburg, MD: Aspen, 2001:282–300.
44. Stewart S, Pearson S, Horowitz JD. Effects of a home-based intervention among patients with congestive heart failure discharged from acute hospital care. *Arch Intern Med* 1998;158:1067–1072.
45. Naylor M, Brooten D, Campbell R, et al. Comprehensive discharge planning and home follow-up of hospitalized elders. *JAMA* 1999;281:613–620.
46. Demakis JG, Beauchamp C, Cull WL, et al. Improving residents' compliance with standards of ambulatory care: results from the VA Cooperative Study on Computerized Reminders. *JAMA* 2000;284:1411–1416.

Chapter 3

Managed Care and Heart Failure

Suzette Cardin, RN, DNSc, FAAN

Heart failure is now considered the single most costly cardiovascular illness in the United States. The forecast for the cost of caring for a patient with heart failure is expected to increase, rather than decrease.[1] There are many factors that affect the cost of caring for patients with heart failure. The purpose of this chapter will be to discuss the perspective of managed care and the effect that this type of health-care financing and delivery system has had and will have on patients who present with heart failure. The cost of health care in the United States and the relationship to the managed care delivery system will be the foundation of the chapter. This chapter will provide an overview of the current status of the managed care delivery system and the impact that this delivery system has had on health-care providers who care for patients with heart failure.

The concept of managed care and its relationship to heart failure patients is a complex one. The complexity results from the economics of the managed care system and the traditional method of caring for patients with heart failure. Current cost containment strategies are aimed at improving the management of the underlying disease process of heart failure, due to the fact that 75% of the hospitalization costs occur within the first 48 h of a hospital admission.[1] Most patients with heart failure are treated using traditional health-care delivery models in which episodic care is delivered during periods of exacerbation of heart failure, with little systematic follow-up. These aspects of traditional care delivery must be changed to improve the increasing incidence, prevalence and economic costs of heart failure. The stimulus for a change from the current treatment patterns to a more comprehensive, integrated heart failure specialty approach is imperative.[2]

From: Jessup M, McCauley KM (eds). *Heart Failure: Providing Optimal Care.* Elmsford, NY: Futura, an imprint of Blackwell Publishing; ©2003.

Perspective of Managed Care

The delivery system of health care in the United States has undergone a dramatic transformation. The past two decades have been challenging and exciting times for health-care providers and recipients of health-care services. Health care is now a business, it is no longer a service. Heart failure as a disease entity and patients with heart failure as a growing part of the elderly population are important aspects within the business of health care. In 1999, heart failure hospitalizations cost $99 billion dollars, which correlates to 5–8% of the federal health-care expenditures.[1] This is a significant statistic when coupled with the fact that the incidence and prevalence of heart failure are expected to grow, primarily because of recent declines in mortality from coronary heart disease and the graying and aging of the United States population at large.

Managed care has come to dominate the health-care finance and delivery system in the United States; how did this happen? It can be postulated from a systems theory perspective that looks at structure, process, and outcome that there is no real "system" of health care in the United States. The current feature in the system is fragmentation. The system presents itself as a kaleidoscope, change is constant, and this change is based on the fact that the delivery, payment, and financing of health care are not consistent throughout the system. There was a lack of control over utilization and payment of health-care services before the dominance of managed care.

In the late 1980s and early 1990s, the health-care delivery system attracted national attention; it was at that time in a state of financial crisis. At that time, private insurers' premiums were rising between 15% and 20% a year, which was almost twice the increase in per capita spending under Medicare. In 1993, the Congressional Budget Office reported that the United States would be spending 20% of the gross domestic product by 2000 and 28% by the year 2010 on health care.[3] This would have bankrupted the Social Security Medicare system. The concept of managed care was a quick solution to this spending curve. In theory, managed care has worked—the initiative has provided a tightening of costs and utilization of services. In a practical sense, however, managed care has created a system that is cumbersome and not very user-friendly. The impact of this failure has been seen in the heart failure population. Guidelines for practice are research-driven, and outcomes are based on interventions that are not fully implemented.

An analysis of the United States health-care system provides a framework for understanding why managed care as a system was not able to effectively reach the goals that were established in the 1990s. The basic character of the health-care delivery system is influenced by external social and physical factors. The factors consist of the following: the political climate of the nation, economic development, technological process, social and cultural values, the physical environment, and population characteristics such as demographic and health trends.[4] The author has also identified ten basic characteristics that differentiate the United States health-care delivery system; this will provide the framework for understanding the current health-care system.

1 *No central governing agency.* A department or agency of the government does not control the United States health-care system. The United States and South Africa are the only two developed countries in the world in which every citizen does not receive a defined set of health-care services. A global budget is established in other developed countries, and the health-care expenditures are within a global type of budget system. The system of health-care delivery in the United States is a private system for both financing and delivery. The delivery of medical services is for the most part done through a private business enterprise system; it is not government-controlled. Private financing, which is predominantly through employees, accounts for 54% of the total health-care expenditures, and the government finances the remaining 46%. The key element is that there is no central agency to monitor total expenditures or to control the availability of services.

2 *Partial access.* Health care is not available to everyone in the United States. Access, for purposes of this discussion, means the ability of an individual to obtain health-care services when needed. Health insurance is the primary means for insuring access—unless it is an emergency illness, in which case anyone can receive care in an emergency room when necessary. Heart failure patients do have access to health care, especially those over 65 years of age; this is due to the fact that Medicare is the mechanism by which the elderly access the health-care system. In this patient population, access does not become the issue, but rather the nonuse of or nonadherence to therapies that have been found to be research- or evidence-based and have a proven success record.

3 *Imperfect market.* The delivery and utilization of health-care services in the United States operates in an imperfect market. The basic tenets of a free market are not met in the current United States health-care system. The health-care system is not a free market where the patients and the providers act independently. The majority of patients are in

health plans; the health plans are the real buyers of the health-care service, not the individual patient. Not all patients have the information they need about availability of services, nor is there information on price and quality for each provider. Patients as consumers do not usually make decisions about the purchase of health-care services; their health plan usually does.

4 *Third-party insurers and payers.* The insurance company functions as an intermediary between those who finance, deliver, or receive health care. The delivery of health care is often viewed as a transaction between the patient and the provider.

5 *Multiple payers.* In the United States, there are multiple health plans and insurance companies, which represent both a billing and collection problem for the providers of services. The managed care system has added to this problem, and the United States consequently has the highest administrative health costs of any country in the world.

6 *No single entity dominates the system.* Many players are involved in delivering health care; these include physicians, hospitals, insurance companies, large employees, and the government. Players have their own economic interests to protect, and the self-interest of different players is often at odds. The forces for changing the health-care system prevent any single entity from dominating the system and also from achieving systemwide reform. Reforms in the health-care system have been typically incremental or piecemeal.

7 *Legal risks.* Providers of health care usually practice a defensive style of medicine. The practice of medicine in the United States is often influenced by the risk of malpractice lawsuits. This has caused additional efforts to be put into the diagnosis and treatment of patients, which in turn has helped to make the current system very costly and inefficient.

8 *High technology.* Patients and providers of health care want the latest and the best, especially when they are covered by health insurance. The resources to finance health care have been shrinking, yet the growth in science and technology has created the opposite effect, which in turn has been passed on to the provider and recipient of health-care services.

9 *Continuum of services.* Health-care services are now delivered on a continuum, and it is no longer confined to the hospitals and physician's office. The changing configuration of

Table 1

Trends in Health Care

Illness	Wellness
Acute care	Primary care
Fragmented care	Managed care
Independence	Integration
Service duplication	Continuum of services

economic incentives has changed the continuum of care, which includes preventive care, primary care, specialized care, chronic care, long-term care, subacute care, acute care, rehabilitative care, and end-of-life care.

10 *Quest for quality.* Providers of health care are now under pressure to develop quality standards and to demonstrate compliance with those standards. Quality is the goal and is now the benchmark for determining where patients receive their health care.

Although the goals of the early 1990s regarding the need for health-care reform were not met, there has been a transformation, and change has occurred in the United States health-care system. The trends in health-care delivery for the most part have been characterized by a fundamental shift in how Americans view health and the type of delivery that can promote health at a lower cost. The trends and directions in health-care delivery are listed in Table 1.

The growth of managed care has been credited with much of the change in the focus on the delivery of health care. An understanding of the health-care delivery system is essential for health-care providers, especially for those who provide services for heart failure patients.

Cost of Health Care

Health-care spending in the United States has grown from a $247 billion in 1980 to $1.3 trillion in 2000; this is up from over 400% in 20 years.[5] Health-care spending is now 14% of the gross domestic product. The average percent increases from 1975 to 1999 are listed in Table 2. Managed care was successful in the mid-1990s; this was also a time of stabilization in the American economy. Increases in the cost of health care are expected to occur as the cost of health care starts to accelerate again. Health-care costs are not expected to reach double-digit increases, but will be significant enough to warrant the attention of providers and consumers.

Table 2

Average Percentage Increases in Health-Care Costs

1975–1980	13.6%
1980–1985	11.6%
1985–1990	10.2%
1990–1995	7.2%
1996–1997	4.8%
1997–1998	5.6%
1998–1999	5.6%
1999–2000	8.3%
2000–2001	8.6%

Annual increases in health-care spending are expected to be 6–7% each year, which is twice the expected growth of the consumer price index over the first 5 years of the new millennium. This prediction is consistent with projections from the United States government.[6] The most important factors driving health-care spending for the next 5 years are as follows:

- *Increasing consumer expectations.* The widespread use of the Internet and drug company advertising will be a major factor that will drive up the cost of health-care spending.
- *New drugs.* There will not be a slowdown to the cost of new drugs and the effect that this will have on health-care expenditures.
- *Technology.* In health care, the application of new technology will continue, and this significantly impacts the cost of health care. In other industries, new technology lowers the cost of care, but in health care this is usually not the case.
- *Aging of the population.* This is an inevitable expense, and will be a very important driver of the cost of health care.
- *Administrative expenses.* The complexity and fragmentation of the United States health-care system makes the overhead costs increase rather than decrease.
- *Surplus of physicians.* This drives up the cost of health care and causes a physician-induced demand situation.

What is Managed Care?

Managed care is defined in a number of ways. The founding principles of managed care are prevention, early detection of disease, coordination of care, and cost-effectiveness.[7] These principles are the foundation for what is now seen as the system of managed care in the United States health-care industry. Managed care is a system of health-care delivery that seeks to achieve efficiencies by integrating the basic foundations of health-care delivery. Managed care uses mechanisms to control or manage utilization of medical services and then determines at which price these services will be purchased. The primary financier of health care is the employer or the government. Health insurance, instead of being purchased through a traditional insurance company, is now purchased through a managed care organization (MCO). Examples of MCOs would be a health-maintenance organization (HMO) or a preferred provider organization (PPO). The MCO then functions like an insurance company and promises to provide health-care services that are contracted under the health plan to the enrollees of the plan. The benefits of an MCO are the following: there is integration of health-care functions into one organizational setting; there is formal control over utilization of services; and the MCO determines the price of services and how much the provider gets paid. The essential features of a managed care system are listed in Table 3.

In a managed care system that is effective, the pros of the system can outweigh what would be considered the cons or the barriers to implementing the system. The goal is to have a seamless system, and if the system is working correctly, that goal can be achieved. The benefits of case management, utilization review, and practice profiling are the hallmarks of a well-run managed care organization. Managed care organizations are increasing the provision of preventive services such as screening immunizations and counseling for high-risk conditions as a means to reduce costs. This shift in focus under managed care from acute services to preventive care has changed who provides health care, as well as how the care is provided.

Table 3

Essential Features of a Managed Care Organization

Essential Features of a Managed Care Organization
Cost containment
Accountability for quality and cost
Measurement of outcomes
Health promotion and prevention
Management of resource consumption
Consumer education
Quality improvement initiatives

The concept of managed care is not fully embraced by many health-care providers and recipients. The consolidation of hospitals and medical groups and health-care plans has been one of the most visible signs of change in health care over the past 20 years, and this is likely to continue. The financial incentives of the health-care marketplace, which is a mix of capitated and fee-for-service payment, continues to be inconsistent, and the hybrid payment system is dysfunctional at the present time. The following factors have had a significant negative effect on the system of managed care:

1 *Gatekeeping.* The fact that someone has to oversee what care is needed before the patient can get the service he/she needs was a radical change for most Americans. In a system where patients got whatever they needed, there was a great deal of resistance to gatekeeping when it was introduced. It was also a very cumbersome process, and it took a while to finally get what you needed. It was not considered very user-friendly.
2 *Restriction in choice.* In a managed care environment, certain choices exist for the enrollees, and this was again a new phenomenon for the American public. Many in the United States see health care as a right, and the fact that choice was restricted or limited was not an easy concept to understand, much less operationalize. The American public wants the best and the biggest, and therefore cost should not be an issue; but with managed care, cost is the underlying theme.
3 *Complex cases.* In the early 1990s, the American public was very skeptical about the type of care that patients who presented with complex problems in MCOs received. Tertiary centers are now commonplace in all states, and the question was always asked: Why should we be denied access to the best care just because we are in an MCO? This practice has been modified on the basis of legal cases that have occurred over the past few years, and there now exists in many MCOs a clause or provision for dealing with complex cases and the fact that complex cases can be referred, treated, and then returned to the original MCO.
4 *Adversarial relationships.* Managed care was introduced at a time when the political fever was quite high over changes in health care, and as a result the change was not seen as a welcome one in many situations. Many enrollees to this day do not feel that they have a say in their health-care coverage and how the MCO manages their medical care needs on a daily basis. Most Americans were used to a system in which they could go to see their health-care provider and spend as much

or as little time as they needed instead of the 10–15 min that is now considered commonplace in most MCOs.

5 *Emphasis only on cost.* This has probably been the major dissatisfier with managed care. Health care is a business, yet it is not seen as that when it is delivered or services are provided. The majority of Americans are still operating under the premise that their employee has to provide health-care coverage, it is their right as a worker in that particular company. As cost shifting continues in health-care coverage and as the American economy begins to decline, this paradigm will become self-evident and health-care coverage will become a focal point as it relates to benefit coverage for employees.

Managed Care and Heart Failure Patients

The spiraling growth in the number of individuals with heart failure can be attributed to several factors, including the aging of the population in the United States and the early successful treatment of acute cardiovascular problems. This has caused a reduced mortality, but has also resulted in large numbers of patients living longer with chronic conditions. Heart failure is now the most frequent discharge seen in the Medicare population, and the incidence increases significantly with age.[8]

In theory, a managed care system is what is needed for heart failure patients. The concerns of patients and families are many, and relate to both the manifestations of heart failure and to the management regimen imposed by health-care providers. The signs and symptoms of acute heart failure are difficult to ignore, yet the subtle increasing symptoms that could warn of impending exacerbation are usually difficult to identify; they are usually subtle and difficult for patients to interpret.[9] In a managed care system where prevention, detection of disease, coordination of care and cost-effectiveness are the cornerstones, patients with heart failure would seem to be a natural choice for inclusion in this group. The Medicare system was chosen to address this issue, but it takes an economic perspective, with the emphasis on managed care programs for those who are currently enrolled in the Medicare program. In this system, there is no emphasis on looking at a specific population such as heart failure patients; rather, the emphasis is on cost-effectiveness measures that can be attained from an overall perspective. Once specific populations are identified in the managed care enrolled population and specific guidelines are adhered to as described in this monograph series, only then will the true benefits of a managed care system be truly manifested.

In the current system, there are many roadblocks that occur when a patient with heart failure is treated in an MCO. The issues revolve around the lack of adherence to heart failure protocols, which need to be implemented in a timely and consistent manner, as described in various chapters throughout this monograph series. The issues of compliance with drug therapy and follow-up also need to be addressed from a protocol perspective. The outcome measures that have been advocated throughout this monograph series are issues that MCOs need to address in order to comprehensively care for heart failure patients. As the management of heart failure patients becomes more sophisticated over time, not only is there an imperative need to continue to identify the most successful best practices and implement them, there is also a pressing need to include more comprehensive data on the range of costs. The evidence is clear that heart failure is a huge health problem with enormous societal and individual costs, and the economic consequences must be addressed.[1]

Future of Managed Care

Health care and the costs associated with caring for individuals who need health care are issues that have now become front-page news on a consistent basis. Earlier in this chapter, it was mentioned that the past 20 years in health care have been the most turbulent and chaotic times in health care to date. What does this all mean to the future of the current managed care system, and how does it relate to the care of the patient with heart failure? These questions have considerable merit, and the answers really depend on whom you talk to and in what part of the country. In response to the question of whether managed care did what it was supposed to do to reduce the cost of health care, Dr. Uwe Reinhardt answered that managed care was successful—it reined in the cost of health care and it controlled the spending curve temporarily, so that it was almost flat, with maybe a 2% increase. In his article in the *Wall Street Journal,* Dr. Reinhardt states that he believes that the health-care system will continue to evolve and will develop into a multitiered system that will be based on ability to pay.[3]

What is the future of managed care at this point in time and where will it go from here? One prediction is that comprehensive health care will be offered to an enrolled population, there will be greater management of risks, and there will be more accountability. The population suited for this is the heart failure population; there is usually a cohort of problems that are present in heart failure patients, since the largest majority are patients who are elderly and present with other problems as well. This will continue to be one of the major challenges that health-care providers will continue to face in the growing numbers of people who are diagnosed with heart failure. Future trends in the health-care delivery system are listed in Table 4. The trends are specific yet far-reaching and

Table 4

Future Trends in Health-care Delivery Systems

- Health care will be converted from a retail market to wholesale transactions
- Price wars will continue
- Providers will contract with a few, large health-care providers
- Health-care plans will acquire their own gatekeepers
- Hospitals and providers will join 3–4 regional networks
- Academic medical centers will be the providers for a limited range of high-tech services
- Demand for in-patient hospital beds will shrink by 15–25%
- 95% of all physicians will join practice groups or managed care networks within 5 years

will continue to affect how health care is delivered in this country. Managed care from a conceptual perspective has evolved through an integration of insurance functions and the need for consumers to have a greater choice in health-care providers. The growth of managed care is one reason why there has been the tremendous amount of consolidation and diversification in the health-care industry. The economics of health care will continue to dominate how care is delivered, and they are now considered to be in an adolescent stage of growth, as compared to where health-care economics was 20 years ago.

Summary

Managed care and heart failure have been discussed in this chapter from an economic and systems perspective. It is critical that these two concepts are discussed from these perspectives; the issues involved are complex and warrant detailed analysis. Heart failure is now considered the single largest health-care expenditure in the United States, and this will continue as the population continues to age and gray at accelerating rates. It is imperative that future work with patients who have heart failure continues to identify the best practices and outcomes; future multidisciplinary interventions must take account of the concepts of economics and the cost of caring for these patients.

References

1. McCauley KM, Naylor, MD. Managing heart failure: economic impact and concerns. In: Moser DK, Riegel B, eds. *Improving Outcomes in Heart Failure.* Gaithersburg, MD: Aspen, 2000:31–40.

2. O'Connell JB, Bristow, MR. Economic impact of heart failure in the United States: Time for a different approach. *J Heart Lung Transplant* 1993;13:S107–S112.
3. Hensley S. Talking about HMOs. *Wall Street Journal* 2001; Wednesday, February 21:R9–R10.
4. Shi L, Singh DA, eds. *Delivering Health Care in America: A Systems Approach*. Gaithersburg, MD: Aspen, 2001:1–32.
5. Coddington DC, Fischer EA, Moore KD, Clarke RL, eds. *Beyond Managed Care: How Consumers and Technology are Changing the Future of Health Care*. San Francisco: Jossey-Bass, 2000:59–72.
6. Coddington DC, Fischer EA, Moore KD, Clarke RL, eds. *Beyond Managed Care: How Consumers and Technology are Changing the Future of Health Care*. San Francisco: Jossey-Bass, 2000:73–88.
7. Coddington DC, Fischer EA, Moore KD, Clarke RL, eds. *Beyond Managed Care: How Consumers and Technology are Changing the Future of Health Care*. San Francisco: Jossey-Bass, 2000:28–54.
8. Dunbar SB, Dracup K, Agency for Health Care Policy and Research. Clinical practice guidelines for heart failure. *J Cardiovasc Nurs* 1996;10:85–88.
9. Moser DK, Riegel B, eds. *Improving Outcomes in Heart Failure: An Interdisciplinary Approach*. Gaithersburg, MD: Aspen, 2001:xv–xvi.

Chapter 4

Defining Heart Failure: Systolic versus Diastolic Dysfunction, Differential Diagnosis, Initial Testing

Mariell Jessup, MD, FACC, FAHA

Definition of Heart Failure

Authors of textbooks struggle with the definition of heart failure even as the pathophysiologic abnormalities that occur in the process are more fully understood. The genetic, structural, neurohormonal, and molecular mechanisms of heart failure are continually updated with the efforts of countless investigators throughout the world; yet we are left with a definition of heart failure that depends on the clinical description of essentially nonspecific symptoms. Thus, the definition of heart failure is a clinical syndrome that results from a structural or functional cardiac disorder that impairs the ability of the ventricle to fill with or eject blood commensurate with the needs of the body. This syndrome, which is a constellation of signs and symptoms, is primarily manifested by dyspnea, fatigue, fluid retention, and a decreased exercise tolerance.

Heart failure may result from disorders of the pericardium, the myocardium, the endocardium or valvular structures, the great vessels of the heart or from rhythm disturbances. From a clinical standpoint, however, we tend to think about heart failure in terms of myocardial dysfunction. This may be because many valvular, pericardial, and arrhythmias are easily amenable to either very effective surgery or other definitive treatments, which go a long way towards correcting the symptoms of heart failure. We are left, then, with patients who have

From: Jessup M, McCauley KM (eds). *Heart Failure: Providing Optimal Care.* Elmsford, NY: Futura, an imprint of Blackwell Publishing; ©2003.

myocardial dysfunction that ultimately accounts for their symptoms of congestion or fatigue.

Abnormalities of the myocardium have been classified in many ways, as has heart failure been variously classified. Probably the most useful classification is to describe the underlying cardiomyopathy, which frequently will suggest etiology as well.[1–4] Some examples of the World Health Organization (WHO) classification include ischemic cardiomyopathy, hypertrophic or restrictive cardiomyopathy, and idiopathic dilated cardiomyopathy. In the United States, the most common cause of heart failure is coronary artery disease,[5,6] causing an ischemic cardiomyopathy. Another practical approach is to divide up patients with heart failure into those with primarily systolic dysfunction and those with diastolic dysfunction. For the clinician, this usually means assessing the patient's left ventricular ejection fraction (LVEF), by a variety of techniques, during the initial evaluation.[7,8] Thus, if a patient has a low LVEF, usually less than 40–45%, their condition is called systolic heart failure. If a patient has symptoms consistent with heart failure but has a preserved or normal LVEF, they are labeled as having diastolic heart failure or diastolic dysfunction. Patients with systolic heart failure typically have a low LVEF, a dilated left ventricular cavity, and a reduced cardiac output because of diminished contractility of the myocardium. In contrast, patients with diastolic heart failure have a normal LVEF, normal contractility, but impaired filling of the heart secondary to a variety of pathophysiologic abnormalities. Table 1 contrast systolic and diastolic heart failure in an outline form, and diastolic dysfunction is discussed later in the chapter.

Table 1

Systolic and Diastolic Heart Failure: Comparison

	Systolic dysfunction	Diastolic dysfunction
Ejection fraction	Below 40%	Above 40%
LV cavity size	Increased	Normal
Age of patient	All ages	Usually elderly
Gender of patient	Primarily male	Primarily female
Presence of S3	Frequently	Uncommon
Associated with hypertension	Sometimes	Frequently
Associated with diabetes	Sometimes	Frequently
Associated with CAD	50–60%	Unclear, but >50%
Frequent hospitalizations	Yes	Yes
Ventricular arrhythmias	Common	Unclear
Atrial arrhythmias	Common	Common

CAD, coronary artery disease; LV, left ventricular.

The Evolution of Heart Failure

Some patients develop heart failure literally "overnight." For example, a previously healthy male cigarette smoker may suffer a massive myocardial infarction and lose enough viable myocardium to progress rapidly to pulmonary edema or cardiogenic shock. If he survives this acute episode, he is usually left with chronic heart failure. A second example is a patient with an acute aortic dissection that causes abrupt aortic insufficiency. This sudden volume overload overwhelms the left ventricle's ability to accommodate to the load, and the patient experiences life-threatening heart failure. However, the majority of patients with heart failure have developed the syndrome in a more gradual manner, making the presentation less dramatic and often more confusing.

It is useful to think of heart failure beginning with an initial insult to the heart. This insult may be as ordinary as an acute ischemic episode, or a transmural myocardial infarction, or involve a more insidious event such as the cumulative toxic effects of a chemotherapeutic drug. Whatever the cause, myocardial tissue is rendered either dysfunctional or destroyed, and a host of compensatory mechanisms begin.[9–12] It is beyond the scope of this text to describe the many pathophysiologic sequences which cause a patient to develop the symptoms of breathlessness and fatigue, or to manifest a decreased cardiac output despite an elevated end-diastolic filling pressure. Moreover, the cellular and biochemical systems that fail are not completely elucidated. Clearly, neurohormonal activation seems to be important, as therapies directed towards these targets have been remarkably successful.[13–16]

The unfortunate fact, however, is that despite our increasingly efficacious therapies for the management of heart failure, morbidity and mortality from the syndrome continue at an alarming rate.[17–19] One could argue that the excessive mortality is primarily related to an underutilization of these treatments by American health personnel. However, even in patients on optimal regimens, the relentless course of the cardiomyopathic process seems to proceed, resulting in progressive heart failure or sudden cardiac death. Most investigators agree that earlier recognition of the syndrome, or better identification of patients at risk for heart failure, may be our best hope for the future reduction of heart failure's death toll. Indeed, this is very analogous to the concerted efforts to screen for and detect cancer at the earliest stages of the malignancy, before the disease can defy therapy.

Unfortunately, progression of myocardial dysfunction is often asymptomatic, and becomes apparent only when a patient is hospitalized, or when testing reveals a deterioration of ventricular function. Yet, all too often physicians treat patients only if their symptoms worsen, and use signs and symptoms as a stimulus to add additional therapy, much of which has been shown to be effective even in the absence of a worsening clinical picture. As an example, a typical clinical scenario is the following: John Jones is a 58-year-old male with type 2 diabetes, hypertension, and hyperlipidemia. He suffered an acute anterior myocardial infarction 2 years ago. At that time he was given an aspirin, a beta-blocker, and a β-hydroxy-β-methylglutaryl coenzyme A (HMG-CoA) reductase inhibitor for long-term management. His physicians failed to recognize that he had suffered a significant loss of myocardium, as they had neglected to perform an echocardiogram prior to his discharge from hospital. (A number of studies have shown that angiotensin-converting enzyme (ACE) inhibitors can prevent adverse remodeling of the left ventricle in such a situation and maintain relatively normal ventricular geometry and function despite the large infarct.) One year later, he had his first episode of congestive heart failure. During that hospitalization, his LVEF was measured at 30% and he had moderate mitral regurgitation on his echocardiogram. His beta-blocker was discontinued, and an ACE inhibitor was started, along with a daily dose of a loop diuretic. The next time Mr. Jones was seen by his physician, there were no signs of heart failure and the patient felt "great." No additional therapy was added. Over the next year, however, his left ventricular size continued to increase and the mitral regurgitation worsened in severity. During this time, the patient reported no specific symptoms, but failed to mention that he had stopped walking in the evening, as had been his custom, because of fatigue. Eventually, 2 years after his initial infarction, he was hospitalized again with severe heart failure. His LVEF was now 15%, and he had pronounced left ventricular dilatation with severe mitral regurgitation.

Mr. Jones might have been spared these hospitalizations, and even the deterioration of his cardiac function, if his physician had recognized that left ventricular (LV) remodeling and myocardial cell loss continue in patients irrespective of symptoms. Possibly the addition of ACE inhibitors and beta-blockers early in Mr. Jones' course might have preserved his LV function, as some studies suggest.[20–24] Moreover, the recognition that LV function worsens over time could have prompted more careful attention to Mr. Jones' diet, blood-pressure control, avoidance of alcohol, and even regular exercise—treatments which have been shown to be effective in many patients to improve symptoms or LV function. To continue the analogy with cancer, physicians have to be ever vigilant that myocardial deterioration progresses, just as cancer can always recur or metastasize.

To address this issue, the updated guidelines for the management of heart failure from the American Heart Association and the American College of Cardiology have created a new classification of stages of heart failure.[25] These stages are the foundation upon which the subsequent discussions of therapy are built.

- *Stage A* represents those patients who are at high risk for developing heart failure. These include patients with hypertension and/or diabetes mellitus, coronary artery disease, or all three diseases. Included in this group are patients with a family history of dilated cardiomyopathy, as the genetic basis of this disease is becoming more clearly elucidated.[26–28] Patients who have been exposed to toxic chemotherapeutic agents are also in this group. Perhaps intensive intervention in Stage A patients will prevent their subsequent development of heart failure symptoms.
- *Stage B* includes those patients who have been found to have left ventricular systolic dysfunction in the absence of symptoms of heart failure. Usually, these patients are discovered coincidentally, often during screening for other problems, such as a preoperative medical clearance. A typical example is a young man who is to undergo orthopedic surgery and is found to have a left bundle branch block (LBBB) pattern on his electrocardiogram. Subsequent evaluation reveals a dilated cardiomyopathy, which has not yet caused symptoms of breathlessness or fluid retention. Other groups of patients who might develop asymptomatic LV systolic dysfunction are those with long-standing hypertension or left ventricular hypertrophy (LVH), an old myocardial infarction, or chronic valvular disease. For instance, some women with chronic mitral valve prolapse and progressive mitral regurgitation can ultimately develop LV dilatation and systolic failure, despite minimal change in their exercise tolerance. There are already some data that have shown a beneficial effect of both betablockers and ACE inhibitors when given to patients at this stage of their cardiac dysfunction.[29,30]
- *Stage C* represents all those patients with current or prior symptoms of heart failure, including those patients who are currently asymptomatic because they have been given appropriate therapy.
- *Stage D* includes those patients with advanced or refractory symptoms of heart failure. These patients have undergone multiple hospitalizations despite all appropriate therapy, or are under consideration for cardiac transplantation or awaiting a donor organ, or those patients who are terminal and require a hospice.

One could argue that since we have defined heart failure as a clinical syndrome, that it is inappropriate to actually label those patients who fall into stages A and B as having heart failure. However, it is possible that by emphasizing the risk for future events of those patients, and with the development of effective therapies to prevent the symptoms of heart failure, this classification will prove useful. Currently, the New York Heart Association (NYHA) functional classification, which has been widely used, does nothing to emphasize the progression of heart failure or to identify individuals at risk. Furthermore, the NYHA has not been helpful to describe patients with asymptomatic left ventricular dysfunction or those patients who have already had an episode of clinical heart failure but are currently symptomatic. In short, an NYHA class I patient—e.g., a patient with no symptoms—may still require a number of medications to prevent further deterioration in LV function or to decrease subsequent hospitalizations. However, the patient's doctor may be lulled into complacency in the absence of symptoms of heart failure. Thus, guidelines keyed to the stages of disease rather than NYHA functional class might prove to be more effective for public health in the future.

Identification of Patients

Patients with heart failure typically present in one of three ways:

- They present with a syndrome of decreased exercise tolerance.
- They present with a syndrome of fluid retention.
- Or their left ventricular dysfunction is incidentally discovered and the patient has been asymptomatic up until that time of discovery.

Each mode of presentation demands a slightly different task on the part of the health professional.

Syndrome of Decreased Exercise Tolerance

In patients who complain of a decreased exercise tolerance, the task is to elucidate the etiology of the decreased exercise ability. Patients with heart failure cannot augment cardiac output during exercise and/or the pulmonary capillary wedge pressure elevates to abnormally high values, and the patient experiences breathlessness and fatigue. Indeed, breathlessness on exertion is usually one of the earliest manifestations of abnormal cardiac function, but many patients attribute this symptom to age or deconditioning and rarely report only this problem. Much has been written about the mechanisms whereby patients with left ventricular dysfunction develop a decreased exercise ability, and most investigators agree that it is undoubtedly multifactorial in nature. However, breathlessness and fatigue during exercise may also be the initial complaints of patients with lung disease as well. Likewise, many elderly Americans rarely exercise regularly, and it is very true that these symptoms develop in some patients who are becoming increasingly deconditioned. Advancing age imparts its own impact on the ability of a human to exercise, and it is only through diligent training that the effects of age can be alleviated.

Syndrome of Fluid Retention

Patients with heart failure may notice peripheral edema, increasing abdominal girth, or have the classic symptoms of paroxysmal nocturnal dyspnea (PND) or orthopnea. The Agency for Health Care Policy and Research (AHCPR) heart failure guidelines have suggested that PND is the most specific symptom in patients with heart failure,[31] and, when present, can help to distinguish a patient's complaints from those of other disease processes. Unfortunately, fluid retention is part of other syndromes besides heart failure, including renal disease and simple venous insufficiency. A typical dilemma is an elderly woman with ankle edema, who has diabetes mellitus, obesity, hypertension, varicosities and normal left ventricular systolic function. It can be challenging to decide if her edema is secondary to diastolic heart failure or as a result of other medical problems and inactivity.

Incidentally Discovered Left Ventricular Dysfunction

Patients in stage B heart failure who have had a documentation of a low LVEF but are apparently asymptomatic are discovered in many ways. Often, however, the clinician must discern whether the patient is truly without symptoms. Frequently, patients have unconsciously decreased their activity so that they do not experience breathlessness. Another manner in which stage B patients may declare their cardiac dysfunction is with a life-threatening arrhythmia. All too often, a patient is resuscitated from sudden cardiac death and subsequently found to have severe LV systolic dysfunction. So while it is true that the patient was asymptomatic with respect to heart failure symptoms, the disease process was already causing havoc.

Identification of Structural Abnormality

Initial Approach

Once a patient is under consideration for the possibility of heart failure, the first step in their management is a *complete history and physical examination*. Key questions in the history should focus primarily on risks

Table 2

Conditions Associated with Diastolic Heart Failure

Conditions
Normal aging phenomena
Increase in systolic blood pressure
Increase in left ventricular hypertrophy
Increase in myocardial interstitial fibrosis
Increase in arterial stiffness
Abnormal beta-adrenergic modulation
Abnormal renal function
Systemic hypertension
Coronary artery disease
Hypertrophic cardiomyopathy
Hypertrophic cardiomyopathy of the elderly
Diabetes
Chronic obstructive pulmonary disease
Chronic renal insufficiency
Aortic stenosis
Atrial fibrillation
Other conduction abnormalities
Obesity
Infiltrative cardiomyopathy
Amyloid
Sarcoid
Sleep apnea

for and/or the presence of coronary artery disease, the possibility of toxic agents such as alcohol or cocaine, any history of valvular disorders, and a detailed family history to detect any other cases of dilated cardiomyopathy. Increasingly, sleep apnea has been associated with heart failure.[32–34] Correction of this syndrome may often improve many of the symptoms of heart failure, so that a detailed sleep history is critical. Concomitant disease processes such as diabetes and hypertension play an important role in diastolic heart failure and need to be screened for during the interview. Other systemic disorders, such as connective-tissue disease, might suggest a possible uncommon cause of an underlying cardiomyopathy.[35–38] Table 2 lists these and other considerations in outline form.

The physical examination may provide many important clues for the subsequent management of the patient. For example, a very young patient with evidence of both right and left ventricular dilatation and an enlarged liver almost certainly has an idiopathic dilated cardiomyopathy, as opposed to an ischemia etiology. A patient with a normal heart size by palpation and a vigorous left ventricular apex will not have significant systolic dysfunction, but is more likely to have a preserved left ventricular ejection fraction. A systolic murmur along the left sternal border which radiates to the neck in an elderly woman with angina and near-syncope should prompt a thorough investigation for aortic stenosis. A patient seen in the emergency department with anasarca, hypotension and cold extremities needs an intensive-care setting and pressor agents. Although all clinicians rely on noninvasive tests to help in the diagnosis and management of heart failure, an adequate job can only be accomplished after a thorough examination. The examination remains the best way to estimate the degree of volume overload; certain aspects of the physical exam can be important for prognostic purposes as well.[39] More about physical examination in the patient with heart failure may be found in Chapter 5.

Some measurement of overall cardiac contractility, or more accurately, the left ventricular ejection fraction, is a cornerstone of the initial assessment of the patient with heart failure. This is most often accomplished by an *echocardiogram,* although a left ventricular ejection fraction (EF) can be measured by nuclear methods or with left ventriculography at the time of catheterization. However, an echocardiogram not only assesses both left and right ventricular size and function, but it can reveal additional information about myocardial hypertrophy, valvular structure, and even the great vessels and pericardium. Moreover, an echocardiogram is safe, readily available and is without major adverse effects.[31] For a variety of reasons, it is useful to classify each patient as having heart failure primarily due to either systolic or diastolic dysfunction. Although many of the medications used for both types of heart failure are similar, the classification helps one to think about etiology and subsequent management.[25,40,41]

Other Testing

Other tests may be a part of the evaluation of the patient with heart failure, and are helpful for the identification of the cardiac structural abnormality which has contributed to the syndrome. A *12-lead electrocardiogram (ECG)* may show evidence of previous myocardial infarctions or acute ischemia as the etiology of the symptoms. The tracing may also suggest left ventricular hypertrophy, significant conduction abnormalities or arrhythmias.

Chest radiography is an important tool, not only to exclude pulmonary disease as a cause of the patient's symptoms, but also to assess the degree of pulmonary congestion.

Other diagnostic tools, which might be utilized in certain patients, are not routine in all patients suspected of having heart failure. These include a *radionuclide ventriculography* for a more objective measurement of the EF. This is occasionally helpful in patients with significant lung disease, in whom adequate echocardiographic images can not be obtained. Often, a radionuclide EF is used in research trials as an endpoint of therapy. Likewise, *magnetic resonance imaging (MRI) or computed tomography (CT) scanning* may be useful in the occasional patient with heart failure in whom pericardial disease or a ventricular mass is suspected to be important. Patients with right ventricular dysplasia may often be detected with MRI scans.

With the aforementioned initial approach to the patient, a clinician should have a very good idea of several issues:

- Possible reasons why the patient's heart has "failed"
- The degree of hemodynamic compromise of the patient, with respect to cerebral and peripheral perfusion, and fluid overload
- The size and contractility of both the right and left ventricles, and the function of the cardiac valves
- Need for hospitalization

Once the patient with heart failure has been stabilized, other issues need to be addressed.

General Laboratory Testing

The blood analyses in a patient with suspected heart failure are, for the most part, routine, designed primarily to assess the current metabolic state of the patient. Tests include: a complete blood count (to exclude infection or anemia as a cause of the patients' symptoms), urinalysis (to exclude infection or renal causes of the presenting syndrome), lipid panel (estimate risk for arteriosclerosis), electrolytes (hyperkalemia and hyponatremia are issues important in heart failure management), renal function (renal disease can mimic heart failure, and its presence can complicate the management of heart failure), hepatic function (severe, or acute heart failure can cause passive congestion of the liver), and thyroid function (both hypo- and hyperthyroid states can reproduce heart failure symptoms). In some patients, more specialized testing may be needed. As an example, patients with symptoms of heart failure and evidence for arthritis or other connective tissue disorders may require a specific analysis for inflammation or complement activation (see above). If primary or secondary hemochromatosis is suggested in the history, laboratory testing for iron stores may be necessary. The majority of these special blood tests will be prompted by the findings of the initial history and physical exam and not by a special mandate to do them in all patients with heart failure.[25]

Evaluation for the Possibility of Coronary Artery Disease as a Cause of Heart Failure

Over the past 10 years, a variety of committees have labored to produce guidelines for the management of heart failure.[31,42–47] Frequently, one of the more contentious issues has been the recommendations regarding the search for and subsequent management of coronary artery disease. Why is this so? It is very clear that nearly one-half or more of patients with heart failure have concomitant, significant coronary artery obstruction.[48] In the patient with preserved systolic function *and* symptoms of heart failure who may or may not also have angina, there has been considerable evidence gathered over the years to guide the management.[49–54] Almost always, revascularization, either through surgery or catheter-based, is indicated. This is also probably true for most patients with systolic dysfunction and angina as well.[55,56] However, in the patient with systolic dysfunction and no symptoms of angina or evidence of ischemia, there are no controlled studies that indicate that revascularization helps to improve the symptoms of heart failure. Indeed, a large, multicenter trial designed to investigate the role of revascularization in a patient with a low EF and significant coronary disease began in 2002. Until that time when the results of the trial are known, it is incumbent upon each clinician to be aware of the high prevalence of coronary disease and ischemia in the patient with heart failure. In addition, any patient with heart failure *and* symptoms of angina will need to have a full assessment of both their coronary anatomy and the pathophysiologic significance of same. The most recent guidelines from the American College of Cardiology/American Heart Association (ACC/AHA) tend to recommend catheterization in many patients, but not all clinicians believe in this approach.[25]

Evaluation for the Possibility of Myocardial Disease

For years, when a patient presented with new-onset heart failure and subsequent catheterization failed to reveal coronary artery obstruction, it was taught that the patient most likely had suffered the consequences of an acute viral infection. It was believed that a sequela of the virus was an intense inflammatory myocarditis that accounted for the rapidity of the onset of symptoms and the occasional complete recovery of these patients and their cardiac function. Although this scenario may still be relevant in selected patients, other causes of myocardial dysfunction have to be considered. Alcohol surely is the culprit in many patients, especially those patients who use significant quantities of beer.[57,58] Cocaine is an unfortunate cause of dilated cardiomyopathy in many young urban patients.[59] Amyloidosis, sarcoidosis, and hemochromatosis are all entities that need to be considered in selected patients. The diagnosis of these systemic diseases can usually be made without the need for endomyocardial biopsy; however, the results of the myocardial biopsy are extremely helpful to have.

Many clinicians ask whether an endomyocardial biopsy is necessary in a patient with stable, compensated heart failure who does not have coronary artery obstruction. In general, the answer is that the information learned from the pathological specimen will not significantly influence the management of the patient. In a patient who has not stabilized, however, or who may be considered for cardiac transplantation, there may be something to be learned from the biopsy material.[60,61] When in doubt, it is perfectly appropriate to call the local heart failure team and ask their opinion. In addition, if an endomyocardial biopsy is going to be done, it is our strong opinion that it be done at a hospital center that has experience both in performing the biopsies and a pathology team experienced in reading them.

Following the Patient with Heart Failure: Which Tests?

Before the components of a follow-up visit for a patient with heart failure are outlined, it is important to note that a great deal of patient education has presumably taken place after the patient is initially stabilized. Patients have been instructed to weigh themselves regularly, if not daily, and have learned which symptoms should be reported and when. Many disease management plans call this information an "action plan." There are numerous ways a patient can become decompensated with heart failure, but almost always noncompliance with the dietary or food regimen is part of the problem. Additionally, many patients do not know how to assess their own increasing manifestations of heart failure, and do not seek medical attention until hospitalization is inevitable. The success of most heart failure management programs rest primarily in keeping the patient out of the hospital.[62–64]

There are three parts to the ongoing clinical evaluation of the patient:

- An assessment of functional capacity
- An assessment of volume status
- A laboratory or noninvasive evaluation

Assessment of Functional Capacity

Apart from the clinician's simple observations of the patient's efforts to walk into the office, get on the examining table, their ability to lie flat on the table, or to speak in long sentences without extra breaths, there are more formal ways to assess functional capacity. The New York Heart Association's (NYHA) functional assessment has been used for many years and still provides a short hand for discussion about the degree of patients' limitations.[65] The limitations of the NYHA classification have been outlined earlier.

Exercise testing can be very useful in many patients with heart failure, particularly in the patient who may be sedentary, or who tends to deny or minimize their symptoms. The testing allows for the clinician to visualize the patient during a form of exercise and compare their performance to published standards. Heart rate, blood pressure and rhythm are also very important variables to observe during the stress. Two commonly utilized methods are the 6-minute walk test,[66–68] and maximal exercise tests while measuring simultaneous oxygen uptake or peak oxygen consumption.[69] Irrespective of the method, serial assessment of functional capacity is critical to the long-term evaluation of the patient. Many treatment options are dependent on the development of symptoms, which serve as the threshold for the next management step. An example might be the timing of replacement of a stenotic aortic valve in a patient with critical stenosis but normal exercise tolerance.

Another way to serially assess functional capacity is to regularly administer a patient questionnaire. Some heart failure centers utilize their own series of questions, and other clinicians like to employ formally developed tools, such as the Minnesota Living with Heart Failure Questionnaire.[70] This survey, which has been validated and used in a series of multicenter trials, provides a score for the individuals' quality of life as it compares to other patients with heart failure.

Assessment of Volume Status

Perhaps the single most important component of the office or hospital visit is to accurately assess the patient's volume status. However, this is also what most clinicians are least adept at doing. This is discussed more fully in other chapters, but apart from the physical exam, there are other markers to help in the assessment. A regular measuring and record of the patient's weight in the office is critical, but frequently omitted. Documentation of neck vein distension, hepatic congestion or peripheral edema in consecutive visits is testimony to inadequate diuretic usage. Finally, an analysis of the patients' home record of weights can often provide an important clue as to their volume status.

Laboratory Evaluation

The majority of patients with heart failure are treated with potent drugs, which are effective, but have attendant adverse effects. In particular, diuretics can cause azotemia, and electrolyte imbalance. Large losses of both potassium and magnesium could impact on the electrical stability of the heart. Therefore, it is necessary for the clinician to assess electrolytes, renal function, digoxin level, and other parameters at any time there has been a change in the patient's volume, clinical stability or weight. This is especially important when initiating drugs such as spironolactone, ACE inhibitors, or angiotensin-receptor antagonists.

How often should a measurement of ejection fraction be made, or a repeat echocardiogram? Certainly, any time the patient's clinical status has changed substantially, consideration should be given to a reassessment of ventricular function. Examples of these instances include a new myocardial infarction, new onset of atrial fibrillation, or the sudden onset of nocturnal dyspnea. However, there is little role for a routine echocardiogram in a stable patient with no change in symptomatic status and no change in medications. With the possible exception of intervention for mitral valve surgery, there is very little therapy for heart failure that is determined by a change in left ventricular dimension or ejection fraction.[71]

Systolic Versus Diastolic Heart Failure

Life has become more complicated for the busy clinician. In the past, if patients complained of breathlessness, fatigue and edema, they had heart failure until proven otherwise. It was always assumed, in the absence of significant valvular murmurs, that the underlying cardiac condition involved a poorly contracting, dilated ventricle; treatment was always the same: bedrest, salt restriction, and digitalis. Potent diuretics were not even routinely prescribed until the last 30 years. Several developments changed this approach. With the advent of widely available, noninvasive techniques to serially assess left ventricular function in patients with heart failure, it became apparent that as many as 50% of patients with heart failure symptoms had preserved left ventricular systolic function.[72–75] Moreover, the era of large, multicenter clinical trials emphasized the clinical characteristics of the patients who might benefit from newer therapies. The implied understanding was that patients without similar clinical indices should not be given the treatment in question. Indeed, many guidelines either chose not to discuss the management of heart failure with normal left ventricular function,[43] or to emphasize that the optimal management of diastolic heart failure had not been defined by large clinical trials.[31]

The dilemma of the patient with heart failure and preserved systolic function is slowly being solved. There are increasing epidemiological studies suggesting the frequency of diastolic heart failure and the comorbid diseases associated with it (Table 2).[74,76–84] Clinical trials are likewise either underway or in the final planning stages. Diagnostic methods for detection, primarily by echocardiography, are being perfected. A simple blood test for B-natriuretic peptide (BNP) may even help in the assessment of the patient with heart failure and preserved left ventricular dysfunction.[85] Most importantly, drugs which have been very important in the management of patients with systolic heart failure are increasingly utilized in diastolic heart failure, even in the absence of evidence-based recommendations. This is especially true of the ACE inhibitors and beta-blockers; even digitalis may become useful in selected patients with normal left ventricular function.[40]

When to Refer to a Cardiologist or Heart Failure Specialist

There are certain patients with the symptoms of heart failure who need to see a specialist interested in the disease sooner rather than later. These include patients with significant valvular disease, including mitral regurgitation, aortic regurgitation and aortic stenosis. Patients with hypertrophic cardiomyopathy and symptoms are another good example. Any patient with continuous atrial or ventricular arrhythmias needs a cardiologist or electrophysiologist. Most clinicians refer a patient with chest pain or significant angina, especially in the setting of heart failure. Any suggestion of significant pulmonary hypertension, or echocardiographic findings of right ventricular dysfunction out of proportion to or greater than left ventricular dysfunction may need a pulmonary specialist or a specialized center for pulmonary hypertension. Finally, if the clinician is not certain about the diagnosis of diastolic heart failure or the management of the condition, referral could be considered.

References

1. Boffa GM, Thiene G, Nava A, Dalla Volta S. Cardiomyopathy: a necessary revision of the WHO classification. *Int J Cardiol* 1991;30:1–7.
2. Goodwin JF. Overview and classification of the cardiomyopathies. *Cardiovasc Clin* 1988;19:3–7.
3. Keren A, Popp RL. Assignment of patients into the classification of cardiomyopathies. *Circulation* 1992;86:1622–1633.
4. Pisani B, Taylor DO, Mason JW. Inflammatory myocardial diseases and cardiomyopathies. *Am J Med* 1997;102:459–469.
5. Massie B, Shah N. Evolving trends in the epidemiologic factors of heart failure: rational for preventive strategies and comprehensive disease management. *Am Heart J* 1997;133:701–712.
6. Wilhelmsen L, Rosengren A, Eriksson H, Lappas G. Heart failure in the general population of men: morbidity, risk factors and prognosis. *J Intern Med* 2001;249:253–261.

7. Gadsboll N, Hoilund-Carlsen P, Neilsen G, et al. Interobserver agreement and accuracy of bedside estimation of right and left-ventricular ejection fraction in acute myocardial infarction. *Am J Cardiol* 1989;63:1301–1307.
8. Ghali J, Kadakia S, Cooper R, et al. Bedside diagnosis of preserved versus impaired left-ventricular systolic function in heart failure. *Am J Cardiol* 1991; 67:1002–1006.
9. Rauchhaus M, Doehner W, Francis DP, et al. Plasma cytokine parameters and mortality in patients with chronic heart failure. *Circulation* 2000;102:3060–3067.
10. Kubota T, Miyagishima M, Alvarez RJ, et al. Expression of proinflammatory cytokines in the failing human heart: comparison of recent-onset and end-stage congestive heart failure. *J Heart Lung Transplant* 2000;19:819–824.
11. Hillege HL, Girbes AR, de Kam PJ, et al. Renal function, neurohormonal activation, and survival in patients with chronic heart failure. *Circulation* 2000;102:203–210.
12. Burger AJ, Aronson D. Activity of the neurohormonal system and its relationship to autonomic abnormalities in decompensated heart failure. *J Card Fail* 2001;7:122–128.
13. Avezum A, Tsuyuki R, Pogue J, Yusuf S. Beta-blocker therapy for congestive heart failure: a systemic overview and critical appraisal of the published trials. *Can J Cardiol* 1998;14:1045–1053.
14. Rich MW, Brooks K, Luther P. Temporal trends in pharmacotherapy for congestive heart failure at an academic medical center, 1990–1995. *Am Heart J* 1998;135:367–372.
15. Brown NJ, Vaughan DE. Angiotensin-converting enzyme inhibitors. *Circulation* 1998;97:1411–1420.
16. Garg R, Yusuf S, Collaborative Group on ACE inhibitor Trials. Overview of randomized trials of angiotensin converting enzyme inhibitors on mortality and morbidity in heart failure. *JAMA* 1995;273:1450–1456.
17. Ho K, Anderson K, Kannel W, et al. Survival after the onset of congestive heart failure in Framingham Heart Study subjects. *Circulation* 1993;88:107.
18. Jaagosild P, Dawson NV, Thomas C, et al. Outcomes of acute exacerbation of severe congestive heart failure: quality of life, resource use, and survival. SUPPORT Investigators. The Study to Understand Prognosis and Preferences for Outcomes and Risks of Treatments. *Arch Intern Med* 1998;158:1081–1089.
19. McDermott MM, Feinglass J, Lee PI, et al. Systolic function, readmission rates, and survival among consecutively hospitalized patients with congestive heart failure. *Am Heart J* 1997;134:728–736.
20. Gibbs CR, Blann AD, Watson RD, Lip GY. Abnormalities of hemorheological, endothelial, and platelet function in patients with chronic heart failure in sinus rhythm: effects of angiotensin-converting enzyme inhibitor and beta-blocker therapy. *Circulation* 2001;103:1746–1751.
21. Hart W, Rhodes G, McMurray J. The cost effectiveness of enalapril in the treatment of chronic heart failure. *Br J Med Econ* 1993;6:91–98.
22. Hart SM. Influence of beta-blockers on mortality in chronic heart failure. *Ann Pharmacother* 2000;34:1440–1451.
23. Lee S, Spencer A. Beta-blockers to reduce mortality in patients with systolic dysfunction: a meta-analysis. *J Fam Pract* 2001;50:499–504.
24. Rodgers JE, Patterson JH. The role of the renin–angiotensin–aldosterone system in the management of heart failure. *Pharmacotherapy* 2000;20:368S–378S.

25. Hunt SA, Baker DW, Chin MH, et al. ACC/AHA guidelines for the evaluation and management of chronic heart failure in the adult: a report of the American College of Cardiology/American Heart Association Task Force on Practice Guidelines (committee to revise the 1995 guidelines for the evaluation and management of heart failure). American College of Cardiology web site, 2001 (http://www.acc.org/clinical/guidelines/failure/hf%5Findex.htm).
26. Mestroni L, Giacca M. Molecular genetics of dilated cardiomyopathy. *Curr Opin Cardiol* 1997;12:303–309.
27. McMinn TR Jr, Ross J Jr. Hereditary dilated cardiomyopathy. *Clin Cardiol* 1995;18:7–15.
28. Keeling PJ, McKenna WJ. Clinical genetics of dilated cardiomyopathy. *Herz* 1994;19:91–96.
29. SOLVD Investigators. Effect of enalapril on survival in patients with reduced left ventricular ejection fractions and congestive heart failure. *N Engl J Med* 1991;325:293–302.
30. SOLVD Investigators. Effect of enalapril on mortality and the development of heart failure in asymptomatic patients with reduced left ventricular ejection fraction. *N Engl J Med* 1992;327:685–691.
31. Konstam M, Dracup K, Baker D, et al. *Heart Failure: Evaluation and Care of Patients with Left-Ventricular Systolic Dysfunction.* Rockville, MD: Agency for Health Care Policy and Research Public Health Service, U.S. Department of Health and Human Services, 1994. (Clinical Practice Guideline No. 11.)
32. Mortara A, Sleight P, Pinna GD, et al. Association between hemodynamic impairment and Cheyne–Stokes respiration and periodic breathing in chronic stable congestive heart failure secondary to ischemic or idiopathic dilated cardiomyopathy. *Am J Cardiol* 1999;84:900–904.
33. Heindl S, Dodt C, Krahwinkel M, Hasenfuss G, Andreas S. Short-term effect of continuous positive airway pressure on muscle sympathetic nerve activity in patients with chronic heart failure. *Heart* 2001;85:185–190.
34. Bradley TD, Logan AG, Floras JS, The CI. Rationale and design of the Canadian Continuous Positive Airway Pressure Trial for Congestive Heart Failure patients with Central Sleep Apnea—CANPAP. *Can J Cardiol* 2001;17:677–684.
35. Deswal A, Follansbee WP. Cardiac involvement in scleroderma. *Rheum Dis Clin North Am* 1996;22:841–860.
36. Kitas G, Banks MJ, Bacon PA. Cardiac involvement in rheumatoid disease. *Clin Med* 2001;1:18–21.
37. Moder KG, Miller TD, Tazelaar HD. Cardiac involvement in systemic lupus erythematosus. *Mayo Clin Proc* 1999;74:275–284.
38. Roldan CA, Shively BK, Crawford MH. An echocardiographic study of valvular heart disease associated with systemic lupus erythematosus. *N Engl J Med* 1996;335:1424–1430.
39. Drazner M, Rame E, Stevenson L, Dries DL. Prognostic importance of elevated jugular venous pressure and a third heart sound in patients with heart failure. *N Engl J Med* 2001;345:574–581.
40. Massie BM, Abdalla I. Heart failure in patients with preserved left ventricular systolic function: Do digitalis glycosides have a role? *Prog Cardiovasc Dis* 1998;40:357–369.
41. Marantz P, Tobin J, Wassertheil-Smoller S, et al. The relationship between left-ventricular systolic function and congestive heart failure diagnosed by clinical criteria. *Circulation* 1988;77:607–612.
42. Gomberg-Maitland M, Baran DA, Fuster V. Treatment of congestive heart

failure: guidelines for the primary care physician and the heart failure specialist. *Arch Intern Med* 2001;161:342–352.

43. Heart Failure Society of America. HFSA guidelines for management of patients with heart failure caused by left ventricular systolic dysfunction: Pharmacological approaches. *J Card Fail* 1999;5:357–382.
44. Northridge D, Penny L. Guidelines on the management of chronic heart failure. *Irish Med J* 1994;87:30–32.
45. Packer M, Cohn JN, Abraham WT, et al. Consensus recommendations for the management of chronic heart failure. *Am J Cardiol* 1999;83:1A–38A.
46. Report of the American College of Cardiology/American Heart Association Task Force on Practice Guidelines (Committee on Evaluation and Management of Heart Failure). Guidelines for the evaluation and management of heart failure. *J Am Coll Cardiol* 1995;26:1376–1398.
47. Teo KK, Ignaszewski AP, Gutierrez R, et al. Contemporary medical management of left ventricular dysfunction and congestive heart failure. *Can J Cardiol* 1992;8:611–619.
48. Gheorghiade M, Bonow RO. Chronic heart failure in the United States: a manifestation of coronary artery disease. *Circulation* 1998;97:282–289.
49. Baker DW, Jones R, Hodges J, Massie BM, Konstam MA, Rose EA. Management of heart failure, 3: The role of revascularization in the treatment of patients with moderate or severe left ventricular systolic dysfunction. *JAMA* 1994;272:1528–1534.
50. Eagle KA, Guyton RA, Davidoff R, et al. ACC/AHA guidelines for coronary artery bypass graft surgery: executive summary and recommendations. A report of the American College of Cardiology/American Heart Association Task Force on Practice Guidelines (committee to revise the 1991 guidelines for coronary artery bypass graft surgery). *Circulation* 1999;100:1464–1480.
51. Jacobson TA. Clinical context: current concepts of coronary heart disease management. *Am J Med* 2001;110:3S–11S.
52. Lee TH, Goldman L. Evaluation of the patient with acute chest pain. *N Engl J Med* 2000;342:1187–1195.
53. Lee TH, Boucher CA. Clinical practice. Noninvasive tests in patients with stable coronary artery disease. *N Engl J Med* 2001;344:1840–1845.
54. Pretre R, Turina MI. Choice of revascularization strategy for patients with coronary artery disease. *JAMA* 2001;285:992–994.
55. Luciani GB, Montalbano G, Casali G, Mazzucco A. Predicting long-term functional results after myocardial revascularization in ischemic cardiomyopathy. *J Thorac Cardiovasc Surg* 2000;120:478–489.
56. Argenziano M, Spotnitz HM, Whang W, Bigger JT Jr, Parides M, Rose EA. Risk stratification for coronary bypass surgery in patients with left ventricular dysfunction: Analysis of the coronary artery bypass grafting patch trial database. *Circulation* 1999;100(19 suppl):II119–24.
57. Evangelista LS, Doering LV, Dracup K. Usefulness of a history of tobacco and alcohol use in predicting multiple heart failure readmissions among veterans. *Am J Cardiol* 2000;86:1339–1342.
58. Schoppet M, Maisch B. Alcohol and the heart. *Herz* 2001;26:345–352.
59. Missouris CG, Swift PA, Singer DR. Cocaine use and acute left ventricular dysfunction. *Lancet* 2001;357:1586.
60. Liangos O, Neure L, Kuhl U, et al. The possible role of myocardial biopsy in systemic sclerosis. *Rheumatology* 2000;39:674–679.
61. Wojnicz R, Nowalany-Kozielska E, Wojciechowska C, et al. Randomized, placebo-controlled study for immunosuppressive treatment of inflamma-

tory dilated cardiomyopathy: two-year follow-up results. *Circulation* 2001; 104:39–45.
62. Whellan DJ, Gaulden L, Gattis WA, et al. The benefit of implementing a heart failure disease management program. *Arch Intern Med* 2001;161:2223–2228.
63. Jaarsma T, Halfens R, Tan F, Abu-Saad HH, Dracup K, Diederiks J. Self-care and quality of life in patients with advanced heart failure: the effect of a supportive educational intervention. *Heart Lung* 2000;29:319–330.
64. Holst DP, Kaye D, Richardson M, et al. Improved outcomes from a comprehensive management system for heart failure. *Eur J Heart Fail* 2001;3:619–625.
65. Gibelin P. An evaluation of symptom classification systems used for the assessment of patients with heart failure in France. *Eur J Heart Fail* 2001;3:739–746.
66. Demers C, McKelvie RS, Negassa A, Yusuf S. Reliability, validity, and responsiveness of the six-minute walk test in patients with heart failure. *Am Heart J* 2001;142:698–703.
67. Mezzani A, Corra U, Baroffio C, Bosimini E, Giannuzzi P. Habitual activities and peak aerobic capacity in patients with asymptomatic and symptomatic left ventricular dysfunction. *Chest* 2000;117:1291–1299.
68. Shah MR, Hasselblad V, Gheorghiade M, et al. Prognostic usefulness of the six-minute walk in patients with advanced congestive heart failure secondary to ischemic or nonischemic cardiomyopathy. *Am J Cardiol* 2001;88:987–993.
69. Weber KT, Kinasewitz GT, Janicki JS, Fishman AP. Oxygen utilization and ventilation during exercise in patients with chronic cardiac failure. *Circulation* 1982;65:1213–1223.
70. Rector TS, Cohn JN. Assessment of patient outcome with the Minnesota Living with Heart Failure questionnaire: Reliability and validity during a randomized, double-blind, placebo-controlled trial of pimobendan. Pimobendan Multicenter Research Group. *Am Heart J* 1992;124:1017–1025.
71. Bonow R, Carabello B, de Leon A, et al. ACC/AHA guidelines for the management of patients with valvular heart disease: a report of the American College of Cardiology/American Heart Association Task Force on Practice Guidelines (Committee on Management of Patients with Valvular Heart Disease). *J Am Coll Cardiol* 1998;32:1486–1588.
72. Brutsaert DL, Sys SU. Diastolic dysfunction in heart failure. *J Card Fail* 1997;3:225–241.
73. Garcia MJ, Thomas JD, Klein AL. New Doppler echocardiographic applications for the study of diastolic function. *J Am Coll Cardiol* 1998;32:865–875.
74. Vasan RS, Larson MG, Benjamin EJ, Evans JC, Reiss CK, Levy D. Congestive heart failure in subjects with normal versus reduced left ventricular ejection fraction: prevalence and mortality in a population-based cohort. *J Am Coll Cardiol* 1999;33:1948–1955.
75. Vasan R, Levy D. Defining diastolic heart failure: A call for standardized diagnostic criteria. *Circulation* 2000;101:2118–2121.
76. Bonow R, Udelson J. Left ventricular diastolic dysfunction as a cause of congestive heart failure: mechanisms and management. *Ann Intern Med* 1992; 117:502–510.
77. Gardin JM, Arnold AM, Bild DE, et al. Left ventricular diastolic filling in the elderly: the cardiovascular health study. *Am J Cardiol* 1998;82:345–351.
78. Lamb HJ, Beyerbacht HP, van der Laarse A, et al. Diastolic dysfunction in hypertensive heart disease is associated with altered myocardial metabolism. *Circulation* 1999;99:2261–2267.

79. Lang CC, McAlpine HM, Kennedy N, Rahman AR, Lipworth BJ, Struthers AD. Effects of lisinopril on congestive heart failure in normotensive patients with diastolic dysfunction but intact systolic function. *Eur J Clin Pharmacol* 1995;49:15–19.
80. Pernenkil R, Vinson JM, Shah AS, Beckham V, Wittenberg C, Rich MW. Course and prognosis in patients > or = 70 years of age with congestive heart failure and normal versus abnormal left ventricular ejection fraction. *Am J Cardiol* 1997;79:216–219.
81. Yip GWK, Ho PPY, Woo KS, Sanderson JE. Comparison of frequencies of left ventricular systolic and diastolic heart failure in Chinese living in Hong Kong. *Am J Cardiol* 1999;84:563–567.
82. Banerjee P, Banerjee T, Khand A, Clark A, Cleland JG. Diastolic heart failure: Neglected or misdiagnosed? *J Am Coll Cardiol* 2002;39:138–141.
83. Senni M, Tribouilloy CM, Rodeheffer RJ, et al. Congestive heart failure in the community: a study of all incident cases in Olmsted County, Minnesota, in 1991. *Circulation* 1998;98:2282–2289.
84. Senni M, Redfield M. Heart failure with preserved systolic function: A different natural history? *J Am Coll Cardiol* 2001;38:1277–1282.
85. Maisel A. B-type natriuretic peptide levels: a potential novel "white count" for congestive heart failure. *J Card Fail* 2001;7:183–193.

Chapter 5

Serial Clinical Assessment of the Patient with Heart Failure

Lynne Warner Stevenson, MD

Knowledge of the accepted medications and lifestyle modifications recommended for heart failure is only the beginning of disease management. For most patients, heart failure is a chronic disease, with a landscape of hills and valleys overlying a gradual decline that may be imperceptible for many years. Individuals vary markedly in their patterns of disease and in their responses to medications. The challenge for effective disease management is to assemble the recommended components of care into a program that can be individualized and redesigned according to the changing needs of each patient.

Initial and ongoing assessment in heart failure can be focused on four areas for specific components of therapy and two additional areas for integration of therapies with individual life patterns (Table 1).[1] First, chronic surveillance should assess potentially reversible contributions to cardiac dysfunction. These may be recurrent activity of the original implicated etiology, such as ischemic heart disease, valvular abnormalities, or toxin exposure, or may be separate exacerbating factors such as anemia or thyroid disease. Second, the current circulatory status should be defined at every encounter.

Resting Hemodynamic Profile

The circulatory status includes the resting hemodynamic profile, and when that is normal, careful evaluation of circulatory reserve. The hemodynamic profile can generally be estimated by careful symptom review and physical examination at each visit, or during daily rounds on a hospitalized patient. Patients can be evaluated as shown in Table 2,

From: Jessup M, McCauley KM (eds). *Heart Failure: Providing Optimal Care*. Elmsford, NY: Futura, an imprint of Blackwell Publishing; ©2003.

Table 1

Ongoing Assessment in Heart Failure

1 Primary cause and contributing factors to cardiac dysfunction
- Examples of primary causes:
  - Coronary artery disease
  - Familial cardiomyopathy
  - Previous adriamycin therapy
- Examples of contributing factors:
  - Tachycardia
  - Anemia
  - Infection
  - Thyroid disease

2 Current circulatory status
- Resting hemodynamic profile:
  - Evidence of elevated filling pressures
  - Evidence of hypoperfusion
  - Cardiorenal limitation
- Cardiovascular reserve:
  - Postural hypotension
  - Routine activity level
  - Exercise capacity
- Potential to improve current status with adjustment of therapy:
  - Decrease diuretics or vasodilators for postural hypotension
  - Increase diuretic dose for evidence of fluid retention if kidney function acceptable

3 Related risks or symptoms
- Dysrhythmias – atrial and ventricular
- Peripheral or cerebral embolic events
- Recurrent ischemic events

4 Behavioral, psychological, and social risks
- Noncompliance and factors threatening compliance
- Anxiety and depression
- Social isolation

5 Appropriate goals for ongoing therapy
- Establishment of clinical stability
- In stable patients, modulation of disease progression:
  - ACE inhibitor doses optimized within total regimen
  - Beta-blockers titrated if no contraindications
- Regular exercise program
- Specific activity goals, such as playing golf, preparing for an important trip

6 Patient preferences regarding therapy and end-of-life decisions

ACE, angiotensin-converting enzyme.

Table 2

Detection of High Left-Sided Filling Pressures (Pulmonary Wedge Pressure ≥22 mmHg) in Chronic Heart Failure

	Sensitivity	Specificity
Right atrial pressure ≥10 mmHg	76%	83%
PA systolic pressure ≥60 mmHg	47%	96%
Tricuspid regurgitation ≥ moderate*	63%	70%
Mitral regurgitation ≥ moderate*	78%	43%

(850 patients with left ventricular ejection fraction 0.22 ± 0.08)

* Echocardiography carried out during same admission. Adapted from Drazner et al.[6]

according to clinical evidence of congestion (wet or dry) and clinical level of perfusion (warm or cold).[1]

Evaluation for Elevated Filling Pressures

Perhaps the most common error in the examination of heart failure patients is failure to recognize elevated cardiac filling pressures. However, chronic elevation of elevated filling pressures usually is not associated with rales, due to chronic hypertrophy of pulmonary lymphatics which drain fluid from the airspaces and keep them clear to examine.[2] Patients are thus frequently misdiagnosed as having no evidence of fluid overload because there are no rales. Reliance upon rales to diagnose fluid overload leads to undertreatment of fluid overload. The residual fluid in the interstitial spaces can nonetheless cause severe dyspnea, particularly in the supine position. For elevated left-sided filling pressures, the most reliable symptom is orthopnea, which should be considered a sign of elevated left-sided filling pressures unless proven otherwise. Third heart sounds are common in patients with reduced ejection fraction, but undetectable in many patients. While the new appearance or increased intensity of the third heart sound suggests higher filling pressures, its initial presence or absence is usually not very helpful. Similarly, the intensity of the regurgitant murmurs of mitral and tricuspid regurgitation often varies with the fluid status, but is of most value when followed serially in an individual patient.

The most common symptom of elevated right-sided filling pressures is edema. It is present, however, in only approximately 25% of patients with chronically elevated filling pressures. It is more common in elderly patients, in whom multiple peripheral factors may cause edema, which is thus less specific for elevated central-filling pressures. Symptoms of abdominal discomfort and anorexia from elevated right-sided pressures are often accompanied by evidence of hepatic enlargement, usually tender and pulsatile. Anorexia in heart failure is most commonly due to elevated hepatosplanchnic filling pressures rather than poor cardiac output. If ascites develops, it is generally late in the course of disease, but may precede edema in younger patients.

Jugular venous pressure is the most sensitive sign of elevated right-sided filling pressures. Assessment of the jugular venous pressure is a skill that has received decreasing emphasis, but it is critical for the effective management of this population.[3] Patients can be examined at any angle from which the top of the venous pulse can be clearly identified. Two wave forms are characteristically identified visually in the venous pulse of a patient in sinus rhythm, helping to distinguish it from prominent carotid pulsations.[4] The wave descents are often accentuated during inspiration, which may in fact make the carotid pulsation less apparent. In some patients with high right ventricular filling pressures, there is a positive Kussmaul's sign in which the venous pressure is actually higher during inspiration. The jugular venous waves are initially accentuated and increased by abdominal or hepatic compression, which can be used to further identify the pulsations. The normal response is for the elevated pressure to fall to normal after about 10–15 seconds of continuous compression as the venous capacitance increases in response.[5] Failure to return to normal in a patient with normal resting pressures indicates borderline volume overload or other cause of venoconstriction limiting venous capacitance.

Concern is frequently raised about the accuracy of estimating jugular venous pressure in the presence of marked tricuspid regurgitation. When primary valve regurgitation exists, such as with rheumatic or postinfectious valvular disease, this is difficult, but an attempt is made to estimate the general height of pressure prior to the regurgitant V wave. However, in patients with chronic heart failure, the most common cause of tricuspid regurgitation is in fact the very elevation of filling pressures that we are trying to ascertain. Thus, severe tricuspid regurgitation itself is a good marker for severely elevated right-sided filling pressures.[6] The exact level of elevation is less important than recognizing severe elevation.

Once identified, the jugular venous pressure height is then measured as the vertical distance between the top of the column and the sternal angle. For general purposes, the sternal angle can be regarded as 5 cm above the right atrium, such that the total height is the height above the sternal angle plus 5 cm.[3] Many observers correctly identify the height but then underestimate the distance in centimeters. It may be helpful for examiners to calibrate their hand span in centimeters in order to correctly measure the height of the jugular venous pressure in centimeters. It reflects the filling pressures on the right side of the heart. Although there is frequent discrepancy between right- and left-sided filling pressures in acute myocardial infarction, the relationship in chronic heart failure is stronger. In a study of 1000 patients undergoing evaluation of chronic systolic heart failure without other obvious confounding diagnoses such as severe pulmonary disease, right atrial pressures and pulmonary capillary wedge pressures were concordant in 79% of patients, analyzing right atrial pressures less than or greater than 10 mmHg and pulmonary capillary wedge pressures less than or greater than 22 mmHg.[6] The most common discordance was a right atrial pressure that was disproportionately high.

Other clinical techniques for evaluation of filling pressures include the blood-pressure response to the Valsalva maneuver.[7] Evaluation of the extent of radiation of the pulmonic component of the second sound can also be useful. When the splitting can be heard left of the parasternal border, pulmonary artery systolic pressure is usually elevated. In chronic heart failure, elevations in pulmonary artery (PA) systolic pressure track closely with elevations in pulmonary capillary wedge pressure, with an approximate relationship of PA systolic equal to twice the pulmonary wedge pressure.[6]

Evaluation for Critical Hypoperfusion

The other part of the classification then relates to the adequacy of perfusion. It should not be assumed that the patient with severe shortness of breath also has severe reduction of cardiac output—particularly in the elderly patient with heart failure in whom systolic function may be preserved. While the symptoms of heart failure decompensation are usually dominated by those of the elevated filling pressures, the efficacy of the plan to reduce elevated filling pressures may be strongly influenced by the degree to which cardiac output is compromised.

It is easy to recognize that cardiac output is severely depressed in a patient with a systolic blood pressure of 60 mmHg, anuria, and acute confusion. While this picture can develop in patients with chronic heart failure, more subtle degrees of hypoperfusion are often underappreciated.

Careful auscultation of the blood pressure is a critical part of the routine physical assessment of patients in the emergency room, hospital, and outpatient settings. Too often measured quickly at a triage desk or by an assistant as part of routine documentation, the blood pressure provides more information to an experienced examiner. The systolic blood pressure is often the focus of casual measurement, and indeed is a strong correlate of outcome in broad populations with systolic dysfunction. However, effective use of angiotensin-converting enzyme (ACE) inhibitors and beta-adrenergic blocking agents often produces systolic blood pressures below 100 mmHg in patients who are well compensated with good perfusion. In patients at risk for hypoperfusion with advanced heart failure, the pulse pressure—the difference between the systolic and diastolic blood pressure—is the most important blood-pressure parameter for determining the adequacy of perfusion. In this population, the proportional pulse pressure (difference between systolic and diastolic pressure divided by the systolic pressure) less than 25% raises concern that cardiac index may be less than $2.2\,L/min/m^2$. This threshold value has not been extensively validated, and has not been validated at all in elderly patients with increased stiffness of the arterial vasculature. The information regarding the pulse pressure for adequate perfusion in advanced heart failure should not be confused with epidemiologic data from large populations without advanced heart failure, in whom a high pulse pressure predicts subsequent cardiac events due to its association with hypertension and noncompliant arterial walls, particularly in elderly populations.

Other information available from the blood pressure includes variation in the systolic level. Patients with pulsus alternans, in which every other beat is at a lower systolic pressure, generally have very compromised perfusion, often more so than might be expected by the height of the systolic blood pressure.[8] Patients in whom very frequent premature contractions produce a systolic blood pressure that is much lower or not detectable may also have poor effective perfusion. Pulsus paradoxus, in which the blood pressure is detectably lower during inspiration, can generally be detected manually at the brachial artery when greater than 10 mm. It is rare in chronic heart failure, however, unless complicated by pericardial effusion or wide respiratory efforts such as due to large pleural effusions. Postural changes in blood pressure are important parameters to follow during adjustment of volume status or drugs with vasodilator actions. Often patients will describe fatigue or leg weakness as limiting their activity, when postural hypotension is the cause despite absence of specific postural dizziness. Measurement of postural vital signs is often relegated to a nursing order, but in fact can instead be quickly performed by the examiner aware of the importance of the findings.

Other evidence for perfusion includes the temperature of the extremities. As hands and feet are often cool as a result of anxiety or individual variation, skin temperature as an index of perfusion is best assessed from palpation of the calves and forearms. Mental status is frequently depressed in patients with low cardiac output. This may be manifest as frequent momentary lapses into apparent sleep while talking or eating. Many patients have poor concentration, lack of interest, and inability to remember common information. These are usually not appreciated until retrospectively, when improved circulatory status leads to

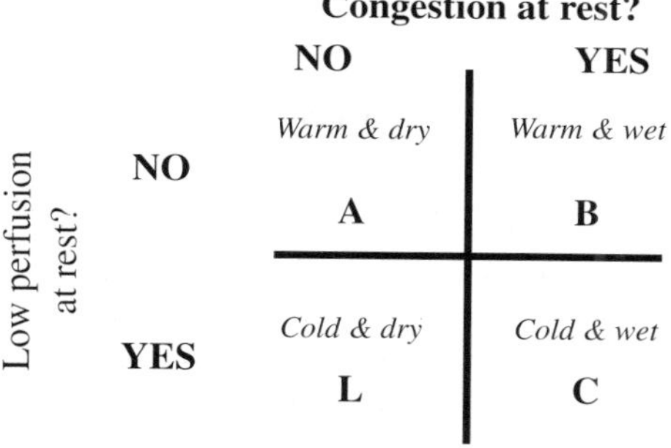

Evidence for congestion

Orthopnea
High jugular venous pressure
Edema
Pulsatile hepatomegaly
Ascites
Radiation of P2 left
Rales (rarely)
Valsalva square wave
Abdomino-jugular reflex

Evidence for low perfusion

Narrow pulse pressure
Cool extremities
May be sleepy, obtunded
Suspect from ACEI hypotension
Suspect from declining serum Na
One cause of worsening renal fn

Figure 1. Simple hemodynamic classification of heart failure by rapid clinical assessment into four profiles. A 2 × 2 table is constructed from the answers to the questions: 1) Is there evidence of elevated filling pressures; and 2) Is there evidence of critical hypoperfusion? This classification helps to guide initial therapy during episodes of decompensation. In practice, some patients are intermediate between profiles B and C.

better perfusion. Hypoperfusion is common and should be suspected in patients with a recent history of inability to tolerate ACE inhibitors due to symptomatic hypotension despite adequate or excessive volume status. Declining urine output in heart failure is due to a complex interplay of neurohormonal and hemodynamic factors, one of which can be poor cardiac output.

The four hemodynamic profiles as shown in Fig. 1 have been useful to define patients at presentation. Initial therapy for acute decompensation may be designed based on these profiles.[9] The prognostic value remains to be determined. When assessed prospectively in a standardized way, the profiles predicted 1-year outcomes for hospitalized patients, with the worst outcome being in profile C, cold and wet.[10] However, retrospective definition of profiles defined from data recorded on case report forms for a large clinical trial showed worse survival in profile C, but the differences did not reach significance.[11]

The dynamic nature of hemodynamic status should be recognized. Fluid status often undergoes wide fluctuations in response to salt and fluid intake and the efficacy of supplemental diuretic therapy. Although congestion is more likely to occur once heart failure is advanced, patients should not assume that an episode of fluid retention heralds an inexorable decline. One of the limitations of the New York Heart Association Classification is that it is sometimes considered to be a permanent progression from which there can be no return, rather than a clinical descriptor that can rapidly be improved. In one study of patients considered to be in New York Heart Association (NYHA) class IV at the time of hospital admission, subsequent survival was found to be closely related to their ability to demonstrate freedom from congestion by 1 month after hospital discharge. By this time, the initial adjustments often required after hospitalization have usually been made to the chronic oral regimen of vasodilators and diuretics. The simple congestion score added one point each for orthopnea, jugular venous pressure over 8 cm, peripheral edema, weight gain or increased diuretic during the immediately preceding week. Patients with a score of 0 had a 2-year survival of 87%, compared to 41% for patients with a score of 3–5 points.[12]

Circulatory Reserve in Heart Failure

Patients with resting hemodynamic abnormalities severe enough to be detected on clinical assessment as described above often have a very limited activity level. Effective therapy to improve the resting hemodynamic profile is the first strategy for improving activity level. When that has been addressed, or addressed to the extent possible, then assessment of activity status becomes more meaningful as a gauge of disease severity, and as a guide to how to improve the patient's perceived quality of life.

The New York Heart Association clinical classes do not provide enough gradation for activity level. The purpose of assessment in clinical practice is not to compare patients to each other but to themselves over time. The initial interview should establish each patient's daily schedule, routine chores, active hobbies, and social activities. For instance, the ability to push a grocery cart, vacuum cleaner, lawnmower, or snow shovel may be a good index for some patients. Hobbies such as golf, fishing, hunting, or antique shopping can easily provide graded information on changing functional capacity. Subsequent assessments can focus on those indicator activities that are both meaningful and vulnerable during a decline in functional reserve.

For many patients, it may be useful to accompany them to directly evaluate their ability to walk short distances or to climb stairs. The distance walked in 6 minutes can classify patients into a general range of compensation, but may not be sensitive for changes in status.[13,14] Watching respiratory rate and pattern can provide key information as to their endurance. Often it is revealed that peripheral claudication, arthritic conditions, or occasionally angina may be the cause of limitation previously attributed to poor cardiac reserve.

Symptoms of Related Risks

The routine interval history should include questions directed at risks related to heart failure beyond the direct limitations of resting circulation or circulatory reserve. Patients may misinterpret or forget to recount symptoms of palpitations, presyncope, or syncope that could reflect serious arrhythmic events. Transient ischemic attacks or minor peripheral embolic events may not be recognized by the patient unless specifically queried. Patients with known coronary artery disease should routinely be asked about symptoms that could be angina or anginal equivalents.

Interval Life History

The clinical assessment should routinely include open questions regarding the patients' current perception of their life. Details may be revealed that influence ability to comply with a complex medical regimen, or with other factors such as depression or decreased social support that increase the risk of adverse events. Patients should also be asked specifically whether they think that they are having problems due to any of their medications, as correct or incorrect attributions of side effects may be compromising compliance. These considerations are reviewed in more detail elsewhere, but should be considered a central part of every ongoing assessment.

Management at a Distance

The value of heart failure disease management has been clearly demonstrated.[15–18] In addition to the serial assessment in heart failure clinics, a central feature of disease management consists of telephone contact with a heart failure team member, in some cases with assistance from computer-based programs. Clinical assessment in this setting is restricted primarily to information that can be provided by telephone, occasionally supplemented with information from other physicians. Changes in clinical status that require expedited intervention relate most often to changes in the hemodynamic profile. In order to correctly identify these, it is necessary to know each patient's symptom spectrum as well as their threshold for observation and concern. For example, some patients develop a cough as the first sign of fluid retention, while others may have abdominal discomfort. A patient with both chronic obstructive pulmonary disease and heart failure cannot automatically be prescribed increased diuretics for any increase in dyspnea.

Routine measurement of blood pressures by patients at home, sometimes with the help of visiting nurses, can provide valuable guidance for advanced heart failure with borderline blood pressures, particularly during titration of newly introduced agents into their regimen. Measurement of blood pressure is helpful also for patients with hypertension, in whom blood pressure control is a key priority. Avoid excessive blood pressure measurements that will yield potentially distracting data and raise unnecessary concerns in patients that are generally stable.

Daily weights are a cornerstone of effective short-term management of heart failure. Most fluctuations in weight that occur over the period of days to a few weeks do reflect changes in fluid that can be used to guide adjustment of diuretics. These changes are of less value over the longer time period, however. Patients with progressive fluid accumulation often have decreased appetite and increased inflammatory markers reflective of altered metabolism. This can lead to loss of true body weight that may mask the simultaneous increase in fluid. Alternatively, patients moving into a phase of stabilization may have improved appetite and renutrition with gradual weight gain. Such patients may take excessive diuretics in an attempt to return to an outdated target weight. Chronic volume depletion may then lead to postural hypotension and activate deleterious reflexes that therapies are designed to inhibit.

Many insurance companies and clinical practice groups are attempting to incorporate features of disease management for their patients with heart failure. However, access to effective disease management is still severely limited, due to lack of reimbursement for the level of individual attention required and scarcity of adequately trained clinical staff with experience and dedication with this population. Multiple experiments are ongoing to identify those components of care that are most essential. Heart failure hospitalizations were not reduced, and actually increased, when patients had ongoing management by a dedicated primary-care physician and nurse in the absence of specific heart failure expertise.[19] Multiple national call centers have arisen that communicate with patients at a distance and provide information to their usual physicians. Current data suggest that these management systems that identify potential problems without integration with active care do not provide the same benefits in terms of decreased hospitalization rate as previously observed with more integrated care teams.[18] In addition, impact is traditionally measured by the hospitalization rate, but should also include functional level and degree of satisfaction with the quality of life achieved. The continued growth of the heart failure population should eventually stimulate the support and training of physicians and advanced practice nurses who can provide an effective standard of disease assessment and intervention.

References

1. Grady KL, Dracup K, Kennedy G, et al. Team management of patients with heart failure: A statement for healthcare professionals from the Cardiovascular Nursing Council of the American Heart Association. *Circulation* 2000; 102:2443–2456.
2. Stevenson LW, Perloff JK. The limited reliability of physical signs for estimating hemodynamics in chronic heart failure. *JAMA* 1989;261:884–888.
3. McGee SR. Physical examination of venous pressure: a critical review. *Am Heart J* 1998;136:10–8.
4. Perloff JK. The veins: jugular and peripheral. In: Perloff JK, ed. *Physical Examination of the Heart and Circulation*. Philadelphia: Saunders, 1982:91–125.
5. Butman SM, Ewy GA, Standen JR, Kern KB, Hahn E. Bedside cardiovascular examination in patients with severe chronic heart failure: importance of rest or inducible jugular venous distension. *J Am Coll Cardiol* 1993;22:968–974.
6. Drazner MH, Hamilton MA, Fonarow G, Creaser J, Flavell C, Stevenson LW. Relationship between right and left-sided filling pressures in 1000 patients with advanced heart failure. *J Heart Lung Transplant* 1999;18:1126–1132.
7. Zema MJ, Restivo B, Sos T, Sniderman KW, Kline S. Left ventricular dysfunction: bedside Valsalva manoeuvre. *Br Heart J* 1980;44:560–569.
8. Kodama M, Kato K, Hirono S, et al. Mechanical alternans in patients with chronic heart failure. *J Card Fail* 2001;7:138–145.
9. Stevenson LW, Massie BM, Francis GS. Optimizing therapy for complex or refractory heart failure: a management algorithm. *Am Heart J* 1998;135:S293–309.
10. Nohria A, Dries DL, Fang JC, et al. Bedside assessment of hemodynamic profiles identifies prognostic groups in patients admitted with heart failure. *J Card Fail* 2000;6 (Suppl. 2): 64.
11. Shah MR, Hasselblad V, Stinnett SS, et al. Hemodynamic profiles of advanced heart failure: association with clinical characteristics and long-term outcomes. *J Card Fail* 2001;7:105–113.
12. Lucas C, Johnson W, Hamilton MA, et al. Freedom from congestion predicts good survival despite previous class IV symptoms of heart failure. *Am Heart J* 2000;140:840–847.
13. Bittner V, Weiner DH, Yusuf S, et al. Prediction of mortality and morbidity with a 6-minute walk test in patients with left ventricular dysfunction. SOLVD Investigators. *JAMA* 1993;270:1702–1707.
14. Lucas C, Stevenson LW, Johnson W, et al. The 6-min walk and peak oxygen consumption in advanced heart failure: aerobic capacity and survival. *Am Heart J* 1999;138:618–624.
15. Rich M. Heart failure disease management: a critical review. *J Card Fail* 1999;5: 64–75.
16. Fonarow GC, Stevenson LW, Walden JA, et al. Impact of a comprehensive heart failure management program on hospital readmission and functional status of patients with advanced heart failure. *J Am Coll Cardiol* 1997;30: 725–732.

17. Hanumanthu S, Butler J, Chomsky D, Davis S, Wilson JR. Effect of a heart failure program on hospitalization frequency and exercise tolerance. *Circulation* 1997;96:2842–2848.
18. McAlister FA, Lawson FM, Teo KK, Armstrong PW. A systematic review of randomized trials of disease management programs in heart failure. *Am J Med* 2001;110:378–384.
19. Weinberger M, Oddone EZ, Henderson WG. Does increased access to primary care reduce hospital readmissions? Veterans Affairs Cooperative Study Group on Primary Care and Hospital Readmission. *N Engl J Med* 1996; 334:1441–1447.

Chapter 6

Treatment Goals for Heart Failure Patients in Critical Care

Anna Gawlinski RN, DNSc, CS, ACNP and Lynne Warner Stevenson, MD

Heart failure affects more than 4.8 million Americans, with more than 1 million hospitalizations annually, most commonly due to exacerbation of chronic heart failure. Heart failure complicates almost as many hospitalizations with other admitting diagnoses such as pulmonary or renal disease. Hospitalizations are increasing due to disease progression in the aging population and the increased survival of patients with acute myocardial infarction, hypertension, and diabetes mellitus.

When heart failure is due to acute myocardial infarction, therapy is dominated by intervention to minimize ischemic injury. When heart failure is due to acute valvular regurgitation, decisions must be made urgently regarding the appropriateness of surgical intervention. Fulminant myocarditis is an uncommon cause of acute heart failure with potentially excellent outcome in almost half of patients, many of whom may require initial high-dose pressor support until mechanical circulatory devices can bridge to recovery. This chapter will focus, however, on the most common hospitalizations, due to acute or subacute decompensation with chronic heart failure (Table 1).

The goals of acute therapy are the relief of symptoms (most of which result from elevated filling pressures—"congestion"), the absence of deleterious events such as arrhythmias or ischemia, and successful transition to an outpatient regimen that will maintain clinical stability after discharge.[1,2]

From: Jessup M, McCauley KM (eds). *Heart Failure: Providing Optimal Care.* Elmsford, NY: Futura, an imprint of Blackwell Publishing; ©2003.

Table 1

When Should Patients Be Admitted to the Hospital for Acute Decompensation of Heart Failure? Adapted with permission from Francis[73]

Onset of acute myocardial ischemia
Pulmonary edema or increasing respiratory distress
Oxygen saturation below 90% not caused by pulmonary disease
Complicating medical illnesses
- Symptomatic hypotension with fluid overload
- Syncope

Heart failure refractory to outpatient treatment
Anasarca
Inadequate outpatient social support system

Initial Assessment of the Hospitalized Patient: Where to Start

This discussion will assume that the underlying etiology of heart failure has been defined where possible, and that specific exacerbating factors are absent or are being addressed concurrently with the hemodynamic derangements. Initial assessment should seek to define the hemodynamic profiles that will guide therapy.[3] Chronic compensatory mechanisms can lead to underestimation of the severity of superimposed decompensation. This may be particularly true when rales are absent despite high ventricular filling pressures, or when vasoconstriction preserves systolic blood pressure despite critically low cardiac output.[4] The severity of hemodynamic compromise is frequently underestimated during triage in emergency departments.[5]

The elevation of filling pressures and the reduction of cardiac output are the central hemodynamic abnormalities, which do not necessarily occur together. The physical assessment of heart failure and the design of the 2×2 table for hemodynamic profiles (Fig. 1) have been discussed in Chapter 5. In the hospitalized patients, congestion is the dominant abnormality associated with most of the symptoms triggering heart failure hospitalization.

Some patients with chronic heart failure may in fact present profile A (warm and dry) when hospitalized. For these patients, hospitalization may be due to related conditions such as recent ischemia or arrhythmias, or unrelated causes such as pulmonary infection. For patients with resting hemodynamic abnormalities at the time of hospitalization for heart failure, profile B (wet and warm) is more common than profile C (wet and cold), even in patients at a referral center.[6] Few patients present with true

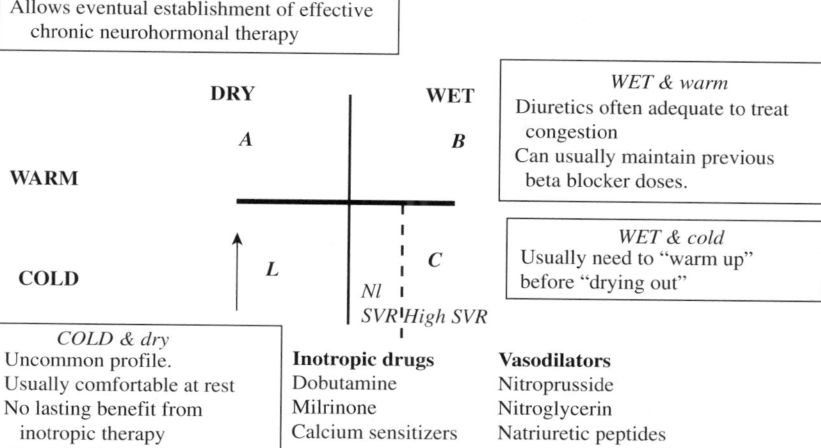

Figure 1. A 2 × 2 table showing schema of heart failure profiles during hospitalization. Factors used in determining profiles are discussed in Chapter 5. Patients who have evidence of congestion without hypoperfusion can often be treated by enhancement of diuretics in addition to their usual outpatient heart failure medications. For patients with both congestion and hypoperfusion, therapy usually needs to improve perfusion ("warm up") in order to achieve effective diuresis ("dry out"). This can generally be achieved with either vasodilator or inotropic therapy. However, for patients in whom baseline systemic vascular resistance is normal or low, inotropic therapy may be necessary to enhance renal blood flow. Patients rarely present for hospitalization with profile L (low perfusion without congestion, "cold and dry") except after aggressive chronic therapy. Acute therapy generally does not lead to chronic improvement in profile L, although beta-blocker therapy may be effective if tolerated. The goal is to relieve congestion and restore good perfusion – a return to profile A. Patients already in profile A at the time of admission generally have admissions related to arrhythmias, ischemic syndromes, or noncardiac conditions. (Reprinted from [28] with permission from Elsevier.)

profile L, dry and cold, at the time of admission for heart failure, most in fact having unrecognized congestion as profile C. Those few patients with profile L after aggressive diuresis often seem less ill than their cardiac output might indicate. Prognosis is better for patients hospitalized with profile B than for profile C (wet and cold),[6] when profiles are defined prospectively, although this may be less reliable when determined retrospectively from recorded findings from a broad range of examiners.[7] Profile L is too uncommon for robust predictions of outcome, but it appears to be better than profile C.

These profiles frame the approach to therapy, which is designed to restore profile A (Fig. 1).[1,8] Earlier institution of therapies to retard disease progression have extended life expectancy with heart failure, and changed the profiles of late heart failure decompensation. This complexity requires refinements of hemodynamic profiles relevant both for adjusting therapy and for predicting outcome. Three refinements are introduced later in this chapter: alteration of the right–left filling relationship, the "lukewarm" perfusion state, and the emergence of the cardiorenal syndrome.[9,10]

Hemodynamic Goals: Where to Go

Reestablishment of profile A, in which filling pressures are not elevated and resting perfusion is adequate, is the initial goal of therapy. Although earlier approaches to heart failure often highlighted improvement of cardiac output, the emphasis has shifted toward reduction of filling pressures as the major target of initial therapy.[8,11] This is the underlying abnormality responsible for heart failure symptoms leading to most hospitalizations. Even when initial and final cardiac output is below average normal levels, tissue perfusion is most often adequate to maintain resting organ function during routine heart failure hospitalization. Cardiac output predictably improves as filling pressures are reduced during therapy with diuretics and vasodilators.[12,13] Comparable increases in cardiac output can frequently be achieved with either vasodilators or inotropic therapy. Even when inotropic therapy to increase cardiac output is occasionally needed to achieve adequate diuresis, the amount of increase required can often be achieved by very modest inotropic support at doses much lower than those previously used to drive cardiac output to maximal levels. Acute studies have in fact shown a deleterious effect of maximizing cardiac output in multiple critical conditions.[14]

During the longer-term follow-up, the multiple hemodynamic, echocardiographic, and clinical correlates of elevated filling pressures have predicted outcomes more consistently than have the indices of cardiac output.[15–18] Thus far, both intravenous and oral therapies intended to improve cardiac output by focusing on improving contractility have been consistently implicated in acceleration of mortality, although many of these studies have used inotropic agents at higher doses than are used currently. At this time, the fundamental goal is acute restoration and chronic maintenance of optimal filling pressures on diuretics and vasodilators without inotropic support. The degree to which this goal can be realized is a critical determinant of the tolerability of longer-term therapy with angiotensin-converting enzyme inhibitors (ACEIs) and beta-blocking agents, and the realization of their benefits to improve subsequent outcomes.

Optimal Filling Pressures—How Far to Go?

Even when initial filling pressures are over 30 mmHg in patients admitted with exacerbation of chronic dilated heart failure, filling pressures can often be reduced to 15–16 mmHg.[12,19] The previous concern that decreased compliance mandated higher filling pressures arose in part from observations made in the relatively nondilated setting of acute ischemia.[20] As high filling pressures are reduced, cardiac output almost always improves. It is not known to what extent this improvement results from an actual increase in contractility as myocardial oxygen consumption decreases and the gradient for myocardial perfusion improves—an improvement in contractility related to decreased systemic vascular resistance and decreased mitral regurgitation. The factor that can most easily be confirmed is decreased mitral regurgitation due to a reduction in the effective mitral regurgitant orifice as left ventricular distention is reduced by small increments.[21–23] The classic study of nitroprusside[24] and more recent studies with combination tailored therapy depict the central role of changing regurgitant flow,[23] which can account for almost all of the improvement in measured cardiac output (which measures forward flow).

The improvement in symptoms during hospitalization relates closely to reduction of pulmonary capillary wedge pressures.[25] Because the initial dramatic relief can occur while filling pressures are still severely elevated, therapy should not stop there. Patients often feel ready for early discharge due to the contrast from the worst symptoms, not realizing that symptoms they may have grown used to can still be further improved. Elevated filling pressures are important determinants of valvular regurgitation, abnormal ventricular filling patterns, pulmonary hypertension, and right ventricular dysfunction, all of which are associated with worse outcomes. Persistently elevated filling pressures are associated with greater activation of the renin–angiotensin and sympathetic nervous systems.[26] The ability to lower filling pressures to near-normal levels predicts survival better than cardiac output responses.[11] Patients who can maintain freedom from congestion at 1 month after hospitalization have a 2-year survival of over 80%, almost twice that of patients with persistent evidence of congestion.[27] It is not clear whether aggressive therapy to establish these lower filling pressures creates survivors or merely improves our ability to identify them.[28]

Patients who have survived longer durations of heart failure present increasing challenges to relief of congestion. Progressive dysfunction of

Table 2

Prediction of Elevated Left-sided Filling Pressures

Finding	For Pulmonary Capillary Wedge Pressure >22 mmHg	
	Sensitivity	Specificity
Right atrial pressure ≥10 mmHg	76%	83%
Pulmonary artery systolic pressure (mmHg)	52 ± 16	41 ± 12
Pulmonary artery systolic pressure ≥60 mmHg	47	96
Tricuspid regurgitation ≥ moderate	78	70
Mitral regurgitation ≥ moderate	78	43

Data derived from Drazner et al.[30]

the right ventricle, leading to a right–left filling ratio that is closer to one than to two limits the ability to reduce filling pressures. This modified profile overlaps with the cardiorenal syndrome,[9,10] in which renal responses limit diuresis below a volume status that is still too high to minimize mitral regurgitation and congestive symptoms. These modified profiles are further discussed below.

Hemodynamic Profiles Guide Approach to Therapy

Filling pressures reflect a complex interplay of circulating volume status, venous capacitance, and arterial vasoconstriction. Apparent abnormalities in diastolic function or chamber compliance result in many cases from excessive filling volume, but also can be due to intrinsic myocardial stiffness. Most patients with high intracardiac filling pressures have some contribution from volume overload. Additional elevations of filling pressures can be caused by marked vasoconstriction, occurring more predictably in patients with low cardiac output or hypertension. The initial approach to therapy is determined by the presenting profile (Fig. 1). Detection of elevated filling pressure is critical (Table 2). The general principles of therapy are discussed first, followed by details of specific medications.

Wet and Warm: Profile B

Patients in whom evidence of congestion occurs without evidence of compromised resting perfusion represent the majority of patients hospitalized for heart failure exacerbation. While this is particularly common for patients who have heart failure with preserved ejection fraction, it also dominates hospitalizations for patients with low ejection fraction. If these patients have previously been well compensated on stable doses of angiotensin-converting enzyme inhibitors and beta-blockers, these medications should be maintained at the same level and diuresis initiated. The doses of these neurohormonal antagonists should not be increased during diuresis, because they may impair diuresis. In addition, tolerability of the vasodilation of ACEI may decline as volume status is restored toward normal.

For patients transferred with chronic decompensation, the average diuresis in several series was approximately 4 L,[27,29] but may be over 15 L in patients with chronic anasarca. Intravenous vasodilator therapy may be used to accelerate symptom relief. This can be effective immediately through venodilation and arterial vasodilation. Diuresis occurs slightly later, as renal blood flow increases due to increase in cardiac output and due to some selective renal vasodilation with natriuretic peptide administration. It is not known whether long-term outcomes are changed by the use of vasodilators in profile B patients. Some of these patients may have "lukewarm" profiles, such that the vasodilation is beneficial. Pharmacologic stimulation of contractility is usually not necessary to generate adequate diuresis. The only controlled data demonstrate increased adverse events during hospitalization with either dobutamine or milrinone, with a trend for worse outcome after discharge.

Cold and Wet: Profile C

Patients in profile C generally need to "warm up" before they can "dry out." Most patients who present with profile C have elevated vascular resistance.[30] Vasodilation serves both to help lower filling pressure and to increase forward cardiac output.[12] The failing ventricle is sensitive to manipulations in afterload, but improvement in ejection fraction with vasodilation is minor when detectable at all. The increase in cardiac output with vasodilators is attributable instead to forward redistribution of mitral regurgitant flow rather than to improvement in total stroke volume. Mitral regurgitant flow frequently consumes half and may consume up to 75% of total stroke volume prior to unloading therapy, after which it may be reduced to 25% or less.[19]

Intravenous inotropic agents stimulate contractility directly, current agents also causing vasodilation, leading to the term "inodilators" (dobutamine, low-dose dopamine, milrinone). Direct comparison often shows similar increases with both inotropic and vasodilating agents when cardiac output is initially low, although the inotropic agents titrated to higher doses can increase cardiac output to a slightly greater degree in this setting.[31] Routine infusion of the inodilator milrinone for patients hospitalized with heart failure with good initial blood pressure caused more hypotension and arrhythmias than placebo infusion, with no benefit for symptom relief, hospital days, or up-titration of ACEI.[32] As hypotension was a common side effect, this agent should not be used when initial therapy causes or is limited by hypotension. Dobutamine has not been compared to placebo in the current therapy era, but clearly increased adverse events when compared to vasodilator infusions. Neither dobutamine nor milrinone showed favorable impact on symptom relief, but the randomized trials were done in populations without severe initial compromise, so their role in more severe decompensation has not been delineated. While low-dose dopamine is often described as "renal-dose," it should be noted that it has systemic effects to increase cardiac output and heart rate even at these levels, so should be considered with the inotropic infusions.

Initiation of therapy with vasodilation is often recommended, with addition of inotropic agents only when compensation cannot be restored with diuretics and vasodilators.

Cold and Dry: Profile L (Low Output)

Patients who appear to be profile L (cold and dry) at presentation often have occult elevation of filling pressures, indicating profile C instead. Most patients who become profile C have been aggressively managed with diuretics and low sodium intake, but a few patients progress to hypoperfusion with relative preservation of volume balance. In the unusual circumstance that filling pressures are lower than optimal for cardiac output—pulmonary capillary wedge pressure (PCWP) <12 or right atrial (RA) pressure <5—a cautious trial of fluid repletion may be considered, with oral fluid replacement off diuretics generally better tolerated than intravenous fluid supplementation, which can rapidly cause pulmonary edema. Unless postural hypotension was present, this approach rarely improves clinical status and may lead to congestive symptoms. Patients with pulmonary capillary wedge pressures in the range of 15 with normal right atrial pressures generally look surprisingly comfortable at rest even if the cardiac output is low, and can usually accomplish activities of daily living slowly. Energy levels and further activity are restricted by the absence of ability to increase cardiac output or to further extract oxygen peripherally. The goals of further therapy depend upon the clinical situation, but options are limited. Further vasodilation may increase resting cardiac output marginally, but will frequently cause symptomatic hypotension. Intravenous inotropic therapy provides only temporary improvement and may be followed by clinical deterioration below baseline, sometimes with new inotropic dependence. Beta-blocking agents initiated cautiously may lead to delayed improvement in systolic function and cardiac output,[33,34] particularly if resting heart rate is high. Titration of beta-blocking agents should proceed only very slowly, over weeks, with frequent reevaluation. When beta-blockers are not tolerated, amiodarone may lead to similar reductions in heart rate and improvement in ejection fraction.

Modified Profiles

Therapy can be initiated in hospital according to the basic profiles, from which many patients can be restored to profile A. As more patients are surviving longer with heart failure, however, some patients present or develop more complex profiles during hospitalization.

Wet and Lukewarm

It can be difficult to define an arbitrary boundary for adequate and critically low perfusion, and indeed this boundary may move during therapy. Most patients admitted with low ejection fraction heart failure have an initial cardiac output that is lower than normal, with compensatory increase in venous oxygen extraction, yielding a lower mixed venous oxygen saturation. A recent study of patients in whom pulmonary artery catheters were considered advisable during heart failure hospitalization showed 60% to have cardiac indices less than 2.2 L/min/m (William Abraham, personal communication). The intravenous vasodilator nesiritide led to accelerated symptom relief compared to placebo.[35] Intravenous nitroglycerin was also effective in many patients. On the other hand, these patients may also respond well after the later onset of effective diuresis alone in conjunction with their usual outpatient heart failure vasodilator regimen. The extent to which borderline low perfusion should be quantified or treated differently has not been established.

Currently, therapy is evaluated on the basis of relief of symptoms, the absence of deleterious events such as arrhythmias or ischemia, and successful transition to an outpatient regimen that will maintain clinical stability after discharge. As for profile C patients, when initial treatment including intravenous vasodilators does not provide effective diuresis and symptom relief, additional therapy with inotropic agents may be needed.

High Right–Left Filling Ratio

Right ventricular dysfunction tends to become more significant with longer duration of left ventricular systolic dysfunction and is associated with worse symptoms and prognosis.[36] Right ventricular dysfunction may clinically dominate in patients with restrictive disease and in young adults with left heart failure. Total fluid accumulation is reflected both in the left and right-sided filling, so it cannot be assumed that more elevation of jugular venous pressure or more edema indicate worsening right ventricular function. The fundamental ratio between right and left-sided filling is best determined *after* diuresis of visible volume as tolerated. This ratio then is an important guide to how vigorously filling pressures can be reduced.

For many patients with chronic heart failure, the left-sided filling pressures are over twice the right atrial pressure, assessed from the jugular venous pressure. This assumed relationship guides diuresis to near-normal left-sided filling pressures, visualizing the jugular venous pressure. When right ventricular function progressively worsens, however, right atrial pressures approach and may come to equal the left atrial pressures. Knowing the precise right–left relationship becomes more critical when the right–left ratio is elevated over normal, when reduction of jugular venous pressure to the usual target level may not be possible without compromise of left-sided filling. Therapy for the "frequent flyers" with multiple hospitalizations may be best adjusted noninvasively according to the documented left–right relationship obtained once invasively. The prevalence of the right–left ratio over one-half seems anecdotally to be increasing, possibly due in part to improving survival of heart failure in mild–moderate stages, during which the right ventricular is exposed to longer duration of overload. The population in whom decompensation has been delayed may ultimately present greater severity of right ventricular dysfunction and resistance to usual interventions during hospitalization. The cardiorenal syndrome may be particularly common in this group of patients.

The Cardiorenal Syndrome

The recently recognized cardiorenal syndrome describes the situation in which renal function declines progressively as diuresis relieves symptoms. In advanced heart failure, a common reason for refractory or recurrent symptoms despite aggressive management is this renal dysfunction. During heart failure hospitalization, aggravated renal dysfunction occurs in approximately 25% of patients undergoing diuresis. It is associated consistently with longer hospital stays and higher mortality.[9,10]

Although often applied, the term *prerenal* does not clarify either the mechanism or the solution. While the declining renal function was at one time assumed to reflect low cardiac output from excessively reduced filling pressures, more thorough observation indicates that this is rarely causative. In fact, filling pressures usually still exceed the optimal levels needed to maintain cardiac output as renal function deteriorates.[9] The duration of heart failure symptoms, perhaps particularly of volume overload, predicts higher likelihood of the cardiorenal syndrome, as though some regulatory process has been readjusted to a deleteriously high volume set-point. Previously demonstrated need for higher diuretic doses seems to predict higher likelihood of the cardiorenal syndrome.[10] This limitation to effective therapy may involve altered balance of vasodilating and vasoconstricting neurohormonal responses during changing fluid status.[37]

Although the cardiac output is often adequate for other needs of resting perfusion, enhancement of cardiac output often helps to override the cardiorenal syndrome. As almost 80% of cardiac output is normally directed to the kidney, this is not surprising. Intravenous inotropic therapy is frequently used to improve renal function while diuresis is being achieved.[38] When diuresis is initially achieved, but followed rapidly by declining renal function, inotropic therapy can improve it temporarily, but the conflict usually recurs once inotropic therapy is weaned. The rate of diuresis may affect the appearance of the cardiorenal syndrome, but it does seem to develop consistently at a given volume level in certain patients. In other patients, renal function may improve over weeks of careful maintenance of a lower volume status. This delayed resetting of the "volume-stat" may occur more often in younger patients.

It may become necessary to discontinue angiotensin-converting enzyme inhibitors when serum creatinine continues to rise above 3 ng/mL and/or blood urea nitrogen levels rise above 80–100 mg/dL. Transition to hydralazine/nitrate combinations or nitrate monotherapy frequently improves renal function. Ultrafiltration for life-threatening anasarca and pulmonary edema may provide short-term relief,[39] but can be associated with progression to hemodialysis in this setting. Inability to maintain adequate renal function on oral therapy is one of the most common reasons for intravenous inotropic infusions in heart failure, both acutely and chronically. In general, however, the initiation of chronic inotropic therapy heralds a downward course in which cardiac output soon becomes limiting for other organ functions as well, and frequent complications from catheter placement are evident. Patients in whom systolic blood pressure and general medical condition are maintained may in rare cases enjoy freedom from congestion on chronic hemodialysis. The advent of specific renal vasodilators may eventually allow a more rational approach to the cardiorenal syndrome.

How Should We Monitor Therapy in Hospital?

There has been considerable debate about the role of invasive hemodynamic monitoring in the diagnosis and management of heart failure during hospitalization. It may be used initially to identify the hemodynamic profile. Individual components of the assessment of filling pressures have been compared to hemodynamic measurements in this population,[4,40,41] but filling pressures are occasionally found to be far above those suspected clinically. The relevance of a lower cardiac output than suspected may be lower, except in the case of evaluation for cardiac replacement therapies in patients who demonstrate severe limitation of exercise capacity. The reliability of the clinical profiles identified by experienced heart failure clinicians remains to be established by the ongoing Evaluation Study of Congestive Heart Failure and Pulmonary Artery Catheterization Effectiveness (ESCAPE) trial.[42] Complex situations in which clinical assessment may be usefully supplemented by hemodynamic measurement include heart failure with concomitant cardiac conditions such as acute ischemia or noncardiac diseases such as intrinsic pulmonary or renal disease. When symptom severity exceeds clinical evidence of hemodynamic compromise, exercise hemodynamic measurements may also be helpful.[43] Pulmonary artery catheterization is currently recommended for the management of patients with clinical heart failure prior to major surgery.

During evaluation for transplantation, pulmonary artery catheterization is routine for determination of pulmonary pressures and reversibility of pulmonary hypertension.[44,45] The most common reason for elevated pulmonary pressures is elevated left-sided pressures, the reduction of which are the main target of therapy to relieve pulmonary hypertension in heart failure. As this frequently requires more than "in and out" pulmonary artery catheter measurement, continued monitoring to guide redesign of therapy over 24–72 h has often been followed by early and prolonged stabilization of these patients without transplantation.[46] This approach has been described as "tailored therapy," to achieve hemodynamic goals of near-normal filling pressures first with intravenous diuretics and vasodilators with subsequent monitored transition to an outpatient oral regimen with the same goals.[28,47] Using this strategy of combined hemodynamic monitoring and clinical assessment as above, the goals are to approach pulmonary capillary wedge pressure ≤16 mmHg and right atrial pressure ≤8 mmHg (Table 3). The systemic vascular resistance range of 1000–1200 (for average-size individuals) guides titration of therapy for reduction of filling pressures, but is no longer considered to be a separate independent target of therapy. Neither is cardiac output a specific goal of this strategy, although it usually improves as loading conditions are optimized.[12,30] Patients with large volume reser-

Table 3

Hemodynamic Goals to Guide for Therapy During Heart Failure Hospitalization

Clinical Assessment	Invasive Monitoring
Relief of orthopnea	Pulmonary capillary wedge pressure ≤15 mmHg
Absence of peripheral edema	Right atrial pressure ≤8 mmHg
Absence of hepatomegaly/ascites	Systemic vascular resistance 1000–1200 dyn · s · cm^{-5}
Absence of Valsalva square wave	Systolic blood pressure ≥80 mmHg
Jugular venous pressure ≤8 cm	*In either approach:*
	Further adjustment of therapy may be required for: Postural hypotension
Warm extremities	Aggravated renal dysfunction
Systolic blood pressure ≥80 mmHg	
SBP – DBP ≥25%	
SBP (proportional pulse pressure)	

DBP, diastolic blood pressure; SBP, systolic blood pressure.

voirs, as in anasarca, require extensive diuresis before adjustment of vasodilators, so hemodynamic monitoring should generally be delayed until later during the hospitalization to guide the chronic oral regimen, rather than to confirm the severity of initial compromise.

Do the hemodynamic goals provide better guide for therapy than goals assessed by clinical assessment? The ongoing ESCAPE trial will compare the two strategies for symptom relief, reduction of mitral regurgitation, natriuretic peptide levels, rehospitalization, and improvement of exercise capacity, quality of life, and patient preference for survival.[42]

The safety of hemodynamic monitoring has been questioned after association with higher mortality in surgical populations, although not with the heart failure population.[48] The results of these retrospective, nonrandomized studies are confounded by the indications for pulmonary catheter insertion, which reflect concern regarding worsening clinical status. There is increasing suspicion that the negative impact of catheters in some studies is related to the adverse effects of inotropic agents titrated in high doses to treat low cardiac output measurements that may not have warranted such aggressive therapy.

In critical situations with progressive cardiogenic shock or rapid downhill course of acute decompensation, hemodynamic monitoring is performed urgently to establish the diagnosis, guide titration of high-dose pressor agents, and evaluate for emergency surgical intervention. If the therapy based on clinical assessment is unsuccessful, hemodynamic monitoring may be performed. In patients who have been labeled as "inotrope-dependent," hemodynamically guided therapy may be particularly helpful to aid adjustment of filling pressures and systemic vascular resistance during weaning of inotropic infusions onto vasodilators. The value of hemodynamic monitoring is less clear in patients developing the cardiorenal syndrome during diuresis, as the hemodynamic values obtained are usually those anticipated from careful clinical assessment.

Development of newer techniques to estimate hemodynamics may guide the individualization of therapy for both acute and chronic therapy for heart failure. Bedside echocardiography may become simple enough to allow adjustment of diuretics and vasodilators to mitral inflow patterns, pulmonary venous flow patterns, and atrioventricular valve regurgitation. Measurement of B-natriuretic peptide (BNP) or pro-BNP levels seems to parallel reduction of volume during diuresis.[49] Better understanding of the physiologic targets to which therapy should be adjusted is necessary in order to select the best tools for monitoring the efficacy of therapy.

Specific Agents used during Hospitalization

Diuretics

Rationale. Intravenous loop diuretics in high doses are indicated in patients with severe heart failure because oral gastrointestinal absorption is impaired by gut edema in patients with decompensated heart failure.[50,51] Furosemide is commonly used as the initial loop diuretic. Intravenous diuretics are administered to reduce preload, or right ventricular end-diastolic volume (RVEDV), left ventricular end-diastolic volume (LVEDV), and myocardial wall tension. The reduction in LVEDV decreases the stretching of the mitral valve annulus and results in less mitral regurgitation. Administration of diuretics should in general be continued until clinical evidence of congestion is resolved (including jugular venous pressure <8 cmHg), or the PCWP, if measured is PCWP ≤15 mmHg and RA ≤7 mmHg.[28,47] When the patient approaches the hemodynamic goal and dry weight, the patient may begin treatment with an oral loop diuretic.

Clinical application. Furosemide is a potent, rapidly acting diuretic that inhibits reabsorption of sodium and chloride in the ascending loop of Henle. Diuresis begins approximately 10 min after intravenous injection; peak effect occurs in about 30 min and lasts for about 6 h.[52] As a general guide, patients are first treated with an intravenous dose that is equivalent to their oral dose, with subsequent doses based on the patient's response (urine output, PCWP and RA). Patients not previously treated with a diuretic can receive a first dose of furosemide (Lasix) 20 mg intravenously.

Diuretics should be given every 6–12 h in an effort to reach the hemodynamic goal, whether assessed clinically or measured directly. For patients who do not respond to high doses of intravenous furosemide, metolazone 5 mg orally can be added 30 min before the intravenous dose of furosemide. Metolazone acts on the proximal and distal loop of Henle and potentiates the diuretic response, as the distal tubular cells have hypertrophied to reabsorb much of the load delivered distally during chronic loop diuretic therapy. Metolazone has a 12-h half-life and should be used only once or twice a day. Metolazone results in marked loss of potassium in the urine. Thus, potassium supplements and monitoring of serum levels of potassium are required. Patients unable to take oral medications may respond similarly to intravenous thiazides to supplement loop diuretics.

Continuous diuretics. When patients do not respond to regularly administered high-dose intravenous loop diuretics with the addition of metolazone, continuous intravenous administration of diuretics should be considered. A continuous infusion may be effective when bolus administration of diuretics does not produce the expected urine output or reduction in PCWP and RA pressure.[53–55] Continuous administration of a diuretic may provide more efficient delivery of the diuretic to the nephron, eliminating compensatory sodium retention or rebound that can occur during a diuretic-free interval. Diuretics that may be used for continuous therapy include furosemide, bumetanide, and torsemide. In general, most patients who do not respond to intravenous furosemide will not respond to equivalent intravenous administration of the other loop diuretics, and further therapy should be undertaken.

The recommended dose for continuous infusion of diuretics varies. Furosemide is often given at a dose of 0.25–1.0 mg/kg per hour. Bumetanide is administered as a continuous infusion at 0.1–0.5 mg/h. Continuous infusion of torsemide is at 5–20 mg/h, although there may be no significant advantage of intravenous torsemide over furosemide, as the major difference is better oral absorption with torsemide.

Intravenous Vasodilators

Nitroprusside

Rationale. Sodium nitroprusside, a potent vasodilator, can be initiated intravenously to decrease high afterload. By vasodilating the venous vessels or peripheral arteries, nitroprusside decreases the preload and afterload, which facilitates greater forward flow (stroke volume) and increases cardiac output, cardiac index, and tissue oxygen delivery. The increased stroke volume is usually sufficient to maintain blood pressure at or only slightly below the pretreatment level.

Numerous studies have reported improvement in left ventricular function, tissue perfusion, cardiac output, and clinical status in patients with low cardiac output and high systemic vascular resistance (SVR).[24,56,57] Nitroprusside reduces PCWP more than dobutamine because of nitroprusside's more potent vasodilating effects and its ability to enhance left ventricular relaxation during diastole.

Clinical application. Continuous infusion of nitroprusside is started at 20 μg/min, and the dose is increased by 10–20 μg/min every 5–10 min until the hemodynamic goal (PCWP <15 mmHg, RA <7 mmHg, SVR <1200 dyn·s·cm^{-5}, while maintaining systolic blood pressure greater than 80 mmHg) is reached. Clinical parameters used to evaluate the effect of nitroprusside include SVR and blood pressure. The maximum dose of nitroprusside is usually 300 μg/min.

Nitroprusside is metabolized by the red blood cells into hydrocyanic acid, which is converted to thiocyanate by the liver and excreted by the kidneys. Therefore, nitroprusside should be used judiciously in patients with hepatic insufficiency, in whom cyanide may accumulate, and renal insufficiency in whom thiocyanate may accumulate over a longer time period.[58] Toxicity is more likely to develop in patients who require prolonged infusions at high doses. Most patients demonstrating irritability, confusion, or nausea as a result of toxicity generally respond to a marked decrease in dose, without the need for specific other therapy.

Nitroprusside versus Nitroglycerin

Rationale. In patients with ischemic heart disease and myocardial ischemia, intravenous nitroglycerin may be preferred over intravenous nitroprusside.[59–61] Early reports suggested that nitroprusside can worsen myocardial ischemia via coronary "steal," especially in patients with acute myocardial infarction, although this has rarely been a clinical problem in patients with acutely decompensated heart failure. For patients with acute (<48 h) myocardial infarction or acute myocardial ischemic syndromes and decompensated heart failure, intravenous nitroglycerin may be preferred to nitroprusside because of nitroglycerin's more favorable effects on coronary blood flow.[24,62]

Intravenous nitroglycerin is a reasonable choice for rapid amelioration of symptoms in any patient with severely elevated filling pressures without severe hypotension. It has been used effectively as initial therapy during heart failure hospitalization. Higher doses of nitroglycerin are usually necessary than for nitroprusside, but many patients improve at doses below 100 μg/min.

Clinical application. For preload reduction, nitrates increase venous capacitance, which relieves congestion (i.e., absence of dyspnea/orthopnea, adventitious breath sounds). When there is significant arteriolar vasoconstrction, nitroglycerin is an effective arteriolar vasodilator also, to decrease afterload. Large doses of nitroglycerin are sometimes required to reduce systemic vascular resistance, and tolerance of nitroglycerin's effect can also develop. Although often titrated to hemodynamic goals of low filling pressures and systemic vascular resistance, nitroglycerin has been used effectively without hemodynamic monitoring. The major side effect is headache, which can be severe enough to limit therapy in some patients.

Nesiritide Use for Decompensated Heart Failure

A new intravenous agent recently approved for therapy during heart failure hospitalization is nesiritide.[35] This agent has been used effectively without dose adjustment or hemodynamic monitoring in many patients studied. It can be given without invasive monitoring, and may have fewer limiting side effects than nitroprusside or nitroglycerin when adjusting hemodynamics with monitoring.

Definition. Nesiritide is human brain natriuretic peptide produced by recombinant DNA technology. Nesiritide produces balanced arterial and venous vasodilatation and results in rapid reduction in ventricular filling pressures and reversal of signs and symptoms of heart failure such as dyspnea. Nesiritide also reduces levels of deleterious neurohormones such as aldosterone and endothelin. Nesiritide has been shown to improve symptoms when added to other standard therapy for decompensated heart failure.[25]

Indications. Nesiritide can be used as indicated for the intravenous treatment of patients with acutely decompensated congestive heart failure who have dyspnea at rest or with minimal exertion. In these patients, the use of nesiritide is expected to reduce PCWP and improve dyspnea.[35] Pulmonary artery pressures may be particularly lowered.

Selection of patients. It is not clear when nesiritide offers additional benefit over diuresis in patients for profile B (wet and warm).[63] The renal vasodilating actions of BNP present theoretical advantage for patients who are refractory to diuretics or demonstrate the cardiorenal syndrome, but have not been specifically studied in these situations. When intravenous vasodilator therapy is desired for treatment of "lukewarm" or profile C "wet and cold" patients, nesiritide presents a therapeutic option with more rapid and sustained hemodynamic profile than other vasodilators without the risk of adverse effects seen with intravenous inotropic therapy such as dobutamine.

Until more clinical experience has been gained with this agent, nesiritide should generally be used under conditions simulating the trials, which included systolic blood pressure of 80–90 mmHg or higher and elevated ventricular filling pressure (20 mHg or higher as shown by pulmonary artery catheter or by clinical estimate).[48]

Patients were excluded from the trials for cardiogenic or other forms of shock, or systolic blood pressure less than 90 mmHg without pulmonary artery catheter or less than 80 mmHg with pulmonary artery catheter in place. Patients with low ventricular filling pressures (PCWP 12 mmHg or less) and systemic vascular resistance <1200 have also been excluded.[35]

Dosage/administration. The recommended initial bolus dose for nesiritide is 2 µg/kg. The bolus dose should be administered over 60 s. After completion of the bolus infusion, begin maintenance infusion of 0.01 µg/kg per minute.[25] If clinically indicated after the first few hours, the dose may be increased to 0.015 µg/kg.

Clinical application. Blood pressure should be checked after initiating the infusion or for any change in dose, every 15 min for the first hour, every 30–60 min for the next 3 h, and every 2–4 h thereafter. Notify the physician if symptomatic hypotension develops or systolic blood pressure is 80 mmHg or lower.

Fluid intake and output should be strictly documented. If urine output is less than 50 mL/h in the first 3 h after treatment with nesiritide is started, notify the physician. The patient's weight should be measured and recorded daily. Improvement of dyspnea is expected. If the patient's respiratory rate or dyspnea do not change or if they worsen during the course of nesiritide therapy, notify the physician.

Inotropic Agents

Rationale. The decision to add an inotropic agent varies among clinicians. The decision should be based on assessment of hemodynamic parameters and physical findings. Measures to improve cardiac output by decreasing PCWP and SVR ("unloading") should in most cases be initiated first. If the patient's cardiac output and cardiac index remain low, and systolic blood pressure is consistently less than 80 mmHg, consider adding dobutamine.[31] Dobutamine is an effective inotropic agent in patients with heart failure and can be used to improve cardiac output and blood pressure by increasing contractility in patients who do not respond well to "unloading" therapy or who require immediate hemodynamic stabilization. Dobutamine is a synthetic catecholamine that stimulates predominantly beta$_1$- and beta$_2$-receptors. It results in increased cardiac contractility and peripheral vasodilatation. Dobutamine is associated with slight increases in heart rate, decreases in PCWP, and increases in cardiac index.[31]

Clinical application. Dobutamine is administered intravenously starting at 2 µg/kg/min, and increased by 1–2 µg/kg/min until the desired clinical or hemodynamic effect is achieved or until adverse effects occur. A lower initial dose and slower titration should be used in patients considered to be at risk for dobutamine-induced ischemia. In general, the lowest dose necessary for the desired clinical response, often only 2–3 µg/kg, should be used. Increasing inotropic agents to treat cardiac output diagnosed from invasive monitoring may be responsible for some of the adverse effects seen with this strategy. The maximum dose likely to improve cardiac output in this setting is 10–15 µg/kg/min, although higher doses are used transiently during stress testing. The half-life is short (2.5–5 min), and the peak effect is within 10 min. Tolerance may develop with extended use due to down-regulation of the beta-receptors. Dobutamine is the inotropic agent of choice in patients with heart failure who have oliguria and renal insufficiency.

Dopamine (Renal Perfusion)

Rationale. Dopamine is classified as an inotropic agent. Low-dose dopamine has dominant dopaminergic effects, producing dilatation of specific vascular beds such as the renal, mesenteric, and cerebral arteries.[64] Although low doses (2–3 µg/kg/min) are often labeled "renal-dose," systemic inotropic and chronotropic effects are frequently evident, in part due to the dopamine-triggered release of norepinephrine.

Clinical application. Low-dose dopamine can be used in conjunction with diuretics to promote diuresis. Urine output frequently increases. Blood pressure may increase, decrease, or stay the same. Heart rate and ventricular tachyarrhythmias occasionally increase. Weaning should be undertaken with the same considerations as for weaning of low-dose dobutamine. When patients demonstrate critical hypotension with imminent compromise of organ and patient viability, increasing dopamine into the pressor range may help for transient stabilization until definitive intervention or other decision can be made.

Epinephrine

Rationale. The most potent inotropic agent available, epinephrine carries tremendous cost in terms of myocardial ischemia and tachyarrhythmias. Prolonged high doses can lead to peripheral ischemia and necrosis. However, in the setting of acute cardiogenic shock, such as sometimes seen with fulminant myocarditis, use of epinephrine can be life-saving until emergency mechanical support can be instituted.

Clinical application. In these settings, epinephrine is started at 1–2 µg/min (not per kilogram), and increased as necessary to keep systolic blood pressure 70–80 mg as other arrangements are being made. Norepinephrine has similar cardiac effects but more profound peripheral vasoconstriction, associated with greater risk of tissue necrosis. It is generally reserved for refractory vasodilatory states in the setting of severe myocardial depression. The use of vasopressin in circulatory collapse may decrease the dose requirement for the catecholamine agonists.

Milrinone

Rationale. Milrinone is used for inotropic support of patients who respond inadequately or develop tolerance to dobutamine. Milrinone blocks the phosphodiesterase III enzyme, thus increasing the intracellular level of cyclic adenosine monophosphate, which enhances cardiac contractility and produces peripheral vasodilatation.[65] The vasodilation is more profound than seen with the other inotropic agents, frequently producing hypotension.[32] Thus, milrinone should *not* be given when the major indication for inotropic support is hypotension. Milrinone has been suggested to have a theoretical advantage over dobutamine in exerting positive inotropic activity when down-regulation of beta-adrenergic receptors occurs as a result of dobutamine use. In practice, most heart failure patients will demonstrate increased cardiac output with dobutamine even in the presence of some beta-adrenergic antagonist activity, which is rarely complete. Milrinone can be used in combination with dobutamine when dobutamine has not adequately increased cardiac output, but considerable care is required when giving milrinone to hypotensive patients, as the additional vasodilation may cause further hypotension.

Clinical application. Milrinone is often started with a 50-µg/kg bolus followed by infusions of 0.20–0.75 µg/kg/min. As with the other inotropic agents, the lowest dose possible should be used. In some patients who are hypotensive, the bolus dose may be eliminated, and continuous infusion may be used alone. Unlike the immediate effects of dobutamine, maximal hemodynamic effects of milrinone are observed at 15 min after initiation of infusion. Because milrinone has a long biological half-life, the hemodynamic effects of lowering the infusion rate or terminating the infusion may not be seen completely until up to 24 h after the action is taken. This is particularly true in the presence of decreased renal function, as milrinone is renally excreted.

Both milrinone and dobutamine affect PCWP, but generally, the reduction in PCWP is more consistent with milrinone than with dobutamine.[65] Milrinone, as with other agents causing vasodilation, is more likely to precipitate hypotension when left ventricular filling pressures (PCWP) are low. Milrinone appears to cause less myocardial oxygen demand than dobutamine. However, milrinone is associated with more ischemic events than placebo therapy in heart failure.

Neurohormonal Antagonism

Angiotensin-Converting Enzyme Inhibitors

Rationale. The beneficial effects of angiotensin-converting enzyme inhibitors (ACEIs) on disease progression, functional status, hospitalization, and mortality warrant treating all patients with left ventricular systolic dysfunction with ACEIs, unless contraindications exist.[66]

Clinical application. Once the hemodynamic goal is achieved and maintained for 12–24 h, the dose of oral ACEI is titrated as the patient is weaned off intravenous nitroprusside, while maintaining optimal hemodynamic parameters. The protocol at University of California at Los Angeles utilizes low doses of short-acting ACEIs such as captopril initially, which are titrated upward to the hemodynamic goal achieved with nitroprusside.[47] The specific doses to use when titrating the dose of captopril upward while weaning patients off nitroprusside are outlined in Table 4. Clinical parameters such as systolic blood pressure, SVR, and serum levels of creatinine and potassium are monitored as treatment is switched from nitroprusside to ACEIs. Nitrates are frequently added to maintain optimal unloading conditions. Hydralazine is used less often.

Initiation of Beta-Blocker Therapy

Rationale. Initiation of beta-blocker therapy is generally delayed until the patient with heart failure has been stabilized. The Carvedilol Prospective Randomized Cumulative Survival (COPERNICUS) trial demonstrated survival benefit when patients with severe heart failure were treated with the beta-blocker carvedilol, suggesting therapy can be safely initiated during hospitalization if there were no recent requirement for intravenous vasoactive therapy and there was no significant fluid retention.[67] Many patients were sufficiently stabilized within the first 4–6 weeks after discharge to begin cautious initiation of beta-blocker therapy. These agents have been demonstrated to improve survival (35% mortality reduction) in patients with class II–IIIB/IV heart failure due to systolic dysfunction. Additional benefits include shorter hospitalization and lower prevalence of myocardial infarction and sudden death.

Table 4

Hemodynamic Management of Cardiomyopathy Patients

1 Right heart catheter placed.
- Hemodynamics are examined.
- If *PCW >16* and/or *cardiac index <2.2 L/min/m²* on two sets of hemodynamic measurements, the catheter remains in place.

2 If *SVR <1300, PCW >20 mmHg, RA >10 mmHg, and CI >2.2 L/min/m²*, then begin diuretics alone and restart previous ACE inhibitors.

3 If the hemodynamics subsequently deteriorate *(SVR >1500)*, discontinue oral vasodilators (except nitrates) and begin nitroprusside.

4 If the *SVR >1300* and *PCW >20* or *CI* <2.2 L/min/m², begin sodium nitroprusside (Nipride) with the following hemodynamic goals:
- SVR <1200, PCW <15 mmHg, RA <7 mmHg, while maintaining SBP >80 mmHg.

5 If the patient has a low cardiac index *(CI <1.4 L/min/m²)*, consider addition of an inotropic agent such as dobutamine.

6 *Sodium nitroprusside (Nipride)* 100 mg in 250 mL D5W.
- Starting dose of *20 μg/min,* titrating upwards by 20 μg/min q 5–10 min to a maximum dose of *300 μg/min*, or until optimum hemodynamics are achieved.
- Diuresis with i.v. *frusemide (Lasix)* should also be initiated.

7 Obtain hemodynamic goals on sodium nitroprusside (Nipride) and i.v. frusemide (Lasix).
- Maintain these optimal hemodynamics for a minimum of *2–4 h* prior to starting oral vasodilators.

8 Start *captopril* as the initial vasodilator in all patients.
- Captopril *6.25 mg*. Increase to *12.5 mg* after 2 h; if tolerated, after an additional 2 h *25 mg*, then increase by *25 mg every 6 h* (e.g., 50 mg, 75 mg, then 100 mg) only as necessary to taper off nitroprusside and match the hemodynamics achieved on sodium nitroprusside (Nipride).
- Maximum captopril dose is *100 mg* p.o. q 6 h.
- Do not continue to titrate captopril dose once off sodium nitroprusside (Nipride), unless specific indication (e.g., SVR ≥1500 or SBP ≥100).
- Avoid hypotension or advancing ACEI dose despite low SVR, due to risk of renal insufficiency.

9 *Isosorbide dinitrate (Isordil)* to be started with initial unloading therapy in patients with coronary artery disease *(10 mg* or their admission dose of nitrates).
- For patients *without* coronary artery disease, once captopril dose has reached 25 mg and still on sodium nitroprusside (Nipride), or for elevated filling pressures despite diuresis, isosorbide dinitrate (Isordil) to be started at *10 mg t.i.d.*
- If tolerated, may be titrated, but only if indicated by high filling pressure or SVR.
- Do not increase nitrates beyond 20 mg t.i.d., unless indicated.
- If tolerated and indicated may increase by *10–20 mg q 8 h*, as tolerated to a maximum of *80 mg t.i.d.*

Continued

Table 4 *Continued*

Hemodynamic Management of Cardiomyopathy Patients
10 If optimum hemodynamics are achieved and sustained for 6–8 h (absolute minimum *4 h*) on captopril or captopril/isosorbide dinitrate (Isordil) regimen, right heart catheter can be discontinued.
11 If optimum hemodynamics are *not* achieved on captopril/ isosorbide dinitrate (Isordil) regimen, or if captopril is not tolerated due to serious side effects (severe symptomatic hypotension, renal insufficiency, allergic reaction), the decision regarding the addition of *angiotensin-receptor antagonist* or *hydralazine* or *doxazosin* should be made by the attending physician in conjunction with the cardiomyopathy staff member. • Continue *captopril* at the greatest tolerated dose (usually *100 mg q 6 h*). • *Hydralazine* is started at *25 mg*, after 2 h *50 mg*, then *50 mg q 6 h*; increase by *25 mg* every 6 h (e.g., 75 mg, 100 mg, then 150 mg) as needed to maximum *150 mg p.o. q 6 h.* Isosorbide dinitrate (Isordil) is to be continued or started.
12 *Digoxin* is indicated if patient remains symptomatic from heart failure. • Start at *0.125 mg* qd or continue outpatient dose. • Check level when at steady state (aim for level 0.5–1.1 ng/mL)
13 Diuresis is of utmost importance in these patients; *Lasix* should be given 2–4 times a day *with supplemental potassium.* • I/O should be closely followed multiple times per day.
14 Potassium and magnesium to be closely followed. • K^+ should be kept 4–4.8 mEq/dL. • Mg^+ should be kept ≥1.8 mEq/dL.
15 Patients should receive a 2-g sodium diet • 1500–2000 mL fluid restriction.

ACE, angiotensin-converting enzyme; ACEI, angiotensin-converting enzyme inhibitor; CI, cardiac index; D5W, 5% dextrose in water; I/O, intake/output; PCW, pulmonary capillary wedge (pressure); RA, right atrial (pressure); SBP, systolic blood pressure; SVR, systemic vascular resistance.

Source: Ahmanson UCLA Cardiomyopathy Clinic.[74]

Clinical applications. Treatment with beta-blockers should be initiated in all patients with heart failure due to systolic dysfunction who have no contraindications or clearly documented intolerance. Beta-blocker therapy should generally not be initiated until after treatment with ACEIs is started. Patients requiring intravenous vasodilators or inotropic agents should have beta-blocker therapy deferred until after the heart failure is compensated, and stability has been demonstrated.

Contraindications. Cardiogenic shock, symptomatic bradycardia without a pacemaker, second- or third-degree heart block and severe bronchospastic pulmonary disease are all contradictions to use of beta-blockers. The recommended starting dose for carvedilol in patients with heart failure is 3.125 mg orally twice a day, with the first dose titration. The starting dose for metoprolol CR/XL is 12.5 mg daily. Beta-blockers should be withheld if systolic blood pressure is <80 mmHg and/or heart rate <50 beats/min. Dose titrations should take place slowly in the outpatient setting, anticipating several months to reach target dose. Many patients with a history of frequent heart failure hospitalization will not tolerate titration to full target dose.

Adjunctive Therapies

Electrolyte Management

Rationale. The risk of electrolyte disturbances is increased in patients with heart failure. Neurohormonal activation, aggressive diuresis, and renal dysfunction all contribute to marked fluctuations in serum levels of electrolytes. Electrolyte disturbances can increase mortality and morbidity by causing arrhythmias, decreased ventricular function, and cardiac arrest. Hospitalized patients with heart failure who undergo aggressive diuresis must have serum levels of electrolytes measured frequently.

Clinical application for potassium. Serum levels of potassium should be maintained between 4.0 and 4.8 mEq/dL. Both hypokalemia and hyperkalemia can affect left ventricular function and result in lethal arrhythmia.[68,69] Potassium supplements should be considered and, in most cases, prescribed. Clinicians must keep in mind that serum potassium levels measured just after an oral dose or an intravenous infusion of potassium do not reflect the potassium level a few hours later. Any new onset of or increase in arrhythmias warrants immediate measurement of electrolyte levels to assess for hypokalemia or hyperkalemia. Hyperkalemia can be life-threatening, and occurs more often in patients on spironolactone.

Clinical application for magnesium. Serum levels of magnesium should be maintained at a level greater than 1.8 mEq/dL.[70] Hypomagnesemia results in lethal arrhythmias such as ventricular tachycardia, ventricular fibrillation, and sudden death. Patients with heart failure who are undergoing aggressive diuresis are at risk for hypomagnesemia. Clinicians must remember that serum magnesium levels do not adequately reflect tissue magnesium levels.

Digoxin

Rationale. Digoxin improves symptoms and functional capacity in patients with heart failure.[71] No effect on mortality has been demonstrated.

Clinical application. Digoxin is indicated in patients with heart failure who remain symptomatic after optimal target doses of ACEIs, beta-blockers, and diuretics.[45] Digoxin levels should be kept between 0.5 and 1.1 ng/mL. Patients with new-onset arrhythmias should be evaluated for possible toxic effects of digoxin. Hypokalemia can potentiate the toxic effects of digoxin. The dose of digoxin should be halved when combined with amiodarone.

Nonpharmacological Therapies

Preparing for Transfer and Discharge

Combining optimization of hemodynamic parameters along with use of nonpharmacological therapies in disease management of heart failure equals the comprehensive approach of heart failure.[29] Discharge criteria should be enforced to decrease risk of rehospitalization (Table 5). Educating patients and their families while they are in the intensive-care unit or cardiac care unit is an important nursing intervention. Patients

Table 5

Discharge Criteria for Hospitalization with Heart Failure. Adapted from Moser and Frazier[72] and Konstam et al.[75]

Clinical status goals
- Achieve dry weight
- Define blood pressure range
- Patient should walk without dyspnea or dizziness

Stability goals
- 24 h without changes in oral cardiac regimen
- ≥48 h off intravenous inotropic agents, if used
- Fluid balance demonstrated on oral diuretics
- Renal function stable or improving

Home maintenance plan
- Patient/family education about:
  Salt restriction
  Fluid limitation, if indicated
  Medication schedule
  Medication effects
  Exercise prescription
- Flexible diuretic plan
- Scheduled call to patient within 3 days
- Patient "call-for" instructions
- Clinic appointment within 7–10 days

have experienced an acute event (hospitalization) and are open and ready for instruction on strategies to prevent rehospitalization and to control disease progression. Detailed topics for education and counseling of patients and their families are listed in Table 6.[72]

During hospitalization, nutritional consultations should be made to

Table 6

Topics for Patient, Family/Caregiver Education and Counseling. Adapted from Moser and Frazier[72] and Konstam et al.[75]

General Counseling
- Cause or probable cause of heart failure
- Explanation of symptoms
- Symptoms of worsening heart failure
- General explanation of treatment/care plan
- Role of family members/other caregivers in the treatment/care plan
- Availability and value of qualified local support group

Self-management
- Importance of compliance with treatment plan
- Clarification of patient responsibilities
- Self-monitoring with daily weights
- Monitoring of symptoms and what to do if they worsen
- Importance of cessation of tobacco use
- Importance of obtaining vaccinations against influenza and pneumococcal disease

Prognosis
- Life expectancy
- Advance directives
- Advice for family members in the event of sudden death

Activity recommendations
- Recommendations for recreation, leisure, and work activity
- Importance of regular aerobic activity
- Recommendations for sexual activity, coping with sexual difficulties

Dietary recommendations
- Sodium restriction
- Avoidance of excessive fluid intake
- Alcohol restriction
- Low fat diet for patients with cardiovascular disease

Medications
- Reasons for medications, dosing and schedule
- Expected effects of medication on quality of life and survival
- Likely side effects and what to do if they occur
- Organizing medications and behavioral strategies (e.g., pill boxes) to coping with complicated regimens
- Availability of lower cost medications or financial assistance

provide patients and their family members with a detailed education on the 2-g sodium diet. Referrals for physical therapy should be initiated for instruction on in-hospital exercises, a progressive home-based walking program, and other exercises to be done at home. Referrals for cardiac rehabilitation should be made as needed.

A fluid restriction of 2 L (64 oz) should be maintained in the hospital and continued at home, with education on monitoring fluid intake for patients with high chronic diuretic requirement. Instruction on the use of a daily weight chart can start in the intensive or cardiac care unit and can be reinforced in the intermediate care unit and upon discharge. Patients should be able to demonstrate proficiency in use of the daily weight chart before discharge. Patients require education on flexible dosing of diuretics based on their daily weight. Because hospitalized patients are weighed daily, this is an excellent teaching opportunity for nurses to test and reinforce patients' knowledge regarding their actions for scenarios of a 2-lb weight gain in 24 h or 4 lb in 4 days. Patients should be able to verbalize actions to double their diuretic dose and increase potassium levels. Patients who are taking high doses of oral furosemide should be instructed on use of metolazone as needed. Further details on the education and counseling of patients and their families are discussed in Chapters 2 and 9.

There are multiple different approaches to heart failure management, both in and out of the hospital. The critical component appears to be continuity between acute and chronic care teams, and the availability of a nurse expert in heart failure management who can facilitate changes in therapy. Call systems that serve merely to register and transfer concerns to a primary provider office have not been effective in decreasing hospitalizations and empowering patients to take responsibility for their health. Regardless of the organizational details, hospitalization provides a critical port from which to launch the course of integrated care for the patient and care team working together.

References

1. Nohria A, Lewis E, Stevenson LW. Medical management of advanced heart failure. *JAMA* 2002;287:628–640.
2. Stevenson L. Management of acute decompensation. In: Mann D, ed. *Heart Failure*. [In press].
3. Grady KL, Dracup K, Kennedy G, et al. Team management of patients with heart failure: A statement for healthcare professionals from the Cardiovascular Nursing Council of the American Heart Association. *Circulation* 2000;102: 2443–2456.
4. Stevenson LW, Perloff JK. The limited reliability of physical signs for estimating hemodynamics in chronic heart failure. *JAMA* 1989;261:884–888.
5. Dao Q, Krishnaswamy P, Kazanegra R, et al. Utility of B-type natriuretic pep-

tide in the diagnosis of congestive heart failure in an urgent-care setting. *J Am Coll Cardiol* 2001;37:379–385.
6. Nohria A TS, Dries DL, Fang JC, et al. Bedside assessment of hemodynamic profiles identifies prognostic groups in patients admitted with heart failure. *J Card Fail* 2000;6:64–68.
7. Shah MR, Hasselblad V, Stinnett SS, et al. Hemodynamic profiles of advanced heart failure: Association with clinical characteristics and long-term outcomes. *J Card Fail* 2001;7:105–113.
8. Stevenson LW, Massie BM, Francis GS. Optimizing therapy for complex or refractory heart failure: a management algorithm. *Am Heart J* 1998;135:S293–309.
9. Weinfeld MS, Chertow GM, Stevenson LW. Aggravated renal dysfunction during intensive therapy for advanced chronic heart failure. *Am Heart J* 1999;138:285–290.
10. Krumholz HM, Chen YT, Vaccarino V, et al. Correlates and impact on outcomes of worsening renal function in patients > or =65 years of age with heart failure. *Am J Cardiol* 2000;85:1110–1113.
11. Stevenson LW, Tillisch JH, Hamilton M, et al. Importance of hemodynamic response to therapy in predicting survival with ejection fraction less than or equal to 20% secondary to ischemic or nonischemic dilated cardiomyopathy. *Am J Cardiol* 1990;66:1348–1354.
12. Stevenson LW, Tillisch JH. Maintenance of cardiac output with normal filling pressures in patients with dilated heart failure. *Circulation* 1986;74:1303–1308.
13. Wilson JR, Reichek N, Dunkman WB, Goldberg S. Effect of diuresis on the performance of the failing left ventricle in man. *Am J Med* 1981;70:234–239.
14. Hayes MA, Timmins AC, Yau EH, Palazzo M, Hinds CJ, Watson D. Elevation of systemic oxygen delivery in the treatment of critically ill patients. *N Engl J Med* 1994;330:1717–1722.
15. Stevenson LW, Couper G, Natterson B, et al. Target heart failure populations for newer therapies. *Circulation* 1995;92:II174–181.
16. Campana C, Gavazzi A, Berzuini C, et al. Predictors of prognosis in patients awaiting heart transplantation. *J Heart Lung Transplant* 1993;12:756–765.
17. Morley D, Brozena SC. Assessing risk by hemodynamic profile in patients awaiting cardiac transplantation. *Am J Cardiol* 1994;73:379–383.
18. Aaronson KD, Schwartz JS, Chen TM, Wong KL, Goin JE, Mancini DM. Development and prospective validation of a clinical index to predict survival in ambulatory patients referred for cardiac transplant evaluation. *Circulation* 1997;95:2660–2667.
19. Stevenson LW, Brunken RC, Belil D, et al. Afterload reduction with vasodilators and diuretics decreases mitral regurgitation during upright exercise in advanced heart failure. *J Am Coll Cardiol* 1990;15:174–180.
20. Rackley CE, Russell RO Jr. Left ventricular function in acute and chronic coronary artery disease. *Ann Rev Med* 1975;26:105–120.
21. Stevenson L, Bellil D, Grover-McKay M, et al. Effects of afterload reduction (diuretics and vasodilators) on left ventricular volume and mitral regurgitation in severe congestive heart failure secondary to ischemic or idiopathic dilated cardiomyopathy. *Am J Cardiol* 1987;60:654–658.
22. Weiland DS, Konstam MA, Salem DN, et al. Contribution of reduced mitral regurgitant volume to vasodilator effect in severe left ventricular failure secondary to coronary artery disease or idiopathic dilated cardiomyopathy. *Am J Cardiol* 1986;58:1046–1050.

23. Rosario LB, Stevenson LW, Solomon SD, Lee RT, Reimold SC. The mechanism of decrease in dynamic mitral regurgitation during heart failure treatment: importance of reduction in the regurgitant orifice size. *J Am Coll Cardiol* 1998; 32:1819–1824.
24. Guiha NH, Cohn JN, Mikulic E, Franciosa JA, Limas CJ. Treatment of refractory heart failure with infusion of nitroprusside. *N Engl J Med* 1974;291: 587–592.
25. Abraham WT, Johnson AD, Wagoner L, Givertz MM, Horton DP. Nesiritide (human BNP) improves symptoms and hemodynamics in NYHA Class III and IV heart failure. *J Am Coll Cardiol* 1999;33:188A.
26. Kaye DM, Lambert GW, Lefkovits J, Morris M, Jennings G, Esler MD. Neurochemical evidence of cardiac sympathetic activation and increased central nervous system norepinephrine turnover in severe congestive heart failure. *J Am Coll Cardiol* 1994;23:570–578.
27. Lucas C, Johnson W, Hamilton MA, et al. Freedom from congestion predicts good survival despite previous class IV symptoms of heart failure. *Am Heart J* 2000;140:840–847.
28. Stevenson LW. Tailored therapy to hemodynamic goals for advanced heart failure. *Eur J Heart Fail* 1999;1:251–257.
29. Fonarow GC, Stevenson LW, Walden JA, et al. Impact of a comprehensive heart failure management program on hospital readmission and functional status of patients with advanced heart failure. *J Am Coll Cardiol* 1997;30:725–732.
30. Drazner MH, Hamilton MA, Fonarow G, Creaser J, Flavell C, Stevenson LW. Relationship between right and left-sided filling pressures in 1000 patients with advanced heart failure. *J Heart Lung Transplant* 1999;18:1126–1132.
31. Leier CV, Webel J, Bush CA. The cardiovascular effects of the continuous infusion of dobutamine in patients with severe cardiac failure. *Circulation* 1977;56:468–472.
32. Cuffe MS, Califf RM, Adams KF, et al. Rationale and design of the OPTIME CHF trial: outcomes of a prospective trial of intravenous milrinone for exacerbations of chronic heart failure. *Am Heart J* 2000;139:15–22.
33. Macdonald PS, Keogh AM, Aboyoun CL, Lund M, Amor R, McCaffrey DJ. Tolerability and efficacy of carvedilol in patients with New York Heart Association class IV heart failure. *J Am Coll Cardiol* 1999;33:924–931.
34. Kukin ML, Kalman J, Charney RH, et al. Prospective, randomized comparison of effect of long-term treatment with metoprolol or carvedilol on symptoms, exercise, ejection fraction, and oxidative stress in heart failure. *Circulation* 1999;99:2645–2651.
35. Colucci WS, Elkayam U, Horton DP, et al. Intravenous nesiritide, a natriuretic peptide, in the treatment of decompensated congestive heart failure. Nesiritide Study Group. *N Engl J Med* 2000;343:246–253.
36. Di Salvo TG, Mathier M, Semigran MJ, Dec GW. Preserved right ventricular ejection fraction predicts exercise capacity and survival in advanced heart failure. *J Am Coll Cardiol* 1995;25:1143–1153.
37. Johnson W, Omland T, Hall C, et al. Neurohormonal activation rapidly decreases after intravenous therapy with diuretics and vasodilators for class IV heart failure. *J Am Coll Cardiol* 2002;39:1623–1629.
38. Cotter G, Weissgarten J, Metzkor E, et al. Increased toxicity of high-dose furosemide versus low-dose dopamine in the treatment of refractory congestive heart failure. *Clin Pharmacol Ther* 1997;62:187–193.
39. Biasioli S, Barbaresi F, Barbiero M, et al. Intermittent venovenous hemofiltra-

tion as a chronic treatment for refractory and intractable heart failure. ASAIO J 1992;38:M658–663.

40. Butman SM, Ewy GA, Standen JR, Kern KB, Hahn E. Bedside cardiovascular examination in patients with severe chronic heart failure: Importance of rest or inducible jugular venous distension. *J Am Coll Cardiol* 1993;22:968–974.
41. Zema MJ, Restivo B, Sos T, Sniderman KW, Kline S. Left ventricular dysfunction—bedside Valsalva manoeuvre. *Br Heart J* 1980;44:560–569.
42. Shah MR, O'Connor CM, Sopko G, Hasselblad V, Califf RM, Stevenson LW. Evaluation study of congestive heart failure and pulmonary artery catheterization effectiveness (ESCAPE): Design and rationale. *Am Heart J* 2001;141: 528–535.
43. Chomsky DB, Lang CC, Rayos GH, et al. Hemodynamic exercise testing: A valuable tool in the selection of cardiac transplantation candidates. *Circulation* 1996;94:3176–3183.
44. Mudge GH, Addonizio GS. Recipient guidelines/prioritization for cardiac transplantation: the 24th Bethesda Conference. *Am J Cardiol* 1993;22: 21–31.
45. Hunt S. Cardiac transplantation. Paper presented at 24th Bethesda Conference. Bethesda, MD, 1992.
46. Stevenson LW, Dracup KA, Tillisch JH. Efficacy of medical therapy tailored for severe congestive heart failure in patients transferred for urgent cardiac transplantation. *Am J Cardiol* 1989;63:461–464.
47. Fonarow GC, Chelimsky-Fallick C, Stevenson LW, et al. Effect of direct vasodilation with hydralazine versus angiotensin-converting enzyme inhibition with captopril on mortality in advanced heart failure: the Hy-C Trial. *J Am Coll Cardiol* 1992;19:842–850.
48. Connors AF Jr, Speroff T, Dawson NV, et al. The effectiveness of right heart catheterization in the initial care of critically ill patients. SUPPORT Investigators. *JAMA* 1996;276:889–897.
49. Maisel AS, Koon J, Krishnaswamy P, et al. Utility of B-natriuretic peptide as a rapid, point-of-care test for screening patients undergoing echocardiography to determine left ventricular dysfunction. *Am Heart J* 2001;141:367–374.
50. Gerlag PG, van Meijel JJ. High-dose furosemide in the treatment of refractory congestive heart failure. *Arch Intern Med* 1988;148:286–291.
51. Vasko MR, Cartwright DB, Knochel JP, Nixon JV, Brater DC. Furosemide absorption altered in decompensated congestive heart failure. *Ann Intern Med* 1985;102:314–318.
52. Biddle TL, Yu PN. Effect of furosemide on hemodynamics and lung water in acute pulmonary edema secondary to myocardial infarction. *Am J Cardiol* 1979;43:86–90.
53. Rudy DW, Voelker JR, Greene PK, Esparza FA, Brater DC. Loop diuretics for chronic renal insufficiency: a continuous infusion is more efficacious than bolus therapy. *Ann Intern Med* 1991;115:360–366.
54. Martin SJ, Danziger LH. Continuous infusion of loop diuretics in the critically ill: a review of the literature. *Crit Care Med* 1994;22:1323–1329.
55. Dormans TP, van Meyel JJ, Gerlag PG, Tan Y, Russel FG, Smits P. Diuretic efficacy of high dose furosemide in severe heart failure: Bolus injection versus continuous infusion. *J Am Coll Cardiol* 1996;28:376–382.
56. Franciosa JA, Limas CJ, Guiha NH, Rodriguera E, Cohn JN. Improved left ventricular function during nitroprusside infusion in acute myocardial infarction. *Lancet* 1972;1:650–654.

57. Chatterjee K, Parmley WW, Ganz W, et al. Hemodynamic and metabolic responses to vasodilator therapy in acute myocardial infarction. *Circulation* 1973;48:1183–1193.
58. Cohn JN, Burke LP. Nitroprusside. *Ann Intern Med* 1979;91:752–757.
59. Ludbrook PA, Byrne JD, Kurnik PB, McKnight RC. Influence of reduction of preload and afterload by nitroglycerin on left ventricular diastolic pressure-volume relations and relaxation in man. *Circulation* 1977;56:937–943.
60. Flaherty JT, Magee PA, Gardner TL, Potter A, MacAllister NP. Comparison of intravenous nitroglycerin and sodium nitroprusside for treatment of acute hypertension developing after coronary artery bypass surgery. *Circulation* 1982;65:1072–1077.
61. Cohn JN, Franciosa JA, Francis GS, et al. Effect of short-term infusion of sodium nitroprusside on mortality rate in acute myocardial infarction complicated by left ventricular failure: results of a Veterans Administration cooperative study. *N Engl J Med* 1982;306:1129–1135.
62. Miller RR, Vismara LA, Williams DO, Amsterdam EA, Mason DT. Pharmacological mechanisms for left ventricular unloading in clinical congestive heart failure: Differential effects of nitroprusside, phentolamine, and nitroglycerin on cardiac function and peripheral circulation. *Circ Res* 1976;39:127–133.
63. Fonarow G. Nesiritide: practical guide to its safe and effective use. *Rev Cardiovasc Med* 2001;2(suppl 2):S32–S35.
64. Goldberg LI. Dopamine—clinical uses of an endogenous catecholamine. *N Engl J Med* 1974;291:707–710.
65. Grose R, Strain J, Greenberg M, LeJemtel TH. Systemic and coronary effects of intravenous milrinone and dobutamine in congestive heart failure. *J Am Coll Cardiol* 1986;7:1107–1113.
66. Hunt SA, Baker DW, Chin MH, et al. ACC/AHA guidelines for the evaluation and management of chronic heart failure in the adult: executive summary. A report of the American College of Cardiology/American Heart Association Task Force on Practice Guidelines (Committee to Revise the 1995 Guidelines for the Evaluation and Management of Heart Failure). *J Am Coll Cardiol* 2001;38:2101–2113.
67. Packer M, Coats AJ, Fowler MB, et al. Effect of carvedilol on survival in severe chronic heart failure. *N Engl J Med* 2001;344:1651–1658.
68. Dargie HJ, Cleland JG, Leckie BJ, Inglis CG, East BW, Ford I. Relation of arrhythmias and electrolyte abnormalities to survival in patients with severe chronic heart failure. *Circulation* 1987;75:IV98–107.
69. Leier CV, Dei Cas L, Metra M. Clinical relevance and management of the major electrolyte abnormalities in congestive heart failure: hyponatremia, hypokalemia, and hypomagnesemia. *Am Heart J* 1994;128:564–574.
70. Gottlieb SS, Fisher ML, Pressel MD, Patten RD, Weinberg M, Greenberg N. Effects of intravenous magnesium sulfate on arrhythmias in patients with congestive heart failure. *Am Heart J* 1993;125:1645–1650.
71. Digitalis Investigation Group. The effect of digoxin on mortality and morbidity in patients with heart failure. *N Engl J Med* 1997;336:525–533.
72. Moser DK, Frazier SK. *The Patient with Heart Failure: Research-Based Protocol.* Aliso Viejo, CA: American Association of Critical-Care Nurses, 2001.
73. Francis GS. Management of acute and decompensated heart failure. In: Hosenpud JD, Greenberg GH, eds. *Congestive Heart Failure*, 8th ed. Philadelphia: Lippincott Williams & Wilkins, 2000: 553–569.
74. Ahmanson UCLA Cardiomyopathy Clinic. *Hemodynamic Management of*

Cardiomyopathy Patients (ACE Protocol). Los Angeles: UCLA Medical Center, 2000 (http://www.med.ucla.edu/champ/ACE%20Protocol.PDF).

75. Konstam M, Dracup K, Baker D, et al. *Heart Failure: Evaluation and Care of Patients with Left-Ventricular Systolic Dysfunction*. Rockville, MD: Agency for Health Care Policy and Research, Public Health Services, U.S. Department of Health and Human Services, 1994 (Clinical Practice Guideline no. 11; AHCPR Publication no. 94–0612).

Chapter 7

Managing Complicated In-Patients: Comorbidities and the Frail Elderly

Lee R. Goldberg, MD, MPH, FACC

Congestive heart failure frequently occurs in the context of a variety of medical illnesses. Many of these illnesses contribute directly to the development or progression of congestive heart failure, while others complicate the assessment or treatment. The common noncardiac comorbidities include diabetes, renal insufficiency, hypertension, pulmonary disease and hyperlipidemia. The common cardiac comorbidities include coronary artery disease and atrial fibrillation. The management of congestive heart failure in the setting of another chronic illness presents both medical as well as psychosocial challenges. A multidisciplinary approach that focuses on clear communication among practitioners and the patient, and careful selection and titration of medications, are critical for success.

An example of where this approach may be of particular benefit is in the management of the elderly with congestive heart failure. This group of patients is often the least aggressively treated, but tends to suffer from the most comorbidities. The elderly are more likely to have frequent hospital admissions and are more likely to experience significant medication side effects. Recent studies have shown that with comprehensive interdisciplinary strategies, the quality of life and clinical outcomes of this population can be significantly improved.

From: Jessup M, McCauley KM (eds). *Heart Failure: Providing Optimal Care.* Elmsford, NY: Futura, an imprint of Blackwell Publishing; ©2003.

Diabetes

One-third of patients with congestive heart failure have concomitant diabetes.[1] Diabetes may be a direct cause of congestive heart failure or may be an indirect cause, as a risk factor for the development of coronary artery disease.[2–4] Retinopathy, nephropathy, and neuropathy as end-organ manifestations of diabetes make the management of heart failure much more challenging.

Patients with heart failure have increased insulin resistance.[5] The development of congestive heart failure may therefore make the management of diabetes more complicated. Worsening insulin resistance may be one explanation of the poor prognosis of patients with both heart failure and diabetes. Given the increased risk of cardiovascular events and progression of heart failure in this population, aggressive strategies are necessary to reduce the risk of morbidity and mortality.[6]

Angiotensin-converting enzyme inhibitors are the cornerstones of both heart failure and diabetes management and risk reduction. Angiotensin-converting enzyme inhibitors have been shown to reduce the risk of death and worsening heart failure for patients with systolic dysfunction.[7–9] This class of drugs has also been shown to be protective against the end-organ damage of diabetes, especially the progression of renal insufficiency. Results of a recent study indicate that the addition of an angiotensin-converting enzyme inhibitor in patients with diabetes can reduce the incidence of cardiovascular events and mortality.[10] For these reasons, any patient with diabetes and heart failure should be treated with an angiotensin-converting enzyme inhibitor unless a clear absolute contraindication is documented.

Angiotensin receptor blockers (ARB) have also been shown to be effective in protecting renal function in patients with type 2 diabetes.[11] In addition, this class of drugs has been shown to be beneficial in patients with heart failure who can not tolerate ACE inhibitors.[12,13] ARB have also been shown to provide vascular protection in animals and humans with atherosclerosis. In a recent study, ARB have been shown to prevent restenosis of stented coronary atherosclerotic lesions.[14] For these reasons, ARB are reasonable alternatives when ACE inhibitors are not tolerated, in particular due to cough, and in the future may become the drug of choice for patients with type 2 diabetes and heart failure. Further studies of the role of ARB in both systolic and diastolic heart failure are underway and will further define the role of this class of drugs.

Angiotensin-converting enzyme (ACE) inhibitors can have several side effects. These include cough, worsening renal insufficiency, hyperkalemia, hypotension, and angioedema.[15–18] Unfortunately, many of these signs and symptoms overlap with those of congestive heart failure. During an acute exacerbation of heart failure, aggressive diuresis may lead to an increase in creatinine or the development of hypotension that is often attributed to an angiotensin-converting enzyme inhibitor. Clinicians then withhold further ACE inhibitors without rechallenging patients when their volume status is under better control. Worsening cough or orthopnea may occur in the setting of fluid overload and may be confused with an ACE inhibitor cough. Due to the impressive benefits of ACE inhibition in this population, all patients should be carefully rechallenged with an ACE inhibitor once they are clinically stable, to confirm an adverse reaction. Exceptions to this would be prior angioedema while taking an ACE inhibitor, or current hyperkalemia. Limiting factors for the use of ACE inhibitors include renal insufficiency and orthostatic hypotension, two problems that frequently occur in the setting of diabetes. Orthostatic hypotension due to venous insufficiency or autonomic neuropathy can often be effectively treated by the use of compression stockings applied to the legs. This mechanical solution may allow the use of this class of drugs and may therefore enable this population to receive the benefits of ACE inhibition with a minimum of side effects.

Angiotensin receptor blockers have similar side-effects to ACE inhibitors but are not usually associated with cough. Angioedema is much less common with ARB and a few case series have been published suggesting that ARB can be used safely in patients with prior angioedema with ACE inhibitors.[19] The risks of recurrent angioedema versus the benefits of ARB use need to be considered on an individual patient basis. The strategy of careful rechallenge with ARB should be considered given the benefit of this class of drugs.

Beta blockers are clearly indicated for patients with congestive heart failure and should not be withheld solely because a patient has diabetes. In the U.S. carvedilol trials, the subgroup with diabetes had a significant reduction in mortality when receiving carvedilol.[20] In the Merit-HF trial evaluating the use of sustained release metoprolol, patients with diabetes also had a trend towards lower mortality.[21] Beta-blockers may worsen glucose control and may theoretically mask some of the symptoms of acute hypoglycemia. For these reasons, whenever a beta-blocker is initiated in a patient with diabetes, more frequent blood glucose monitoring should be performed. The nonselective beta-blocker carvedilol may have an advantage over the more selective agents in the diabetic population with heart failure. Recent studies have shown that the nonselective beta-blockers through their alpha blocking effect do not worsen glucose control when compared to a more selective beta-blocker.[22] For patients with orthostatic hypotension, however, the alpha-blocking effect of the nonselective drug may worsen symptoms of orthostasis. Compression stockings or conversion to a selective beta-blocker may help to ameliorate some of these challenges. There have now been several studies that have shown that if there is intolerance to one class of beta-blockers, conversion to the other class is frequently tolerated. As with ACE inhibitors, rechallenge and perseverance are necessary to give every patient the opportunity to receive the long-term mortality benefits of beta-blockade.

Oral agents that are used to treat diabetes, in particular the thiazolidinediones, may significantly increase salt and water retention and lead to an acute heart failure exacerbation.[23] Although these drugs have a variety of beneficial nonendocrine effects, especially on endothelial function, in a select group of patients the volume expansion is not well tolerated.[23,24] It is important to take a thorough medication history whenever a patient presents with an exacerbation of heart failure to determine if any of these agents have been recently added or adjusted. Increased diuretic dosage may help to minimize the impact of salt and water retention. Despite augmented diuretics, however, in some patients these agents will need to be withdrawn.

Metformin is a drug that needs to be used with caution in patients with both diabetes and heart failure. One serious side effect of metformin is the development of lactic acidosis, which can be life-threatening. The reported cases have occurred in patients with changing renal function that impairs the clearance of metformin. Therefore, metformin should be avoided in patients with renal insufficiency or in those in whom the renal function is likely to be changing. Examples include unstable heart failure, heart failure decompensation, and patients undergoing procedures with iodinated contrast.[25,26] Most clinicians avoid metformin in the heart failure population, but if used, metformin should be stopped during an acute heart failure exacerbation or at the time of any procedure that may acutely worsen renal function.

Diabetes concomitantly with heart failure may be an opportunity to help focus a patient on the importance of lifestyle changes. Diet, exercise, medication compliance and daily monitoring are the keys to success in both diseases and an approach that educates about diabetes and heart failure together may be more successful and less overwhelming to a patient and their support system.

Renal Insufficiency

Renal insufficiency is also a common problem for patients with heart failure. The etiology of renal insufficiency is usually multifactorial but has its root causes in the same risk factors that lead to heart failure. Longstanding hypertension, diabetes, or vascular disease may lead to intrinsic renal insufficiency. In the setting of heart failure, renal function tends to suffer as renal perfusion falls. Differentiating between prerenal azotemia due to low renal blood flow or over diuresis and intrinsic renal disease can be challenging. In many instances, optimal treatment of heart failure may improve renal function, but unfortunately significant intrinsic renal disease complicates and limits effective heart failure management.

Worsening renal function may increase the risk of toxicity of both digoxin and spironolactone.[27] Previously tolerated doses of ACE inhibitors or ARB may lead to hyperkalemia as renal function changes. Careful monitoring of renal function is necessary leading to the appropriate dosage adjustment or withdrawal of heart failure medications.

Loop diuretics may be less effective as renal function deteriorates and the use of the aldosterone blocking agent spironolactone becomes contraindicated.[28] ACE inhibitors and ARB are often withheld due to poor renal function, but a controlled rechallenge is often indicated to confirm that renal function is negatively influenced. Worsening renal function to ACE inhibitors especially in the setting of hypertension and heart failure may indicate the presence of renal artery stenosis. As there are now effective methods to noninvasively diagnose and percutaneously treat this disease, renal artery stenosis should be considered in patients with the appropriate clinical picture and risk factors. Treatment of bilateral renal artery stenosis can markedly simplify the management of patients with heart failure and allow the use of proven mortality benefit therapies.

In selected patients, hemodynamic monitoring to confirm adequate renal perfusion may be necessary to assist in management. Careful hemodynamic monitoring will assure adequate preload as well as adequate cardiac index. The use of inotropes to improve renal blood flow may help to differentiate intrinsic renal disease from poor renal perfusion. Renal function that is worsening without obvious cause may be a marker of worsening end-organ perfusion. This should prompt a repeat evaluation of the status of the patient to rule out the presence of a low cardiac output state or volume contraction.

Asymptomatic increases in blood urea nitrogen or creatinine should be tolerated in patients with heart failure and renal disease provided that electrolyte balance is maintained, there is no evidence of uremic symptoms, and a low cardiac output or low volume state have been ruled out.[17] As renal function deteriorates, heart failure medications become less effective.[29] As the creatinine rises above 3.0 mg/dL standard heart failure drugs become less effective.[30] As the creatinine rises above 5.0 mg/dL dialysis may be necessary to control fluid status, uremia and electrolytes. The initiation of dialysis often allows the use of ACE inhibitors in a patient who previously had not been considered a candidate for this class of drugs. Dialysis also may make volume management less complicated in a patient previously suffering from significant renal insufficiency. Rarely, the placement of a dialysis access can lead to worsening heart failure by creating an arterial–venous fistula, thus shunting blood away from the organs and directly back into the venous system.

The use of alternative vasodilators may be necessary for patients with renal insufficiency. Nitrates and hydralazine have proven benefit and may be reasonable substitutes when ACE inhibitors or ARB are not tolerated.[31,32] Angiotensin-receptor blockers have similar renal effects to the ACE inhibitors and therefore have the same limitations as ACE inhibitors in this population.

The use of digoxin in the setting of renal insufficiency should be undertaken with caution. In patients with changing renal function, digoxin should be withdrawn or the dose decreased until renal function has stabilized. More frequent monitoring of digoxin levels is important to avoid potentially life threatening toxicity.

Renal disease can lead to the development of anemia that can worsen heart failure and lead to symptoms of fatigue. Aggressive treatment of anemia with blood products and erythropoietin, if indicated, can improve these symptoms and reduce the physiologic strain of anemia on the heart. Additional studies on the role of anemia in heart failure are ongoing and may lead to additional recommendations for the management of this common problem.

Hypertension

Two-thirds of patients with congestive heart failure have a past or current history of hypertension.[1] Hypertension is associated with worsening heart failure and increased risk of cardiovascular events and strokes. The management of hypertension in the context of heart failure follows the same general guidelines: ACE inhibitors, beta-blockers, and diuretics. In general, calcium-channel antagonists should be avoided, due to their negative inotropic effects and potential for worsening heart failure outcomes. The one exception may be amlodipine, which may be safe in selected patients who remain hypertensive despite maximum doses of ACE inhibitors or ARB and beta-blockers. Amlodipine should only be used when other classes of drugs with proven mortality benefit are not tolerated or when adequate blood pressure control is not achieved by these agents.

Beta-blockers that have intrinsic sympathomimetic effects should also be avoided. These drugs have in increased risk of mortality when compared to placebo. In addition, direct vasodilators like minoxidil may cause impressive salt and water retention that can make heart failure very difficult to manage. Hypertension is also a significant risk factor for diastolic heart failure. Aggressive treatment of the hypertension can help to reduce the symptoms of volume overload and potentially protect against the progression to systolic dysfunction. Additional clinical trials are needed for patients with diastolic heart failure in order to determine the optimal management strategies. Current data suggest that ACE inhibitors or angiotensin receptor blockers may be the preferred agents in this large population of patients.

Pulmonary Disease

The symptoms of pulmonary disease often overlap with those of heart failure. Cough, dyspnea on exertion, fatigue, and shortness of breath at rest occur with both disease processes. To further complicate the management of these patients, the physical findings of the two diseases also overlap. Wheezing or "crackles" can be appreciated in patients with either heart failure or pulmonary disease. Peripheral or abdominal edema may occur in the setting of right heart failure due to pulmonary hypertension and may be mistaken for left ventricular systolic dysfunction. Jugular venous pulsation may be prominent when tricuspid regurgitation is present due to high right ventricular pressures in the setting of pulmonary hypertension. Pulmonary symptoms such as cough may be mistaken for ACE inhibitor cough, further confounding the ability to maximally treat the heart failure. Amiodarone may also be withheld due to the fear of worsening the pulmonary status in a patient with both lung and heart disease.[33]

The key to managing this very challenging population is to maximize the treatment of both the lung and heart disease. Educating patients to monitor their daily body weight may help to differentiate shortness of breath due to volume overload from an exacerbation of underlying lung disease. If the patient's weight is elevated in the setting of worsening symptoms then augmentation of diuretics may be helpful. If, on the other hand, the weight is unchanged then augmentation of pulmonary medications may be useful.

A new marker for the presence of heart failure is B-natriuretic peptide (BNP). This compound is present in elevated amounts in the serum of patients with heart failure. Recent studies have suggested that the use of BNP levels can differentiate heart failure from other causes of dyspnea.[34] Further studies in this area may help clarify the role of BNP and may enable clinicians to have a more precise clinical test to define heart failure.

In selected patients in whom the usual clinical markers cannot help differentiate pulmonary from cardiac causes of symptoms, a right heart catheterization may yield useful diagnostic information. In the setting of dyspnea and cough, a normal pulmonary capillary wedge pressure suggests a pulmonary etiology to the symptoms. On the other hand, an elevated wedge may implicate heart failure as a cause. Monitoring the patient with the pulmonary artery catheter indwelling may enable titration of heart failure medications and maximization of cardiac status. Obtaining the weight of the patient at a time when the pulmonary capillary wedge pressure is known not be elevated can be extremely useful in the longitudinal management of the patient. Occasionally, cardiopulmonary exercise testing can be used to help determine the etiology of exercise intolerance in a patient with both heart and lung disease. In very challenging cases, exercise hemodynamic studies can also be used to understand cardiac function during exercise.[35] Adequate augmentation of cardiac output without increase in pulmonary capillary wedge pressure in the setting of dyspnea may implicate pulmonary disease as the major component of exercise intolerance. Arterial oxygen hemoglobin desaturation with exercise in the setting of a normal pulmonary capillary wedge pressure is indicative of a pulmonary etiology. Exercise hemodynamic studies may also be particularly useful in the setting of valvular heart disease, where resting studies often underestimate the degree of dysfunction.

The use of beta-blockers in patients with pulmonary disease may be problematic but most patients with chronic obstructive lung disease can tolerate beta-blockers.[33] In this population, a selective beta-blocker that avoids blockade of $beta_2$-receptors may be better tolerated. A careful challenge with a low dose of a selective beta-blocker is indicated in most patients without a documented history of bronchospasm. If tolerated, slow up-titration to target doses will enable the majority of these patients to enjoy the mortality and symptomatic benefits of beta-blockade in heart failure.

Sleep apnea is also a common problem for patients with congestive heart failure.[36] Sleep apnea can take two forms, and both can have negative consequences on the progression of heart failure as well as quality of life.[37] Obstructive sleep apnea occurs when the upper airway becomes lax during sleep, causing a mechanical obstruction to airflow. Patients typically are obese, snore loudly, and have multiple cardiovascular risk factors, including hypertension and diabetes. Obstructive sleep apnea leads to hypoxia and disruption of sleep. It is associated with pulmonary hypertension, systemic hypertension, increased risk of cardiac arrhythmias, and increased risk of cardiovascular events. Patients often complain of fatigue and the need for frequent naps. This is a common complaint in patients with heart failure and may be difficult to differentiate from the symptoms of obstructive sleep apnea. Treatment of obstructive sleep apnea through continuous positive airway pressure (CPAP), weight loss, or surgery improves sleep, decreases pulmonary hypertension, decreases fatigue, improves quality of life and reduces cardiovascular risk.[38] Some preliminary studies suggest that there may be a mortality benefit of the treatment of obstructive sleep apnea.

Central sleep apnea in heart failure has recently become an area of intense clinical research. Central sleep apnea occurs when the brain, respiratory muscles, and circulation fail to effectively regulate respiration and maintain homeostasis of the blood gases. Classically, patients will develop Cheyne–Stokes respiration, in which the respiratory pattern oscillates between hyperventilation and apnea. Central sleep apnea is associated with increased catecholamines, fatigue and worsening heart failure. Treatment of central sleep apnea improves sleep and fatigue as well as exercise capacity and ejection fraction.[39,40] The impact on mortality has not been defined, although there is preliminary evidence that reductions in adrenergic neurohormones may improve outcomes. Two large-scale clinical trials are evaluating the treatment of central sleep apnea in heart failure. The results may help to define an effective treatment that will stabilize or improve heart function and improve quality of life.

Atrial Fibrillation

Atrial fibrillation is the most common arrhythmia effecting patients with congestive heart failure. The etiology of atrial fibrillation in this population is very variable and is often multifactorial, but may result from chronic volume and pressure overload of the atria. Consideration should be given to worsening valvular heart disease as a cause of new onset atrial fibrillation. Valvular heart disease may be amenable to surgical correction in selected patients in order to stabilize ventricular function over time. Regardless of the causes, atrial fibrillation can acutely lead to decompensated heart failure and chronically to worsening ventricular function. Atrial fibrillation leads to decreased exercise capacity and a worse prognosis.[41,42] Both the tachycardia and loss of the atrial contribution to ventricular filling may account for the worsening symptoms. Chronic tachycardia may lead to deteriorating ventricular function, partially explaining the overall worse prognosis. Even if the heart rate is controlled at rest, many patients experience significant increases in their heart rate with activity which may lead to significant reductions in exercise capacity.

Atrial fibrillation in the setting of heart failure is a significant risk factor for the development of thromboemboli.[43] Strokes are common in this population making chronic anticoagulation with warfarin indicated. Special consideration is necessary prior to electrical or chemical cardioversion, to rule out the possibility of atrial thrombi. This can be accomplished by a suitable period of anticoagulation before cardioversion or by the use of transesophageal echocardiography just prior to cardioversion.

Lack of rate control is the most common management problem.[44] The typical drugs used for acute rate control are difficult to use in patients with heart failure, particularly when they are in a decompensated state. Intravenous beta-blockers and calcium-channel blockers can acutely worsen left ventricular function and lead to increased symptoms of heart failure. For this reason, these agents should be used with caution. Digoxin is effective in controlling heart rate for patients with atrial fibrillation only at rest, and is rarely effective in the acute setting. With exercise, heart rate rapidly increases. In combination with beta-blockers, digoxin provides good rate control both at rest and with exercise. In patients who are not decompensated, a reasonable strategy would be to start digoxin and a low dose of oral beta-blocker. The beta-blocker dose can then slowly be titrated over time in order to provide better exercise heart rate control as well as the benefits of beta-blockade in heart failure. Calcium-channel blockers should be avoided in patients with heart failure if possible.

In certain instances, the atrial fibrillation cannot be managed medically. Patients who have severe decompensation of their heart failure or are hypotensive should be urgently electrically cardioverted. The use of an antiarrhythmic such as amiodarone may be necessary to maintain sinus rhythm and hemodynamic stability. Rarely, rate control can not be achieved with drugs over time. In these instances, an ablation of the atrioventricular node and placement of a permanent pacemaker will at least provide rate control without the side effects of medications.

There is some controversy over the benefit of attempting to maintain long-term sinus rhythm in patients with heart failure who have developed atrial fibrillation. Amiodarone, an effective antiarrhythmic in this population, has numerous side effects when used long-term, and despite appropriate therapy, atrial fibrillation often recurs. This needs to be balanced against the theoretical benefits of normal rhythm. On the other hand, many clinicians will perform a cardioversion at least once to attempt to reestablish normal rhythm and improve cardiac performance. Amiodarone may significantly increase the likelihood that a cardioversion will be successful. Amiodarone has numerous drug interactions with other agents commonly used in the management of congestive heart failure. Levels of digoxin and further prolongation of the international normalized ratio (INR) with warfarin are the most common. Dosage adjustment of warfarin and digoxin is critical upon initiating therapy with amiodarone. Due to the presence of structural heart disease, most antiarrhythmic drugs, with the exception of amiodarone, are contraindicated in heart failure. In many patients, adequate rate control and anticoagulation may be the only option to manage atrial fibrillation and heart failure.

Hyperlipidemia

Hyperlipidemia is common in patients with heart failure. Fasting lipids should be obtained in all patients with other risk factors or known cardiovascular disease, in order to identify those patients who may benefit from intervention. Recent studies have shown that treatment of abnormal lipids can prevent initial and subsequent cardiovascular ischemic events. In addition, treatment may also prevent the progression of heart failure by protecting the myocardium from additional ischemic events. The management of hyperlipidemia in the setting of heart failure is no different than that in other clinical settings; β-hydroxy- β-methylglutaryl coenzyme A (HMG-CoA) reductase inhibitors or statins are the mainstay of therapy. Careful monitoring for side effects, including myositis and liver abnormalities, should be routinely performed. Elevated liver enzymes in a patient with heart failure and statin therapy can have multiple causes. It is important to rule out worsening heart failure as a cause, but other concurrent medications—including amiodarone or diabetic agents—may also be responsible.

Heart Failure in the Elderly

The elderly represent the largest population with heart failure.[45] With advancing age, diastolic dysfunction becomes a much more common cause of congestive heart failure symptoms. Unfortunately, there are few studies of diastolic heart failure and little data upon which to base recommendations.

Elderly patients tend to suffer more adverse effects and are less likely to respond to diuretics or inotropes. They are more likely to suffer from orthostatic hypotension and are commonly treated with medications that may exacerbate heart failure. The elderly are more likely to suffer from the comorbidities described above, and end-organ dysfunction in multiple organ systems is more common.

Psychosocial issues, including social isolation and depression, may complicate the management of older patients. Depression, an independent risk factor for mortality in several populations of patients with heart disease, may be more common in the elderly, especially those that are isolated. Recognition and treatment of depression may not only improve quality of life, but also may improve compliance and decrease mortality.

Disease management strategies have been shown to be effective in minimizing hospital admissions and improving the quality of life and clinical outcomes of elderly patients with congestive heart failure.[46] The hallmark of these strategies is the use of a multidisciplinary model that includes physicians, nurses, social workers, and other allied health professionals. Frequent monitoring and reassessment of the status of these patients has been shown to improve clinical outcomes. Incorporating available community resources often provides the support and structure these patients require in order to be successful in the management of their heart failure.

References

1. Solang L, Malmberg K, Ryden L. Diabetes mellitus and congestive heart failure: Further knowledge needed. *Eur Heart J* 1999;20:789–795.
2. Galderisi M, Anderson KM, Wilson PW, Levy D. Echocardiographic evidence for the existence of a distinct diabetic cardiomyopathy (the Framingham Heart Study). *Am J Cardiol* 1991;68:85–89.
3. Sahai A, Ganguly PK. Congestive heart failure in diabetes with hypertension may be due to uncoupling of the atrial natriuretic peptide receptor–effector system in the kidney basolateral membrane. *Am Heart J* 1991;122: 164–170.
4. Zarich SW, Nesto RW. Diabetic cardiomyopathy. *Am Heart J* 1989;118:1000–1012.
5. Swan JW, Anker SD, Walton C, al e. Insulin resistance in chronic heart failure: Relation to severity and etiology of heart failure. *J Am Coll Cardiol* 1997; 30:527–532.
6. Shindler DM, Kostis JB, Yusuf S, et al. Diabetes mellitus: A predictor of morbidity and mortality in the Studies of Left Ventricular Dysfunction (SOLVD) Trials and Registry. *Am J Cardiol* 1996;77:1017–1020.
7. The CONSENSUS Trial Study Group. Effects of enalapril on mortality in severe congestive heart failure. Results of the Cooperative North Scandinavian Enalapril Survival Study (CONSENSUS). *N Engl J Med* 1987;316:1429–1435.
8. The SOLVD Investigators. Effect of enalapril on survival in patients with reduced left ventricular ejection fractions and congestive heart failure. *N Engl J Med* 1991;325:293–302.
9. Garg R, Yusuf S, Collaborative Group on ACE Inhibitor Trials. Overview of randomized trials of angiotensin converting enzyme inhibitors on mortality and morbidity in heart failure. *JAMA* 1995;273:1450–1456.
10. Yusuf S, Sleight P, Pogue J, Bosch J, Davies R, Dagenais G. Effects of an angiotensin-converting enzyme inhibitor, ramipril, on cardiovascular events in high-risk patients. The Heart Outcomes Prevention Evaluation Study Investigators. *N Engl J Med* 2000;342:145–153.
11. Viberti G, Wheeldon NM. MicroAlbuminuria Reduction With VALsartan (MARVAL) Study Investigators. Microalbuminuria reduction with valsartan in patients with type 2 diabetes mellitus: a blood pressure-independent effect. *Circulation* 2002;106(6):672–678.
12. Maggioni AP, Anand I, Gottlieb SO, Latini R, Tognoni G, Cohn JN, Val-HeFT Investigators (Valsartan Heart Failure Trial). Effects of valsartan on morbidity and mortality in patients with heart failure not receiving angiotensin-converting enzyme inhibitors. *J Am Coll Cardiol* 2002;40(8):1414–1421.
13. Cohn JN, Tognoni G, Valsartan Heart Failure Trial Investigators. A randomized trial of the angiotensin-receptor blocker valsartan in chronic heart failure. *N Engl J Med* 2001;345(23):1667–1675.
14. Peters S, Gotting B, Trummel M, Rust H, Brattstrom A. Valsartan for preven-

tion of restenosis after stenting of type B2/C lesions: the VAL-PREST trial. *J Invas Cardiol* 2001;13(2):93–97.

15. Israili ZH, Hall WD. Cough and angioneurotic edema associated with angiotensin-converting enzyme inhibitor therapy: A review of the literature and pathophysiology. *Ann Intern Med* 1992;117:234–242.
16. Packer M, Kessler PD, Gottlieb SS. Adverse effects of converting-enzyme inhibition in patients with severe congestive heart failure: Pathophysiology and management. *Postgrad Med J* 1986;62:179–182.
17. Packer M, Lee WH, Medina N, Yushak M, Kessler PD. Functional renal insufficiency during long-term therapy with captopril and enalapril in severe chronic heart failure. *Ann Intern Med* 1987;106:346–354.
18. Packer M, Lee WH, Medina N, Yushak M, Kessler PD, Gottlieb SS. Influence of diabetes mellitus on changes in left ventricular performance and renal function produced by converting enzyme inhibition in patients with severe chronic heart failure. *Am J Med* 1987;82:1119–1126.
19. Sica DA, Black HR. Current concepts of pharmacotherapy in hypertension: ACE inhibitor-related angioedema: can angiotensin-receptor blockers be safely used?. *J Clin Hyper* 2002;4(5):375–380.
20. Packer M, Bristow MR, Cohn JN, et al. The effect of carvedilol on morbidity and mortality in patients with chronic heart failure. *N Engl J Med* 1996;334: 1349–1355.
21. MERIT-HF Study Group. Effect of metoprolol CR/XL in chronic heart failure: Metoprolol CR/XL randomized intervention trial in congestive heart failure. *Lancet* 1999;353:2001–2007.
22. Jacob S, Rett K, Wicklmayr M, Agrawal B, Augustin HJ, Dietze GJ. Differential effect of chronic treatment with two beta-blocking agents on insulin sensitivity: the carvedilol-metoprolol study. *J Hypertens* 1996;14:489–494.
23. Mudaliar S, Henry RR. New oral therapies for type 2 diabetes mellitus: The glitazones or insulin sensitizers. *Ann Rev Med* 2001;52:239–257.
24. Schoonjans K, Auwerx J. Thiazolidinediones: an update. *Lancet* 2000;355: 1008–1010.
25. Bailey CJ, Turner RC. Metformin. *N Engl J Med* 1996;334:574–579.
26. DeFronzo RA. Pharmacologic therapy for type 2 diabetes mellitus. *Ann Intern Med* 1999;131:281–303.
27. Steiner JF, Robbins LJ, Hammermeister KE, Roth SC, Hammond WS. Incidence of digoxin toxicity in outpatients. *West J Med* 1994;161:474–478.
28. Risler T, Schwab A, Kramer B, Braun N, Erley C. Comparative pharmacokinetics and pharmacodynamics of loop diuretics in renal failure. *Cardiology* 1994;84:155–161.
29. Vasko MR, Cartwright DB, Knochel JP, Nixon JV, Brater DC. Furosemide absorption altered in decompensated congestive heart failure. *Ann Intern Med* 1985;102:314–318.
30. Philbin EF, Santella RN, Rocco TAJ. Angiotensin-converting enzyme inhibitor use in older patients with heart failure and renal dysfunction. *J Am Geriatr Soc* 1999;47:302–308.
31. Loeb HS, Johnson G, Henrick A, et al. Effect of enalapril, hydralazine plus isosorbide dinitrate, and prazosin on hospitalization in patients with chronic congestive heart failure. The V-HeFT VA Cooperative Studies Group. *Circulation* 1993;87:V178–V187.
32. Cohn JN, Archibald DG, Ziesche S, et al. Effect of vasodilator therapy on mortality in chronic congestive heart failure: Results of a Veterans Administration Cooperative Study. *N Engl J Med* 1986;314:1547–1552.

33. Singh SN, Fisher SG, Deedwania PC, Rohatgi P, Singh BN, Fletcher RD. Pulmonary effect of amiodarone in patients with heart failure. The Congestive Heart Failure Survival Trial of Antiarrhythmic Therapy (CHF-STAT) Investigators (Veterans Affairs Cooperative Study No. 320). *J Am Coll Cardiol* 1997;30:514–517.
34. Cabanes L, Richaud-Thiriez B, Fulla Y, et al. Brain natriuretic peptide blood levels in the differential diagnosis of dyspnea. *Chest* 2001;120:2047–2050.
35. Weber KT, Wilson JR, Janicki JS, Likoff MJ. Exercise testing in the evaluation of the patient with chronic cardiac failure. *Am Rev Respir Dis* 1984;129:S60–62.
36. Javaheri S, Parker TJ, Liming JD, et al. Sleep apnea in 81 ambulatory male patients with stable heart failure: Types and their prevalences, consequences, and presentations. *Circulation* 1998;97:2154–2159.
37. Ferguson KA, Fleetham JA. Sleep-related breathing disorders, 4: Consequences of sleep disordered breathing. *Thorax* 1995;50:998–1004.
38. Bradley TD, Floras JS. Pathophysiologic and therapeutic implications of sleep apnea in congestive heart failure. *J Card Fail* 1996;2:223–40.
39. Javaheri S. A mechanism of central sleep apnea in patients with heart failure. *N Engl J Med* 1999;341:949–954.
40. Javaheri S. Treatment of central sleep apnea in heart failure. Sleep 2000;23: S224–227.
41. Dries DL, Exner DV, Gersh BJ, Domanski MJ, Waclawiw MA, Stevenson LW. Atrial fibrillation is associated with an increased risk for mortality and heart failure progression in patients with asymptomatic and symptomatic left ventricular systolic dysfunction: A retrospective analysis of the SOLVD trials. Studies of Left Ventricular Dysfunction. *J Am Coll Cardiol* 1998;32:695–703.
42. Pardaens K, Van Cleemput J, Vanhaecke J, Fagard RH. Atrial fibrillation is associated with a lower exercise capacity in male chronic heart failure patients. *Heart* 1997;78:564–568.
43. Shivkumar K, Jafri SM, Gheorghiade M. Antithrombotic therapy in atrial fibrillation: A review of randomized trials with special reference to the Stroke Prevention in Atrial Fibrillation II (SPAF II) Trial. *Progr Cardiovasc Dis* 1996;38:337–342.
44. Crijns HJ, Van den Berg MP, Van Gelder IC, Van Veldhuisen DJ. Management of atrial fibrillation in the setting of heart failure. *Eur Heart J* 1997;18:C45–49.
45. Rich MW. Epidemiology, pathophysiology, and etiology of congestive heart failure in older adults. *J Am Geriatr Soc* 1997;45:968–974.
46. Rich MW. Heart failure disease management: A critical review. *J Card Fail* 1999;5:64–75.

Chapter 8

Transition from Hospital to Home: Interdisciplinary Management Models

Sara Paul, RN, MSN, FNP and Kathleen M. McCauley, PhD, RN, CS, FAAN, FAHA

Heart failure (HF) is a chronic condition characterized by frequent exacerbation of symptoms requiring acute care visits, emergency department treatment, or hospital readmission. There is evidence that the transition time from hospital to home is particularly problematic for patients and families as they adjust to altered medications and dosage schedules, diminished functional status, and a greater need to understand and adhere to treatment regimens.[1] Several models of managing patients across this transition from hospital to home will be addressed in this chapter, including advance practice nurse transitional care models, collaborative nurse–physician practice models, and heart failure-specific visiting nurse programs. Specific ways that patient and family needs can be addressed through these models and issues related to implementing these programs will be discussed.

Patients with HF are hospitalized more than 2 million times annually and generate over 11 million outpatient visits each year, resulting in annual costs in excess of $38 billion.[2] Most hospital readmissions are due to preventable causes, with the most common being sodium retention.[3,4] Bennett and colleagues found that sodium retention leading to volume overload was identified as a precipitant of decompensation in 59% of 585 HF-related hospital admissions.[5] The next most common reason for decompensation, increasing angina or acute myocardial infarction, was found less than half as frequently. Ghali and colleagues found

From: Jessup M, McCauley KM (eds). *Heart Failure: Providing Optimal Care*. Elmsford, NY: Futura, an imprint of Blackwell Publishing; ©2003.

Table 1

Patients at Risk for Rehospitalization with a Diagnosis of Heart Failure

The presence of one or more of the following:

- Older age
- Polypharmacy
- Presence of one or more comorbidities
- One or more hospitalizations in previous 6–12 months for heart failure
- Or multiple hospitalizations for any reason
- Lack of or inadequate social support
- Moderate to severe functional impairment
- History of noncompliance
- Depression and other psychological problems
- Impaired sensory function

that noncompliance with medication or diet therapy was a major reason for hospital readmission.[6] These findings were supported by a qualitative analysis of data from a randomized clinical trial where problems with obtaining a supply of medications, dietary nonadherence, and poor general health behaviors contributed to rehospitalization.[7] Table 1 outlines a list of patients at risk for rehospitalization in the presence of heart failure.

Prospective payment systems are responsible for shorter hospital stays, while the number of elderly patients discharged with unresolved health problems is increasing.[8] As a result of shorter stays, an acute exacerbation of a chronic illness may not necessarily be resolved at the time of hospital discharge. Furthermore, some patients are being discharged with care needs too complex for their families to manage alone.

In addition to factors already cited, inadequate discharge follow-up, failed social support mechanisms, general medication nonadherence, and failure to obtain medical assistance when symptoms increase have also resulted in preventable rehospitalization. Elderly patients with HF are at increased risk for early rehospitalization, with readmission rates ranging from 29% to 47% within 3–6 months.[6,9,10] Data demonstrate that the incidence of medication noncompliance and inadequate medication knowledge are extremely high in patients just released from a hospitalization, even though they receive medication education before discharge.[11]

In an unpublished graduate research study, patient and spouse satisfaction with discharge instructions at discharge and 2 weeks following discharge from the hospital after coronary artery bypass surgery were evaluated.[12] The results showed that, although patients and their spouses were very satisfied with discharge instructions, they did not understand them, remember them, or adhere to them once they went home from the hospital. If this is true for a one-time hospitalization, such as for coronary bypass grafting, it may be even more critical for patients with a chronic illness such as those who are repeatedly hospitalized and must manage complex medication, dietary, and symptom management regimens. Elderly patients may particularly become confused, with too much information delivered over a shortened period of time as lengths of stay decrease. Simply discharging patients from the hospital with a set of self-care instructions does not guarantee that they will successfully care for themselves once they are at home. Without appropriate outpatient follow-up and support, the likelihood of readmission increases. Situations that are linked to exacerbation of heart failure symptoms and subsequent rehospitalization include adequacy of the discharge plan, patient and caregiver understanding of the discharge plan, adequacy of essential resources (i.e., money), and environmental health threats.

Disease Management Models

In order to decrease repeated hospitalizations and encourage patients to make appropriate lifestyle changes, numerous models have been developed to manage heart failure patients in an outpatient setting (Table 2). The interventions range from very basic actions, such as mailing educational information to patients after discharge, to more complex programs where interdisciplinary teams contribute to the care of the patient. Interestingly, all of these models have been shown to successfully decrease hospitalizations, cost, and in some cases, increase the patient's quality of life.[13] The common factor among each of these outpatient programs is communication. Whether communicating with the patient via postal service, telephone, clinic visit, or home visit, the important issue is

Table 2

Disease Management Models for Heart Failure

- Mailings
- Telemonitoring
- Inotropic infusion clinics
- Home visitation nurses
- Short-stay observation unit in hospital emergency departments
- Hospital-sponsored cardiac rehabilitation programs
- In-patient subacute specialty unit for heart failure
- Physician-run/nurse educator clinics
- Nurse practitioner coordinated clinics
- Multidisciplinary roles in heart failure clinic

that the patient is not left at home without support or follow-up after discharge from the hospital.

Mailings

Serxner and colleagues hypothesized that education alone could significantly affect outcomes.[14] They sent direct educational mailings to 109 recently discharged HF patients randomized to control or education intervention groups. The subjects in the intervention group were mailed patient education materials every 3–4 weeks, as well as a heart failure video. Control patients received normal and customary education in the hospital, but no special information once they were discharged. Specially trained nurses conducted preintervention and postintervention telephone surveys with all subjects. There was no difference between the two groups on the preintervention survey. On the postintervention survey, more patients in the intervention group reported that a low-sodium diet was important in managing their health; they indicated that they were making positive dietary changes; and they reported cooking differently because of their HF. Additionally, the intervention group weighed themselves significantly more often. Although the intervention group continued to forget to take medications at same rate as before the intervention, the control group doubled the number of times they forgot to take medications. The intervention patients were significantly more confident than the control group patients in their ability to manage their condition, and when asked to rate their health, the intervention group rated their health as better than the control group. Fewer patients in the intervention group had to be readmitted to the hospital. Among the subjects with hospital readmissions, those who participated in the intervention group were readmitted less often. The total cost of the program was $50 per patient. The researchers estimated that if the program had been applied to all HF admissions in their hospital during the 6-month study period, the savings would have amounted to $172,790 after the cost of the program was deducted. This represented an $8 : $1 return on investment to the hospital.

Telemanagement

West and coworkers implemented a program called Multifit, which was a physician-supervised nurse mediated home-based system.[15] Patients with HF who met the inclusion criteria had an initial visit, during which a nurse educated them about their disease state and diet, medications, when to call their health-care provider, and other appropriate lifestyle changes. The patient's confidence to comply with diet and pharmacologic therapy was assessed with a self-efficacy questionnaire. There were three objectives of the Multifit system: (1) to optimize doses of angiotensin-converting enzyme inhibitor or isosorbide dinitrate (Isordil)/hydralazine therapy; (2) to promote sodium intake below 2000 mg/day; and (3) to evaluate for symptoms and laboratory evidence of worsening heart failure. Nurses communicated with patients on the telephone to promote dietary and medication adherence, and to hear the patient's self-report of symptoms and weight. The nurse phoned or faxed the patient's primary physician data about the patients. After the initial visit, the nurse phoned patients weekly for 6 weeks. If any problems were detected, this prompted weekly calls for another 6 weeks. Patients were referred to the emergency department (ED) or their primary physician if problems arose, according to protocols. Stable patients continued with nurse contact at 8, 10, 12, 16, 20, and 24 weeks. Patients completed food-frequency questionnaires at 2, 4, 8, and 12 weeks that were used to generate a computerized report of the patient's sodium intake, identify foods with excessive sodium, and provide instructions for limiting these foods. Data were evaluated before and 6 months after entry into the program. Functional status and health-related quality of life were evaluated at baseline and 3 and 6 months. Fifty-one patients participated in the program for about 138 days. Functional status varied from New York Heart Association (NYHA) class I to IV. General care visits decreased 23% (39–30 visits), cardiology visits decreased 31% (16–11 visits), ED visits for HF decreased 67% (six to two visits), and total ED visits declined 53%. Hospitalization rates for HF declined 87% and total hospitalization rates declined 74%. Functional status and symptomatic status improved, and Duke Activity Status Index scores improved 249–265 at 3 and 6 months. The physical component from the health-related quality of life scores improved 352–406 and the mental component scores improved 475–512. Target doses of HF medications increased and sodium intake decreased 38%.

Home Visits

Kornowski and colleagues initiated a home-monitoring program with physician home visits in Tel Aviv.[16] Forty-two elderly patients in NYHA class III and IV HF (mean ejection fraction was 27%) were enrolled in a home-care surveillance program consisting of weekly home visits. The physician interviewed the patient and family, performed a physical exam, maintained medical charting, reviewed the patient's medications and prescribed medications as needed. Intravenous medications such as diuretics were administered if needed, and nurses were available to draw blood, etc. If the patient had problems, an extra home visit was given.

Physiotherapy and home oxygen were available. Mean total hospitalizations were reduced from 32 ± 15 hospitalizations/year to 12 ± 16 hospitalizations/year. Cardiovascular hospitalizations were reduced from 29 to eight hospitalizations per year (72% reduction). Hospital duration reduced from 26 to 6 days per year (76% reduction) and cardiovascular admission days decreased from 23 to 4 days per year (83% reduction). Global functional status index (scaled 1–4) increased from 14 to 23 at the end of 1 year of follow-up. This score was determined by the physician using the following scale: Score 1, patient confined to bed; 2, needs assistance for daily activities; 3, independent with daily activities but housebound; and 4, independent in daily activities.

Programs using home visits as an intervention are more likely to use nurses as providers. Lasater implemented a program known as "Follow-up Nursing" (FUN) at a south-eastern medical center, using staff nurses from the cardiac step-down unit to make home visits to patients following discharge from the hospital.[17] Eighty patients were enrolled in a 6-month pre- and postintervention comparison trial. All patients diagnosed with HF who were discharged to a tri-county area surrounding the hospital had at least one home visit from a staff nurse who had cared for patients while they were in the hospital. At each visit, the nurse reviewed diet and medication information, and adjusted diuretic therapy based on the patient's weight and other findings. Over the 6 months of follow-up, patients received an average of averaged 37 home visits. Results revealed that there were 14% fewer readmissions, a 22% shorter length of hospital stay (73–57 days), and a 32% reduction in total hospitalization days. These changes reduced hospitalization costs by $500 per patient.

In a similar program, Stewart and coworkers initiated a home based intervention program in Australia.[18–20] Ninety elderly HF patients were randomized to home visits from a nurse and pharmacist team versus usual care (no home visits). Intervention patients received an in-patient educational visit from the nurse, and were visited within a week of hospital discharge by a nurse and a pharmacist who assessed the patient's medical knowledge, compliance, and physical status. Patients received reinforcement of educational information, a pillbox to organize medications, medication information and reminder card, and referral to a community pharmacist for additional attention. The nurse and pharmacist communicated with the patient's primary-care doctor about the patient's status. Six-month follow-up compared to the usual care group showed 42% fewer hospitalizations and hospital days among the intervention group and lower hospitalization costs that were not statistically significant. The researchers extended follow-up to 18 months and found fewer out-of-hospital deaths and unplanned readmissions among the treatment group. Additionally, the treatment group required fewer days of hospitalization and ED visits than usual care patients. The authors conducted another study with a similar intervention, where 200 patients received home visits from a nurse only. After 6 months, significantly more patients in the intervention group remained event-free, and there were 40% fewer readmissions and out of hospital deaths. Hospital costs were lowered by nearly half in the intervention group. In evaluating Stewart's results, differences in the health-care systems must be considered.

Community-Based Management

Naylor and associates developed an interdisciplinary transitional care model, which evaluated the impact of discharge planning and home care delivered by advanced practice nurses (APNs).[13,21,22] The program was initially developed to enable earlier hospital discharge of vulnerable patients, such as low birth weight infants, but grew to focus on improving post-discharge outcomes for high-risk, high-cost, high-volume patient groups. Funded by the National Institute of Nursing Research (NINR), the intervention consisted of comprehensive discharge planning and home follow-up to address problems of high-risk elders. The researchers conducted several studies.

The first study was a randomized clinical trial to compare the effectiveness of a comprehensive discharge planning protocol for hospitalized elders implemented by gerontologic APNs compared to general discharge planning procedures. Two hundred and seventy-six patients with medical or surgical cardiac problems were randomized to a control or intervention group. Control group patients received standard discharge planning, while the intervention group received standard care plus a comprehensive discharge planning protocol that extended from hospital admission through 2 weeks post-discharge. Patients received a visit from an APN while in the hospital and telephone calls after discharge. Results from the first 6 weeks after discharge revealed decreased readmissions, fewer total days of rehospitalization, lower readmission charges, and lower charges for health-care costs after discharge for the medical intervention patients.[23]

Data from this study were used to develop a high-risk profile of hospitalized elders that defined the inclusion criteria for a second study of 363 patients with a medical or surgical problem randomized to control or APN intervention. High-risk patients were those with one of the following characteristics: inadequate support systems, multiple chronic health problems, history of depression, moderate to severe functional impairment, multiple hospitalizations during the past 6 months, hospitalization in the past 30 days, fair or poor self-health rating, history of nonadherence to therapeutic interventions, or greater than 80 years of age. The intervention consisted of APN discharge planning and an expanded 1-month follow up including home visits and telephone calls. Results at 6 months showed decreased hospital readmissions and hospitalization days, and decreased time to first readmission in the intervention group. It is interesting to note that for elderly patients with HF, benefits of the intervention ended after 6 weeks. There were estimated savings of $600,000 for the intervention group (about $3000 per patient). However, there was no significant difference between groups in post-discharge acute care visits, functional status, depression, or patient satisfaction.[1] In order to determine if the transitional care model can be effective in HF patients, this team of researchers has completed a randomized clinical trial with an expanded 3-month home follow-up intervention guided by a protocol targeted specifically for patients with heart failure. Findings have been submitted for publication.

Another study that incorporated a home visit component used community case managers (CCM) to optimize the care of HF patients at risk for repeated rehospitalizations or high health-care resource utilization.[24] This program consisted of identification of high-risk hospitalized patients, discharge planning, and home visits to evaluate physical status and the social environment, provide patient and family education and define advance directives. The CCM helped the patient establish links to health-care providers and community services, and provided emotional support. Care maps driven by the patient's NYHA functional status guided the intervention and addressed issues of adherence, improved health behaviors, enhanced self-efficacy and self-management. CCMs followed a set visit protocol of high intensity at the beginning (one to three times per week), decreasing in frequency over the next 6 months. The hospital absorbed the $80 per visit cost, and the 6-month evaluation showed a 70–80% reduction in HF rehospitalizations, with a total cost of rehospitalization reduction of 50–60%.

Collaborative Practice Models

Rich and colleagues conducted a prospective, randomized trial to evaluate the effect of a nurse-directed multidisciplinary team intervention on 282 patients 70 years of age or older.[25] Patients with heart failure were included in the study if they had risk factors for early readmission. The participants received either standard care or intervention, which consisted of comprehensive patient education by a geriatric cardiovascular nurse, detailed medication review by a geriatric cardiologist, social services consultation for discharge planning and transition into the home, dietary teaching from a registered dietician, and close follow-up after discharge with home visits and telephone contact. Patients were followed for 1 year, with the primary endpoint of readmission-free survival at 90 days. This endpoint was achieved in 91 of the 142 patients in the treatment group and 75 of the 140 patients in the control group. The number of readmissions for heart failure was reduced by 562% in the treatment group, while multiple readmissions were more frequent in the control group. There was a total of 444% fewer admissions in the treatment group, and the total number of days of hospitalization was reduced from 865 in the control group to 556 in the treatment group. Intervention patients had a significant improvement in quality of life, and the overall cost of care was higher in the control group by $460, or an average of $153 per patient per month.

The notion of a collaborative comprehensive HF clinic was investigated by Fonarow and colleagues, who evaluated its impact on functional status, hospital readmission rate and estimated hospital costs.[26] Medications were optimized, a heart failure Clinical Nurse Specialist educated patients about diet and lifestyle changes in groups and individually, and patients were taught to adjust their diuretic dose as needed. Patients were seen 3 days after hospital discharge and weekly until they were stable. The patients received phone calls 2 days after any major medication change and at routine intervals between 2 and 8 weeks post-discharge. Patient data 6 months before clinic entry were compared to 6 months after clinic entry. Cardiopulmonary exercise testing (CPT) was done at baseline and at 6 months. The researchers found that at 6 months after entry into the clinic, NYHA functional class improved in 49% of the patients. CPT showed an increase in oxygen consumption of 11 ± 36–152 ± 44. Admissions decreased from 92% in the 6 months prior to clinic entry, to 26% in the 6 months after clinic entry. For the whole group (179 patients), hospitalization costs were $3,157,000 before patients entered the specialized clinic, and $312,000 in the 6 months after.

Smith and coworkers, who studied the effect of a nurse practitioner (NP) and cardiologist practice in a cardiomyopathy clinic at a Veterans Administration medical center, further examined the effectiveness of specialty clinics.[27] Study data included CPT, echocardiogram, and radionuclide left ventriculogram prior to the patient's first clinic visit, the Minnesota Living with Heart Failure Questionnaire (MLHFQ), history and physical exam findings and laboratory work. Heart failure medications were optimized, and the frequency of visits was determined by the severity of the patient's illness or symptoms. Patients received education about their medications, diet, activity, and the importance of daily weights. The NP was available by telephone to answer questions or resolve patient problems related to their heart failure. Six months after joining the clinic, echocardiogram, radionuclide left ventriculogram, CPT and MLHFQ were repeated. The numbers of HF clinic and emergency department visits and hospital admissions were reviewed for the 6 months before and after joining the clinic. Sample size was a limitation of the study with only 20 patients completing data collection. However, NYHA class improved from 2.6 to 2.2, and MLHFQ scores improved 23 points. Exercise time increased from 67 to 88 min, but oxygen consumption was unchanged. Ejection fraction improved from a mean of 24–36%. Emergency department visits and hospitalizations decreased more than 80%. It is important to note that patients were excluded from the study if they had severe valve disease, pulmonary disease, pulmonary hypertension, or any noncardiac condition that impaired exercise performance or life expectancy. Patients were also excluded if they lived a long distance from the clinic, making regular follow-up difficult.

Paul described outcomes from a multidisciplinary outpatient heart failure clinic at a south-eastern medical center.[28] Data were collected on hospital readmissions, ED visits, length of stay, charges and reimbursement for 15 patients from the 6 months before and the 6 months after joining a heart failure clinic. In the clinic, patients were seen by a clinical pharmacist, a nurse practitioner, a physician, and if needed, a dietician or social worker. Patients were managed closely via telephone calls and frequent clinic visits. Total hospital admissions in this group of patients were reduced from 38 (151 hospital days) to 19 (72 hospital days) after entering the clinic. Lengths of stay and ED visits were decreased, although they were not statistically significant. Mean in-patient hospital charges decreased, while reimbursements (as measured by the percent collection rate) increased.

Initiating a Heart Failure Management Program

A common theme of all of these management strategies is post-discharge follow-up to enhance patients' ability to understand and manage the chronic illness of heart failure and its expected exacerbations. Connection to a consistent provider is essential—whether this is an APN or case manager working with a variety of physician providers, or a multidisciplinary team managing patients within their own practice. The same approach will not work in every health-care setting, but each program must be individualized to work within a given environment and community. Before a heart failure management program is developed, careful consideration must be given to the goals of the program. Does an existing physician practice have a large number of heart failure patients with recurrent rehospitalizations and suboptimal outcomes? Are frequent visits to the clinic feasible for the patient population? Can APNs be recruited to practice collaboratively with the physicians to develop a comprehensive program? Do existing home-care agencies have the capability of establishing an effective home-care component with nursing providers who have established expertise in heart failure? Is the HF program part of a service contract for a managed care corporation? If insurance reimbursement is not feasible, can other payment options be defined, given strong documentation of cost savings due to prevented rehospitalizations? Is the goal of the HF program to generate revenue for a hospital or community practice? Once the goals have been identified, it is important to plan, organize, implement, and evaluate the program.

Planning

Data gathering is the starting point for any HF management program. Information about HF readmissions, lengths of stay, costs and reimbursement will emphasize the need for the program if the hospital or practice is losing revenue from repeated HF admissions. The estimated cost of the program should include equipment (such as computers and transcription machines), staff, telephone expenses, patient education materials, scales to support patient adherence with daily weights, secretarial costs, and any other expenses that will be incurred. If an APN will be involved, billing issues and insurance reimbursement rules should be investigated. The costs of the program should be balanced against revenue generated via an expanded patient caseload with improved outcomes. Hospitals and insurance carriers may be more willing to support the costs of the program when they realize the savings to be gained by reduction in unnecessary readmissions. Commitment from the institution's administration is imperative before moving forward with further planning.

Resources, such as physical space to examine patients or review patient education materials, should be identified if the plan is to start a HF clinic. Access to equipment for procedures such as inserting intravenous lines, obtaining an electrocardiogram or echocardiogram, applying a Holter monitor, or administering medication should be readily available. Staff—who triage the patient, obtain vital signs, and maintain the flow of patients—should be somewhat knowledgeable about heart failure in order to support patient education. For home follow-up programs, travel costs as well as APN communication strategies (i.e., cellular telephones to facilitate patient or physician contact while on the road) must be considered.

Many different models of HF programs exist around the country. It would be helpful for the nurse implementing a HF program to contact colleagues who have already established a successful program.[29] Experienced HF nurses can answer questions, predict barriers and offer solutions to overcome obstacles. They can also offer copies of protocols, policies, and patient education information that will help decrease the amount of work in developing the program.

Organization

Frequent interaction with HF patients has been shown to decrease hospitalizations. Systems for following patient information help the health-care provider to track changes or alterations in the patient's clinical status, particularly when the number of patients in the HF program increases. Documenting demographic data and tracking vital signs, weights, medication changes, and patient-related telephone conversations is imperative. The nurse must develop a system to keep up with current patient information in order to make informed decisions about HF management.

Many states require APNs to practice with a set of protocols for patient care. Protocols may be developed by the individual APN or purchased in a prepublished book or manual. If the APN is practicing with a physician, collaboration between the two professionals when developing the protocols will ensure that appropriate patient care is administered and that the standards of care are comparable between the disciplines.

Telephone management, or telemanagement, is commonly used to maintain communication with patients and identify problems that may arise between clinic visits. In this manner, exacerbation of HF can often be avoided and the patient can be managed without requiring hospitalization. Furthermore, patients have a sense of well-being when they know that a health-care provider is concerned for them and is available to assist them as needed. There are many systems that can be purchased to monitor patients in their home. Some very sophisticated systems can measure vital signs, weight, and other physiologic parameters, and transmit that information to the heart failure office via the Internet. Other systems may have the patient answer a series of questions about their heart failure symptoms and then transmit that information to the heart failure office. Most HF programs, however, use a very old and reliable system, with a nurse who manually telephones the patient to ask a series of questions to ascertain the patient's current heart failure status. In this manner, human contact is made, the patient has an increased sense of well-being, and the nurse hears the patient's own words describing symptoms. The nurse managing the HF program will need to create a system to keep up with patients and may need to set aside specific time during the week for telephone contact with patients.

Participation from other disciplines can add valuable services to the HF program. Pharmacists are well informed of medication interactions, appropriate dosages, cost of medications, and maneuvers to help streamline the patient's medication list. The pharmacist can be particularly helpful in determining whether a bothersome symptom is due to a medication side effect or interaction, or the underlying disease. They are also helpful with patient education in the home, the clinic or the hospital setting. A dietician offers expertise in teaching patients how plan their diet. This is particularly helpful if the patient has concomitant diseases, such as diabetes, hypertension, coronary artery disease, or renal failure. The dietician can also help patients create a sodium restriction or weight loss plan that is specifically tailored to the patient's food preferences. A social worker provides community resources and financial information for patients who are economically challenged.

Before implementing a heart failure program, it is important to have patient education materials such as easy-to-read pamphlets, videos, cassette tapes and other media. The volume of information that is given to patients about HF and lifestyle changes can be overwhelming. Therefore, they need to have access to written information to review at home. As patients become more familiar with Internet information sources, they may need help in identifying sites that contain accurate information versus those that are misleading.

Implementation

Once the program is ready to proceed, the roles of each provider should be clearly delineated. The nurse's role may involve patient education, home visits, communication with the patient's physician, clinic examination and determination of the patient's disposition, or all of these activities. An advantage of home-care programs is that the nurse has the ability to observe directly how the home environment, support systems, and patient behaviors interact to either enhance or hinder effective management of HF. Whatever the nurse's role is in the HF program, expectations must be clearly stated so that each person involved in the program is aware of their role and how they will interact with other members of the HF team. Conflict may arise if role delineation is not clear. Hours of operation and on-call hours and responsibilities need to be written as policies. Occasionally, these details are not clear until the program has been functioning for a short time. Policies, responsibilities and details may need to be adjusted once the process has been underway, and problems or conflicts rise to the surface.

Evaluation

Once the HF program is actively functional, data should be gathered to evaluate the effectiveness of the program, including patient outcomes and satisfaction of patients and team members. Systems for managing patients should be reviewed, and any necessary changes should be made. Collection of cost data in terms of actual costs of care delivery with this system and changes in health-care resource utilization, such as prevented rehospitalizations, may be critical to ongoing program support.

Summary

Clearly, when HF patients face the transition from the hospital setting to home, they need follow-up to prevent deterioration and preventable exacerbation of their disease. Many studies have shown positive outcomes when the patient is closely managed as an outpatient. In the vast majority of these studies, nurses are the health-care providers who interact with the patient and follow their clinical status, using a team approach to manage the patient's care. A criticism of many of these studies is the use of a pre- versus postintervention measurement rather than a randomized clinical trial design. However, the fact that such varied interventions and designs consistently result in improved outcomes, and often at reduced costs, points to the serious problem that patients and providers face in managing this complex illness. Although the incidence of HF is increasing, hospital readmissions can be controlled and quality of life can be improved if the patient is closely managed—ideally by a multidisciplinary team with specialized knowledge.

References

1. Naylor M, Brooten D, Campbell R, et al. Comprehensive discharge planning and home follow-up of hospitalized elders: A randomized clinical trial. *JAMA* 1999;281:613–620.
2. O'Connell J, Bristow M. Economic impact of heart failure in the United States: time for a different approach. *J Heart Lung Transplant* 1994;13:S107–S112.
3. Bennett S, Saywell R, Zollinger T, et al. Cost of hospitalizations for heart failure: Sodium retention versus other decompensating factors. *Heart Lung* 1999;28:102–109.
4. Vinson JM, Rich MW, Sperry JC, Shah AS, McNamara T. Early readmission of elderly patients with congestive heart failure. *J Am Geriatr Soc* 1990;38:1290–1295.
5. Bennett S, Huster G, Baker S, et al. Heart failure decompensation: Precipitants and strategies for case management. *Am J Crit Care* 1998;7:168–174.
6. Ghali J, Kadakia S, Cooper R, Ferlinz J. Precipitating factors leading to decompensation of heart failure: Traits among urban blacks. *Arch Intern Med* 1988;148:2013–2016.
7. Happ MB, Naylor M, Roe-Prior P. Factors contributing to re-hospitalization in elderly patients with heart failure. *J Cardiovasc Nurs* 1997;11:75–84.
8. Rogers W, Draper D, Kahn K, et al. Quality of care before and after implementation of the DRG-based prospective payment system: A summary of effects. *JAMA* 1990;264:1989–1994.
9. Rich MW, Freedland KE. Effect of DRGs on three-month readmission rate of geriatric patients with congestive heart failure. *Am J Public Health* 1988;78:680–682.

10. Gooding J, Jette A. Hospital readmissions among the elderly. *J Am Geriatr Soc* 1985;33:595–601.
11. Naylor M. A decade of transitional care research with vulnerable elders. *J Cardiovasc Nurs* 2000;14:1–14.
12. Paul S. Patient and spouse satisfaction with discharge instructions following coronary artery bypass graft surgery at the time of discharge and two weeks after discharge [unpublished graduate research, University of Alabama School of Nursing]. Birmingham, AL: University of Alabama at Birmingham, 1986.
13. Rich M. Heart failure disease management: A critical review. *J Card Fail* 1999;5:64–74.
14. Serxner S, Miyaji M, Jeffords J. Congestive heart failure disease management study: A patient education intervention. *Congest Heart Fail* 1998;4:23–28.
15. West J, Miller N, Parker K, et al. A comprehensive management system for heart failure improves clinical outcomes and reduces medical resource utilization. *Am J Cardiol* 1997;79:58–63.
16. Kornowski R, Zeeli D, Averbuch M, et al. Intensive home-care surveillance prevents hospitalization and improves morbidity rates among elderly patients with severe congestive heart failure. *Am Heart J* 1995;129:762–766.
17. Lasater M. The effect of a nurse-managed CHF clinic on patient readmission and length of stay. *Home Healthc Nurse* 1996;14:351–356.
18. Stewart S, Marley J, Horowitz JD. Effects of a multidisciplinary, home-based intervention on unplanned readmissions and survival among patients with chronic congestive heart failure: a randomised controlled study. *Lancet* 1999;354:1077–1083.
19. Stewart S, Pearson S, Horowitz J. Effects of a home-based intervention among patients with congestive heart failure discharged from acute hospital care. *Arch Intern Med* 1998;158:1067–1072.
20. Stewart S, Vandenbroek AJ, Pearson S, Horowitz JD. Prolonged beneficial effects of a home-based intervention on unplanned readmissions and mortality among patients with congestive heart failure. *Arch Intern Med* 1999;159: 257–261.
21. Naylor M, Brooten D, Campbell R, et al. Comprehensive discharge planning and home follow-up of hospitalized elders. *JAMA* 1999;281:613–620.
22. Naylor M, McCauley K. The effects of a discharge planning and home follow-up intervention on elders hospitalized with common medical and surgical cardiac conditions. *J Cardiovasc Nurs* 1999;14:44–54.
23. Naylor M, Brooten D, Jones R, Lavizzo-Mourey R, Mezey M, Pauly M. Comprehensive discharge planning for the hospitalized elderly. *Ann Intern Med* 1994;120:999–1006.
24. Moser D, Macko M, Hackett F, Hutchins M. Community case management models of heart failure care. In: Moser D, Riegel B, eds. *Improving Outcomes in Heart Failure: An Interdisciplinary Approach.* Gaithersburg, MD: Aspen, 2001: 282–300.
25. Rich MW, Beckham V, Wittenberg C, Leven CL, Freedland KE, Carney RM. A multidisciplinary intervention to prevent the readmission of elderly patients with congestive heart failure. *N Engl J Med* 1995;333:1190–1195.
26. Fonarow GC, Stevenson LW, Walden JA, et al. Impact of a comprehensive heart failure management program on hospital readmission and functional status of patients with advanced heart failure. *J Am Coll Cardiol* 1997;30:725–732.

27. Smith L, Fabbri S, Pai R, Ferry D, Heywood J. Symptomatic improvement and reduced hospitalization for patients attending a cardiomyopathy clinic. *Clin Cardiol* 1997;20:949–954.
28. Paul S. Impact of a nurse-managed heart failure clinic: A pilot study. *Am J Crit Care* 2000;9:140–146.
29. Paul S. Implementing an outpatient congestive heart failure clinic: The nurse practitioner role. *Heart Lung* 1997;26:486–491.

Chapter 9

Living with Heart Failure: Promoting Adherence, Managing Symptoms, and Optimizing Function

Nancy M. Albert, MSN, RN, CCNS, CCRN, CNA and Sara Paul, RN, MSN, FNP

As in many other chronic medical conditions, living with left ventricular systolic dysfunction or heart failure (HF) is often easier said than done. After the diagnosis is made, there are many hurdles to overcome to optimize functional capacity and improve quality of life. When the condition is asymptomatic or mild, as represented by a New York Heart Association (NYHA) functional class of I or II (Stage B), consensus recommendations for self-management are less stringent. When the condition exhibits worsening symptoms of a moderate to advanced state and the NYHA functional classification is III or IV (Stage C and D), the medication regimen increases and lifestyle changes are more extreme (Table 1).[1,2] Current HF-specific lifestyle recommendations emphasize a low-sodium diet, daily weight monitoring, regular aerobic exercise, and communication with the health-care provider for new or worsening symptoms reflecting HF decompensation. Unfortunately, current guidelines do not facilitate active patient-mediated steps to minimize or alleviate symptoms that may positively alter left ventricular remodeling and/or neuroendocrine activation. This shortcoming does not assist patients and their significant others to help themselves to their fullest potential.

This chapter will emphasize active patient involvement in promotion of adherence, managing symptoms, and optimizing function. Instead of focusing on patient "compliance" with therapies, which im-

From: Jessup M, McCauley KM (eds). *Heart Failure: Providing Optimal Care.* Elmsford, NY: Futura, an imprint of Blackwell Publishing; ©2003.

Table 1

Lifestyle Changes Required in the Self-Management of Heart Failure

Functional class I and II:
- 3000 mg sodium diet

Functional class III and IV:
- 2000 mg sodium diet
- Routine preventive strategies, as below, plus:
  - Assess herbal/alternative therapies for interactions with heart failure medications
- Fluid management: fluid intake restriction

All functional classes:
- Regular aerobic exercise: low to moderate intensity
  - Do not lift objects greater than 25 pounds
  - Allow for periods of rest during the day between activities
- Daily weight monitoring
- Routine preventive strategies
  - Annual flu shot
  - Scheduled follow-up examinations
  - Smoking cessation
  - Weight control
  - Elimination of alcohol
  - Optimum treatment of endocrine abnormalities and other comorbidities
  - Stress management
  - Reduce fat & cholesterol in diet if coronary disease present
- Learn signs and symptoms of worsening condition and report problems immediately, such as:
  - Weight gain >2 pounds overnight or 3 pounds in 1 week
  - Pressure or pain in the chest, neck, jaw, arm, or shoulder
  - Increased shortness of breath or fatigue
  - Dizziness or syncope
  - Swelling in feet, ankles, legs, or abdomen
  - Palpitations, racing heart, new onset of heart rate >120 beats/min

plies health-care personnel authority and power and denies patients decision-making in their care, we will emphasize "self-management" and personal responsibility for one's life. We will also offer strategies to increase the self-efficacy of specific target interventions, with emphasis on meeting individual patient needs.

Lessons Learned in Managing Symptoms and Optimizing Function: The Continuum of Heart Failure

Primary-care practitioners, emergency-care center physicians, and even most hospital physicians use an acute episodic approach in managing patients. When patients develop symptoms, they seek medical advice. When there are no symptoms, it is assumed that the patient is stable and not in need of new or more aggressive therapies. When people seek emergency or hospital care for HF symptom relief and the symptoms are alleviated, insurance companies expect them to be discharged and treated in an ambulatory setting. This management approach gives the illusion that HF is a series of discrete events and that patients are either "in" or "out" of it, based on symptoms. The problem with this approach is that patients do not learn the impact of HF pathophysiology on their overall state of well-being, and they assume that lack of, or stabilization of, symptoms equals a steady state. Through HF pharmacological therapy research and the long-standing Framingham Study, we have learned that elimination of or improvement in symptoms (with diuretics and direct-acting vasodilators) does not equal prolonged life and improved life quality; in fact, symptomatic improvement does not necessarily correlate with disease improvement.[3] It is for this reason that up-titration of angiotensin-converting enzyme inhibitors and beta-blocker agents to target dosages are encouraged, even when symptoms have diminished or been alleviated at a lower drug dose.

Patients with HF must be taught that it is a chronic and ongoing condition that has a continuum of signs and symptoms ranging from asymptomatic (NYHA functional class I) to symptoms at rest (NYHA functional class IV). This paradigm shift encourages introduction of education content related to HF pathophysiology of ventricular remodeling and neurohormonal stimulation. People living with HF need to understand that ventricular reshaping may occur even though they are asymptomatic and that medication therapies need to be given at doses that have been shown to cause attenuation or modulation of this process. When patients understand that there are many silent processes of HF (left ventricular dysfunction and remodeling, low ejection fraction and pump failure, arrhythmias, and neuroendocrine activation) and silent risk factors that worsen HF (coronary artery disease, hypertension, valve dysfunction and cardiomyopathy), they may be more likely to actively listen to educational messages of the treatment plan. Education related to silent processes of HF and the continuum of HF will not only help patients understand the necessity of frequent office visits for drug optimization, but it will also facilitate understanding of adherence of nonpharmacologic therapies.

A paradigm shift from episodes of HF to a continuum of HF may help patients living with the condition realize that reliance on diuretics to manage symptoms of fluid overload may not be the best option in overall health promotion. While diuretics are considered the cornerstone of symptomatic HF treatment, they are also known to stimulate the renin–angiotensin–aldosterone and sympathetic nervous systems.[4] The hormone surge that is associated with an aggressive dose of loop diuretics to treat HF exacerbation from volume overload may remain in the systemic circulation for days to weeks and ultimately worsen the HF condition.[5] While it is important to alleviate acute, threatening symptoms with aggressive diuretic dosing, it may be equally important to teach patients *not* to assume that this same therapy is the primary means of relieving distress associated with dietary or medication nonadherence. It is true that the patient's distress will be relieved with volume removal following diuretic administration, but the lesson the patient living with HF ultimately learns from this action is that it is OK to "cheat" on sodium restrictions, since a pill will fix the problem.

A paradigm shift away from double or other aggressive diuretic dosing regimens when low level fluid overload occurs requires that patients be educated in not just weight monitoring, but also actions to take when their weight increases slightly, so that they can use nonpharmacological means to reduce it. For this paradigm shift to be truly understood, patients require knowledge of the effects of increased weight on the cardiovascular system and heart function, even when symptoms have not changed. They need to understand the term "dry" or "ideal" weight as it pertains to their volume status, so that incremental increases in weight are taken seriously. Patients need to learn how to adjust their daily sodium and fluid intake and how to properly manage thirst so they can actively influence their volume load and potentially eliminate or decrease the incidence of episodic decompensation. Table 2 offers suggestions related to self-management of food and thirst. Future research is needed in this area to increase support for nonpharmacological management of fluid overload, especially since this approach takes more time and effort for the health-care team to implement and for the patient to comprehend.

Management Issues and Ongoing Communication

There are many factors that influence patient adherence to medications, dietary restrictions, fluid management monitoring (daily weight and fluid intake monitoring), self-management actions, and a routine exercise schedule. Before we can expect a patient to adhere to guideline recommendations, health-care providers must take the time to understand common barriers and individual issues that impact adherence to the treatment plan. In most cases, patients do not purposely choose to ignore or neglect care recommendations, but oftentimes their behaviors do not coincide with medical advice due to factors in which health-care providers must intervene (Table 3).

The patient's knowledge level of HF pathophysiology and management approaches is a major factor that must be assessed to assure self-management of lifestyle changes and proper medication administration.

Table 2

Self-Management of Low-Sodium Diet and Fluids

Diet

- Instruct in reading labels for sodium content and serving size for all processed foods
  - Many foods that do not taste salty (pancakes and other boxed flour mixtures) have a high sodium content since sodium is used as a preservative
  - Smoked meats and fish are high in sodium (used in the smoking process)
  - Deli meats, pickled foods, and canned foods/soups are high in sodium
- Focus on what *can* be chosen instead of only focusing on what not to eat
- Always talk about milligrams (i.e., 2000 mg) of sodium, not grams; food labels are marked in milligrams
- Learn ethnic and cultural food tastes of patients; give specific instructions that reflect low-sodium diet choices
- Do *not* place emphasis on only eating food items with a "very low" sodium content (i.e., choosing foods that are 200 mg or less in sodium content per serving). This may discourage patients from following their diet. Rather, focus on the total daily sodium content and the need for flexibility
- Encourage comparison shopping for food items of high interest, since different brands of a product may have different sodium content
- Give tips for eating out in restaurants:
  - Order salad dressing, sauces and gravies on the side; dip fork in the mixture, then spear the fork in the food. This will give the food flavor without increasing the sodium content of the food to a great degree
  - Typically, heart-healthy foods are low in fat and cholesterol, but may be very high in sodium, since sodium is often used to give low-fat foods flavor
  - Fried foods are high in sodium, since sodium is an ingredient of the breading mixture
- Encourage creativity with nonsodium-based spices when cooking

Fluids

- Generally, 2000 mL (approximately 8 cups) of fluids per day is recommended as a limit
  - This volume limit may be decreased by 1–2 cups (to 2500 mL) if work or outdoor activity creates volume loss through sweat
  - This volume limit may be increased by 1–2 cups (to 1500 mL) if the serum sodium level is below 135 mmol/L or the patient is on high-dose diuretics (>80 mg twice daily)
- Thirst should be managed without drinking fluids or relying on ice chips
  - Thirst-quenching ideas are to suck on frozen strawberry or banana bites or individual grapes; suck on hard candy or a sucker; chew gum (sugarless)
- Milk and milk-based products (ice cream) often increase thirst

Self-management in minor volume overload (slight weight gain of <3 pounds in one day or less than 7 pounds in 1 week):

- Decrease daily sodium intake by 200 mg per day for 1–3 days and fluid intake by 2 cups per day for 1–3 days and observe closely for a decrease in weight
- Keep a diary of everything ingested for 2–3 days to determine if one type of food is at fault or if intake was high in juicy fruit, other fluids, or high-sodium-content foods

Table 3

Common Factors Influencing Adherence to the Plan of Care

Medication issues
- Confusion over generic versus trade names
- Inadequate/incomplete instructions (may be taking medications that have been discontinued)
- Poor eyesight/cannot read label
- Lack of funds
- No transportation to pharmacy
- Managed care: nonformulary medications ordered by physician
- Frequent medication and/or medication dose changes
- Forgotten doses
- Medication side effects
- Self-prescription of medications to decrease cost; i.e., if blood pressure is "low", will hold "antihypertension" medication

Dietary issues
- Knowledge of low-sodium diet in general
- Belief that using a salt shaker to prepare meals (when cooking) is OK, as long as the salt shaker is avoided when eating
- Unable to read nutrition labels
- Home delivery from grocery store
- Use of canned and boxed products to preserve shelf life; not fresh (especially when the budget is limited)
- Additional dietary restraints (low fat and cholesterol, diabetic or renal failure diet)
- Relies on eating out or meals-on-wheels program
- Patients often feel as though there is no control in the sodium content of foods served; must eat what they are given
- Limited funds/inability to pay for fresh or low-sodium foods (which are more costly)
- Belief that piercing food to let juices out or rinsing canned food will decrease sodium content
- Belief that substituting low-sodium-content additive (Salt Sense, Lo Salt or Lite Salt) or removing salt from the table is adequate

Fluid management issues
- Unsure of how to measure fluids or what a fluid is
- Thirsty from diuretics and renin angiotensin system activation; patient assumes thirst is a signal for them to drink and replenish fluid loss
- Misconception: "I should drink plenty of water to flush out salt and impurities"
- Mixed messages from physicians and health-care providers about drinking fluids

Daily weight issues
- No scale, or scale does not work properly (especially when on carpet)
- Unable to read scale numbers
- Fear of weight values (often seen in females with unsupportive husbands)
- Weight not obtained at same time each day
- Fear of falling (chair bound) during the weight procedure
- Forget to record numbers

Continued

Table 3 *Continued*

Common Factors Influencing Adherence to the Plan of Care

- Perceived lack of value for the daily process
- When they notify the health-care provider of an increase in the value, a treatment change is not made
- Do not want to bother their health-care provider with a small weight change, especially in the absence of new or worsening symptoms

Exercise issues

- Symptomatic. Afraid exercise will worsen their overall condition, or that they may die after carrying out exercise
- Comorbid conditions: gout, arthritis, COPD/asthma, other "pain" problem prevent exercise
- Lack of ambition or enthusiasm
- Sedentary lifestyle
- Assume they have to "buy" equipment to exercise
- May not be able to walk outdoors in extreme heat or cold

Other issues

- Family members use hospitalization as a respite measure
- Winter months: missed appointments

COPD, chronic obstructive pulmonary disease.

Health-care providers may make broad statements to patients, such as "remove salt from your diet" or "weigh yourself every day." The three aspects of education that are often left out of the conversation are the reason why it is important to carry out specific actions, specific details so that the message is interpreted as the health-care provider intended, and examples of how to go about achieving lifestyle changes. People learn best through different methods. The health-care team must find the best way to communicate on an individual basis, then offer the patient options so that the message can be reinforced. Common methods of communication are: verbal persuasion, written education handouts, refrigerator magnets, videos, nutrition classes, a cardiac rehabilitation program, and reputable Internet information sites (American Heart Association and the Heart Failure Society of America). Some of these methods promote learning through personal mastery, observation, and emotional or physical arousal. These learning modes have been shown to strengthen self-efficacy perceptions and ultimately influence thought patterns, actions, and emotional arousal related to individual behaviors.[6,7]

Many groups have studied HF disease management programs in an effort to manage symptoms and optimize function. In a systematic review of 11 randomized HF trials of disease management programs, McAlister and colleagues found that these programs decreased costs and hospitalizations, but not all-cause mortality.[8] These programs offered ongoing follow-up in different forms that spanned a spectrum of services and also a spectrum of health-care personnel involvement, from written communication through mailers (without health-care personnel intervention) to specialized outpatient services and home health-care programs involving physician and/or nurse caregivers. Of all the types of programs included in this systemic review, only trials that employed telephone contact with improved coordination of primary-care services failed to significantly improve patient outcomes.[8] Current research does not single out a specific form of follow-up that is better than another; rather, it appears that any form of vigilance monitoring that includes multidisciplinary team collaboration may be used to achieve the goal of improved quality of life and functional status.

Follow-up monitoring interventions may have many differing key components; however, observational (trials with a before–after design) and randomized programs that consistently reported benefits had an educational component.[9] Some examples of HF disease management vigilance programs are: regularly mailed handouts which encourage self-management, nurse-mediated home care, patient support/education via regular telephone calls, monthly HF support education group sessions, and web-based or other telemonitoring programs (may be fully computerized or involve patient–health-care provider interaction). In addition, case manager telephone follow-up and nurse-on-call programs may be beneficial if they are integrated with a specialized HF team and involve more than just data gathering. The goal of follow-up programming is to reach out to patients and their families on a regular basis and offer support (physical, emotional, psychosocial), encouragement in self-management, ongoing education, symptom management, and a reliable source of general HF follow-up. Even when patients are told to contact their health-care team for worsening symptoms, they often ignore this advice because they do not want to bother the physician for a problem they consider minimal (i.e., slight weight gain without symptoms). An ongoing follow-up program teaches patients the importance of early communication of symptom changes and also rewards them for their assertive communication through collaborative fine-tuning of the pharmacologic and nonpharmacologic plan of care.

Over-the-Counter and Prescription Medication Therapies

When managing symptoms related to HF decompensation, it is important to assess and reassess the patient's current medication profile. Heart failure is associated with aging and involves many risk factors, some of which may be treated with agents that could worsen the HF syndrome (i.e., first- or second-generation calcium-channel blockers for angina or hypertension). Comorbid conditions may be treated with medications that cause sodium and fluid retention, vasoconstriction, proarrhythmia, or negative inotropy (i.e., treating arthritis with nonsteroidal anti-inflammatory agents). Over-the-counter agents and herbal therapies used to treat common ailments or boost energy may interact with HF prescriptions or worsen the HF condition (i.e., decongestants taken for a common cold cause vasoconstriction and increased afterload). Patients with HF may be receiving therapies (over-the-counter or prescription) that could negatively impact the HF condition.

In addition to the issues above, drug companies have targeted their marketing efforts directly to customers through television and print media. Health-care consumers are more likely to use herbal therapies and make requests to their health-care providers for medications. Since many health supplements can be purchased at food and drug stores, consumers do not think of herbal therapies and supplements as medications that could interact with prescription therapies. Primary-care providers may not be aware of medication actions and interactions that could possibly cause cardiotoxicity and worsening of HF. The damage caused by some cardiotoxic agents can be cumulative and hard to decipher without obtaining a cardiac biopsy.[10] The HF team must act as patient advocates by communicating information about potentially harmful medications and supplements. In turn, this will improve patient self-management and may facilitate ongoing dialogue with other health-care providers (Table 4). In addition, the HF team should offer alternative therapies whenever possible so that a patient does not have to live with a debilitating condition.

Patients with moderate to advanced HF take five to ten medications for their HF condition and HF risk factors. Primary agents include a vasodilator, beta-blocker, loop diuretic, aldosterone inhibitor, digoxin and electrolyte supplements (potassium and magnesium). Other agents associated with risk factors or comorbid cardiac conditions are statins for hypercholesterolemia, low-dose aspirin for secondary prevention of coronary artery disease, warfarin for atrial fibrillation, and amiodarone for ventricular and/or atrial tachyarrhythmias. These agents are in addition to medications used in the treatment of chronic comorbid conditions, such as diabetes, chronic obstructive pulmonary disease (COPD), hypertension and arthritis.

The multiplicity of prescription medications can easily lead to confusion and medication errors. Elderly patients may have difficulty reading labels, may have lost the manual dexterity to deal with multiple vials of medications, or may be taking two drugs with the same "class" of actions—e.g., enalapril (Vasotec) and benazepril (Lotensin). In addition, monthly medication costs might prompt decisions about how to spend a

Table 4

Medications/Supplements to Avoid, and Alternatives

Condition	Avoid	Alternatives
Indigestion, gas pain	• Sodium-based antacids	• Nonsodium-based antacids
Colds with runny nose or sinusitis	• Decongestants: Neo-Synephrine or Sudafed (phenylephrine; pseudoephedrine; epinephrine; ephedrine); catecholamines	• Antihistamines; vaporizer; saline nose drops • Inhale steam; hot shower; warm damp cloth over nose
Arthritis	• NSAIDs, including COX-2 inhibitors	• Tumor necrosis factor inhibitor (etanercept or infliximab; with caution), arthritis-strength Tylenol, or glucosamine; capsaicin cream; encourage healthy weight, regular exercise, good posture; apply heat or cold packs to stiff joints; warm baths; short-term use of a mild narcotic or pulsed steroid treatment, if necessary
Hypertension	• 1st- and 2nd-generation calcium blockers	• 3rd-generation calcium-channel blockers: amlodipine (Norvasc) or felodipine (Plendil)
Tachyarrhythmias	• Class 1a and 1c antiarrhythmics Class 3 antiarrhythmics with high risk for prolongation of QT or QTc interval leading to ventricular tachycardia or *torsades de pointes* (dofetilide; ibutilide) or 1st- and 2nd-generation calcium-channel blockers	• Amiodarone or 2nd- or 3rd-generation beta-blockers studied in heart failure (bisoprolol, metoprolol or carvedilol); implantable converter–defibrillator

Glaucoma	• 1st-generation beta-blocker eye solutions (timilol, carteolol) or epinephrine solutions (dipivefrin; Epifrin; Epinal) or pilocarpine solutions	• Acetazolamide (Diamox); dorzolamide (Trusopt)
Aches; pains	• Aspirin >325 mg/day • NSAIDs	• Tylenol (regular or extra strength); regular exercise; good body mechanics
Type 2 diabetes	• Thiazolinediones: (Actos, Avandia) and 1st-generation sulfonylureas	• Metformin (Glucophage); acarbose (Precose) and 2nd-generation sulfonylureas (glyburide, glipizide, and glimepiride)
Other	• Black licorice • Germanium compounds – e.g., ginseng • Echinacea (if not taken intermittently) • Ginkgo • Ephedra (high doses) • Cobalt • Lead • Lithium • Adriamycin • Cocaine • Alcohol • Amphetamines	• Artificial licorice-flavored candies

COX-2, cyclooxygenase-2; NSAIDs, nonsteroidal anti-inflammatory drugs.

fixed income. Due to these and other issues listed in Table 3, it is important for the health-care team to thoroughly assess all medications and determine if the patient's regimen can be minimized or altered. Questions to ask are:

- Is this the right medication for patient's current condition(s) and functional class, based on current research and HF consensus guidelines?
- Is it the right time to add or delete medications?
- Is the patient having symptoms despite current therapies, requiring additional medication or device (cardiac resynchronization) therapies?
- What alternatives can be employed to prevent discontinuation of medications that are known to modulate cardiac remodeling (e.g., continuing beta-blocker use when symptoms of hypervolemia appear)?
- Can a medication that was discontinued when it failed initially be reinstituted now that the patient's condition is different (e.g., failed angiotensin-converting enzyme inhibitor due to symptomatic hypotension when serum sodium was below 130 mmol/L or failed beta-blocker due to hypervolemia when initiated)?

Moving Forward

There have been many lessons learned in managing symptoms and optimizing function of patients with HF. Clearly, a three-tiered regimen that incorporates the right drugs at the right doses, self-management of lifestyle expectations, and open ongoing education, communication and vigilance monitoring are important strategies that ultimately decrease morbidity and mortality associated with HF.

Concept of Change and Barriers to Changing Behavior

Self-management of HF means controlling factors that may relieve or prevent symptoms. Certain behaviors, such as eating a low-sodium diet, exercising regularly, taking medications properly, and calling a health-care provider when symptoms arise, are critical for living with HF (Table 1). For most patients, these behaviors involve lifestyle changes that are significantly different from previous habits. Changing one's lifestyle behaviors is 50% of the management of HF; medications alone cannot maximize a patient's clinical status. For instance, patients who consume a high-sodium diet can often expect to suffer symptoms of fluid retention, despite increased use of diuretics. It is the *combination* of a low-sodium diet and diuretic use that may prevent or relieve symptoms of fluid overload. Unfortunately, the behaviors that require changing are usually lifelong habits that are quite difficult to alter.

Most patient education programs for HF present all of the lifestyle changes that need to be incorporated into the patient's behaviors during one educational session, regardless of where patients are in their readiness to make changes in their life. They are told to make these significant changes all at once. Instead of making change in phases, patients are expected to give up cigarettes, alcohol, and dietary sodium, and they are instructed to begin an exercise program right away. For some people, each one of these changes alone takes great inner strength to endure, much less making numerous significant changes in one's life virtually overnight. Admittedly, there are a few patients who are motivated to incorporate these changes in their lifestyle immediately. However, most people are unprepared or unwilling to make large changes in their lives. In fact, fewer than 20% of a problem population are prepared for change action at any given time; yet, more than 90% of behavior change programs are designed with this 20% in mind.[11]

Consider a lifestyle habit that one would want to change by choice. It may be to lose 20 pounds, improve a tennis game, increase the amount of exercise, spend more time on oneself, etc. How good are people at making this change? Imagine making changes that are imposed, not by choice. Where is the source of motivation for making such a change? Many lifestyle habits, such as eating certain foods, are associated with memories from childhood or happy times in one's life. If patients are told to give up foods that are associated with pleasant memories, what is the likelihood of successful change? For example, Sunday dinners in the South consisting of chicken fried steak with gravy, buttermilk biscuits, buttered mashed potatoes, and green beans baked with pork fat conjure up happy memories of family gatherings for many people. How is a health-care provider supposed to break food and lifestyle habits that have been passed down through the generations? These are lifelong behaviors that we are asking patients to change. How can we promote lifestyle changes in such a way that patients will adhere to them?

Any activity that you initiate to help modify your thinking, feeling, or behavior is a change process. The primary determinants of behavior and behavior change have been identified by Fishbein and coworkers[12] as:

1 Intention—does the patient have a commitment to perform the behavior?

2 Environmental constraints—what external conditions could facilitate or be a barrier to the behavior? (E.g., economics, insurance carrier, caregiver issues, social isolation, living with a smoker.)
3 Ability—does the patient have the necessary skills (depression, elderly, frail, homebound)?
4 Anticipated outcome—do the pros for performing the behavior outweigh the cons? Does the patient feel bad enough to *want* to change?
5 Norms—what are the social pressures to perform the behaviors (e.g., repeated hospitalizations, impact on the family)?
6 Self-standards—is the new behavior consistent with the patient's self-image (such as men who are forced to take on dependent roles, or are no longer working)?
7 Emotion—does the patient have a positive reaction to performing the behavior?
8 Self-efficacy—does the patient perceive that he/she is capable of performing the behavior?

Promoting Adherence: Evaluating the Patient's Readiness to Change

James Prochaska is a practicing clinical psychologist and university professor who, along with several colleagues, developed the transtheoretical model to evaluate readiness for change. This model originated from analysis of 18 systems of psychotherapy that identified common processes of change.[13] Prochaska and colleagues looked at successful self-changers, and evaluated the processes these people went through to achieve permanent change. Most of their work was in the domains of smoking cessation, alcoholism, and weight loss. After reviewing the commonalties of these successful self-changers, Prochaska and colleagues narrowed the change process down to six stages:

- *Stage 1—precontemplation.* Patients have no intention of changing behavior in the foreseeable future (defined as the next 6 months) and typically deny having a problem. They resist change. This brings to mind a young patient with a relatively new diagnosis of systolic heart failure, who, during an initial clinic visit, told this author "I only eat food because it makes my salt taste good."
- *Stage 2—contemplation.* Patients acknowledge that they need to change behavior, and they begin to think about making changes; but not within the next 6 months.

- *Stage 3—preparation.* Patients plan to take action sometime in the near future (within a month); may have instituted some small behavior changes (e.g., decreasing the number of times they eat at fast-food restaurants, removing salt shaker from table, reading food labels). They may announce the intended change—"I'll really start watching what I eat after the holidays." They are committed to action, but have not necessarily resolved their ambivalence. It is important to note that if the preparation stage is cut short—such as someone who stops smoking "cold turkey," there is less chance of successful change in behavior. During this phase, the health-care provider should help the patient develop a plan of action and must ensure that the patient is well educated about the necessary changes. During the preparation stage, the patient making the change must:
  (a) Make the choice to change
  (b) Take small steps; not changing everything at once
  (c) Set a date to begin
  (d) Go public; tell others
  (e) Create a personal plan of action with the assistance of their health-care provider. The patient may wish to talk with other HF patients and ask how they made changes. Then patients will need help adapting the ideas into their own lifestyle.
- *Stage 4—action.* Patients modify actions and surroundings (e.g., read labels and decrease salt in diet, participate in smoking cessation program or a weight loss program). This is a recent change that requires time and energy. The patient has engaged in the actions less than 6 months.
- *Stage 5—maintenance.* Patients struggle to prevent relapses; maintaining change for at least 6 months. Without strong commitment, the patient will not continue with the change. The goal of maintenance is a permanent change that becomes part of the patient's personality. During the maintenance stage, patients must:
  (a) Keep a healthy distance from temptations; control their environment (e.g., having no salt in the house, not going to break room at work if people are smoking there)
  (b) Create a new lifestyle; develop new ways to cope with stress (instead of smoking or overeating); exercise and relaxation are key
  (c) Check their thinking. Denial, distortion, and rationalization are the enemies of maintenance.

- *Stage 6—termination.* Patient is no longer tempted by high-sodium foods, no longer smokes cigarettes, has an established exercise walking program, etc. They have made successful changes in their lifestyle, and may offer support to other HF patients who are making lifestyle changes. Similar to Alcoholics Anonymous, the last step involves helping others. Patients should share stories and ideas at support group meetings or with someone who has been diagnosed with HF. This is key to maintaining change.

Change is sometimes conceptualized as linear, but "spiral" or "circular" is a better description. The patient may recycle up and down the stages. It is important to remember that a single lapse is not a relapse. The patient should turn to helping relationships for support (this is why family involvement is important). If the patient does relapse, contemplation, preparation and action usually follow before getting back to the maintenance stage.

Determining the Patient's Level of Readiness to Change

The only way to determine the patient's readiness to change is through self-assessment. The patient's answers to direct questions such as "Do you seriously intend to quit smoking in the next 6 months?" and "Do you plan to quit in the next 30 days?" will determine the level of readiness. For instance, if patients answer "no" to both questions, they are not contemplating any change to their life and are therefore in the precontemplation stage. If, however, they answer "yes" to the first question and "no" to the second, they are in the contemplation stage. If they answer "yes" to both questions, they are in the preparation stage and plan to make a change (in regard to cigarette smoking) in the next 30 days. If patients have quit smoking within the past 6 months, they are in the action stage. If they have quit smoking for over 6 months, but are occasionally tempted to resume smoking, they are in the maintenance stage. If patients have quit smoking and are free of temptation to resume smoking, they have achieved termination.

Developing a self-assessment tool to determine the patient's level of readiness to change consists of asking a series of questions that relate to the behaviors to be changed. For instance, an example of one question would be: "Do you consistently avoid eating high-sodium (salty) foods in your diet?"

1 Yes, and I have been for more than 6 months
2 Yes, but I have been for less than 6 months

3 No, but I intend to in the next 30 days
4 No, but I intend to in the next 6 months
5 No, and I do not intend to in the next 6 months

Obviously, if patients answer with choice #1, they are at least in the maintenance stage. If they answer with choice #2, they are in action; #3 in preparation; #4 in contemplation; and #5 represents the precontemplation stage. Questions can be created from all of the areas of behavior that should be changed in HF patients. To take it one step further, a questionnaire such as this may help identify varied levels of readiness for change among the different behaviors. For instance, a patient may be at the maintenance stage when it comes to eating a high-sodium diet, but they may still be in the contemplation stage regarding smoking cessation.

Developing a Program to Help Patients Achieve Self-Management Based on their Level of Readiness to Change

In order to assist patients in achieving lasting behavior change, it is important to first determine their level of readiness for change, as discussed earlier. Patient and family interventions toward change should be developed to target each level of readiness. For instance, it would not be appropriate to prescribe a nicotine patch for a patient who is still in the precontemplation stage for smoking cessation. A more appropriate intervention for this stage would be to inform the patient of the specific hazards of smoking and perhaps encourage nonsmoking family members to share their feelings about the patient's smoking (e.g., causing cigarette odors to linger in the house and in their clothing, expressing concern over second-hand smoke, etc.). These interventions do not offer information that the patient is not ready to hear (such as specific techniques for smoking cessation), but rather, simply serve to enforce the importance of considering the change in the future. Later, when the patient is in the preparation stage and close to taking action, specific smoking cessation techniques will be meaningful and useful to the patient. Patient education must be tailored to meet the patient's level of readiness for successful and permanent change.

The Role of the Heart Failure Nurse

The most important role of the nurse caring for HF patients is to educate, educate, educate! Patients cannot make changes in their behavior if they do not know which behaviors to change or how to change them. Furthermore, it is critical that the patients understand *why* it is important to make lifestyle changes and how these changes will benefit them. Another important role for the HF nurse is that of providing a helping relationship. When the patient is faced with temptation to return to old hazardous habits, the nurse must offer support and help the patient keep on track. It is important not to criticize when a lapse leads to hospitalization or worsening of symptoms. The nurse must help the patient get back on track toward maintenance.

Developing a program of education and intervention that corresponds with the patient's level of readiness to change will increase the likelihood that the changes will be long-lasting. For patients who are in the precontemplation stage, simply giving them some broad information about the lifestyle changes may be enough. Once the patient is ready to start contemplating change, they may need more detailed information. When they are ready to prepare for change, they will be most ready to hear pertinent information and begin a course of action for change. The nurse must continue to reinforce information and behaviors during the maintenance stage in order to prevent the patient from lapsing into previous unhealthy behaviors. With the appropriate time and energy invested, patients living with HF can expect to feel better, and even possibly live longer. The role of the nurse in managing heart failure cannot be overstated, particularly when the nurse helps the patients achieve self-efficacy.

References

1. Uretsky BF, Pina I, Quigg RJ, et al. Beyond drug therapy: Nonpharmacologic care of the patient with advanced heart failure. *Am Heart J* 1998;135:S264–S284.
2. American College of Cardiology/American Heart Association Task Force. ACC/AHA guidelines for the evaluation and management of chronic heart failure in the adult: Executive summary. *J Am Coll Cardiol.* 2001;38:2101–2113.
3. Remme WJ. Prevention of worsening heart failure: future focus. *Eur Heart J* 1998;19(suppl B):B47–B53.
4. Lechat P. Prevention of heart failure progression: Current approaches. *Eur Heart J* 1998;19(suppl B):B12–B18.
5. Agostoni P, Marenzi G, Lauri G, et al. Sustained improvement in functional capacity after removal of body fluid with isolated ultrafiltration in chronic cardiac insufficiency: Failure of furosemide to provide the same result. *Am J Med* 1994;96:191–199.
6. Bandura A. Self-efficacy mechanism in human agency. *Am Psychol* 1982;37: 122–147.
7. Strecher VJ, DeVellis BM, Becker MH, Rosenstock IM. The role of self-efficacy in achieving health behavior change. *Health Educ Q* 1986;13:73–91.
8. McAlister FA, Lawson ME, Teo KK, Armstrong PW. A systematic review of randomized trials of disease management programs in heart failure. *Am J Med* 2001;110:378–384.

9. Rich MW. Heart failure disease management: A critical review. *J Card Fail* 1999;5:54–75.
10. Olivari MT. Behavioral and environmental factors contributing to the development and progression of congestive heart failure. *J Heart Lung Transplant* 2000;19:12–20.
11. Prochaska JO, Norcross JC, DiClemente CC. *Changing for Good: A Revolutionary Six-Stage Program for Overcoming Bad Habits and Moving your Life Positively Forward*. New York: Avon Books, 1994.
12. Fishbein M, Bandura A, Triandis HC, et al. *Factors Influencing Behavior and Behavior Change: Final Report—Theorists' Workshop, October 3–5, 1991*. Rockville, MD: National Institute of Mental Health, 1992.
13. Prochaska JO, DiClemente CC. Transtheoretical therapy: Towards a more interactive model of change. *Psychother Theory Res Pract* 1982;19:276–288.

Chapter 10

Pharmacologic Management: Achieving Target Doses and Managing Interactions

David Rabin, MD, FACC

Our understanding of the pathophysiology of congestive heart failure (HF) has progressed dramatically over the past decades. We now know that the development of the dilated, dysfunctional ventricle is caused by a complex interaction of activated neurohormonal systems, namely the renin–angiotensin–aldosterone system (RAAS) and the sympathetic nervous system (SNS). Our pharmacopeia now includes agents which interrupt and block the activity of the RAAS and SNS, including angiotensin-converting enzyme inhibitors (ACEIs), angiotensin-receptor blockers (ARBs), beta-blockers (BBs), spironolactone, digoxin, hydralazine, and nitroglycerin.

Much emphasis has been placed, and much attention has been paid recently, to achieving "target" doses of these agents, particularly ACEIs.[1–4] Trials demonstrating the effectiveness of ACEIs all used high doses (captopril 150 mg/day, enalapril 20 mg/day),[5–9] yet multiple studies and surveys have revealed that ACEIs were not prescribed as widely as they should be and when they were prescribed, they were at far lower doses than the "target" doses used in the trials.[10–16] A major question has been "Are ACEIs effective at less than *target* doses?" A recent major trial (Assessment of Treatment with Lisinopril and Survival, ATLAS) focused on just this question, and returned mixed results, concluding that "the difference between intermediate doses and high doses of an ACE inhibitor (if any) is likely to be very small."[4] Therefore, instead of focusing on one drug in particular and pushing it to a "target" dose, it may be more important to attack the neurohormonal systems at multiple targets with

From: Jessup M, McCauley KM (eds). *Heart Failure: Providing Optimal Care*. Elmsford, NY: Futura, an imprint of Blackwell Publishing; ©2003.

multiple agents, each at perhaps a lower dose than those used in the trials. To do this safely requires monitoring electrolytes, renal function, weights, blood pressures, diet, and knowledge of the other prescription and over-the-counter drugs the patients are taking.

The medical regimen for the HF patient has expanded significantly from the digoxin and diuretic era. Currently, there are four agents which have been shown to significantly effect morbidity and mortality. These are the "cornerstones" of therapy and include: ACEIs, ARBs (for those patients who do not tolerate ACEIs), BBs, and spironolactone. Hydralazine/nitroglycerin has been shown to improve exercise tolerance as well as having a modest effect on survival.[17,18] Digoxin continues to be a controversial agent, but withdrawal of digoxin may result in exacerbation of HF symptoms and hospital readmissions.[19,20] Addition of digoxin has not been shown to improve survival, but even in patients in sinus rhythm, it may reduce symptoms and hospitalizations for HF.[21] Loop diuretics are virtually always part of the regimen, to prevent and/or relieve congestion.[22,23] It is beyond the scope of this chapter to review the evidence and pathophysiological basis for all of these agents. Instead, the focus will be on the initiation and upward titration of these agents and how to monitor not only the direct effects of the agents on the patient, but also how these agents may interact with each other as well as with other prescription and nonprescription agents the patient is taking.

Angiotensin-Converting Enzyme Inhibitors

These are first-line agents in all patients with HF and ejection fraction (EF) less than 40%.

Initiation

Initial dosing should begin with a low dose of any one of a number of agents. In the in-patient setting, when the patient is monitored with frequent vital signs, captopril 6.25 mg t.i.d. can be started and titrated up quickly to 25 mg t.i.d. within 48–72 h if the patient tolerates the agent. Alternatively, lisinopril 2.5–5 mg/day or trandolapril 0.5 mg/day can be initiated and titrated up after 48–72 h to 5–10 mg of lisinopril or 1 mg of trandolapril. The patient's symptoms, potassium, and renal function should serve as guides to titration, as opposed to arbitrary blood pressure cut-offs. Given that both cost and dosing schedule are important to insure compliance, patients should be discharged to home on inexpensive and easy-to-take agents such as trandolapril, moexipril, and lisinopril. Trandolapril has a very good trough-to-peak ratio, which gives the patient a more even level of drug throughout the day and avoids high peaks that can precipitate hypotension.[24] An initial "target" dose is equivalent to 10 mg of lisinopril (1 mg of trandolapril, 25 mg t.i.d. of captopril, 15 mg of moexipril, etc.). There are times when patients do not tolerate increasing doses of the long-acting ACEIs. These patients many times do well switching to a short-acting agent such as captopril. These patients may need transient escape from suppression of the RAAS/SNS at the trough level of the short-acting agent. One can often get to relatively higher doses of the shorter-acting agent than one could by pushing the long-acting drug, and reduce the symptoms of lethargy and fatigue.

Contraindications

Absolute contraindications to ACEI include: bilateral renal artery stenosis, serum creatinine greater than 3.0 mg/dL, elevated baseline potassium (greater than 5.5 mmol/L), systolic blood pressure less than 80 mmHg, rash, angioedema. A relative contraindication is severe to critical aortic stenosis, as vasodilatation in the setting of a severe fixed stenosis can precipitate hypotension. Cough is a common problem occurring in about 5–15% of patients. It can be variable, ranging from an occasional dry "tickle" to a relentless, hacking dry cough. If the cough is minimal, and not really an issue, the drug should be continued; otherwise it should be stopped.[25]

Monitoring

Serum electrolytes, blood urea nitrogen (BUN), creatinine, and blood pressure should be checked within a week after any upward titration of an ACEI dose. Rarely do patients need supplemental KCl, since they tend to retain potassium secondary to ACEIs' effects on aldosterone production. As the ACEI dose is titrated upward, diuretic dose can, and should be cut back, as the ACEI should help limit sodium and fluid retention, thus decreasing the need for high-dose diuretic. High-dose diuretic with increasing ACEI dose can result in hypotension and prerenal azotemia, thus exacerbating the nephrotoxicity of ACEI. Some increases in serum creatinine (up to about 2.5 mg/dL) and potassium (5.5 mmol/L) are acceptable.[25,26]

Drug Interaction

As stated above, diuretics need to be adjusted as ACEIs are titrated. If spironolactone is part of the regimen, careful attention needs to paid to serum potassium as both agents inhibit the effects of aldosterone.

Digoxin levels also need to be monitored. Other non-HF medications need to be reviewed on a consistent basis.

Antibiotics, such as trimethoprim, which can adversely effect renal function have significant ramifications. An example of such an interaction is a case of a patient who was begun on spironolactone, in addition to an ACEI. The potassium was checked within a week and was within normal limits. At this point, the patient developed a urinary tract infection, and the patient's internist began trimethoprim. The patient began to feel poorly, and several days later had her renal function and electrolytes checked. She was in renal failure, with a potassium of 7 mmol/L. She was summoned to the hospital, where she suffered cardiac arrest in the parking lot and was fortunately successfully resuscitated.

Nonsteroidal anti-inflammatory drugs (NSAIDs) are another class of drugs which interfere with the actions of ACEIs by negating one of the major proposed beneficial effects of ACEIs on bradykinin-mediated prostaglandin synthesis.[25] Notably, the new cyclooxygenase-2 (COX-2) inhibitors (celecoxib and rofecoxib) are extremely potent in this regard. The addition of one of these agents alone can be responsible for marked increases in blood pressure and can lead to exacerbations of congestive heart failure (in patients with systolic or diastolic dysfunction). Patients need to be aware of the potential dangers of these agents and alert both the prescribing physician and their cardiologist. The use of aspirin (acetylsalicylic acid, ASA) in patients on ACEIs is fairly controversial.[27–29] Retrospective subgroup analyses of the Cooperative North Scandinavian Enalapril Survival Study II (CONSENSUS II), Studies of Left Ventricular Dysfunction (SOLVD) and Global Use of Strategies to Open Occluded Arteries I (GUSTO I) studies have shown a negative interaction. On the other hand, Leor *et al.*,[30] actually showed a beneficial effect in patients with HF and coronary artery disease (CAD). The answer to the acetylsalicylic acid (ASA)/ACEI issue is being addressed in the ongoing Warfarin–Antiplatelet Trial in Chronic Heart Failure (WATCH). This trial will look at patients taking ACEIs and randomly assigned to ASA, clopidogrel, or warfarin.

Angiotensin-Receptor Blockers

Given the results of the Evaluation of Losartan in the Elderly II (ELITE II) and Valsartan–Heart Failure Trial (Val-HeFT) studies, ARBs are probably the drug to turn to if ACEIs are not tolerated (due to allergic reaction, cough, etc.).[31] ELITE II, despite limitations, demonstrated no difference between losartan and captopril in all-cause mortality, sudden death, and resuscitated death.[32] Val-HeFT recently has shown significant benefit with the ARB valsartan compared to placebo. This was most markedly seen in those patients not on ACEIs (only 7% of the study population), but was also prominent in those patients in those patients taking BBs.[31,33]

Initiation

There are fewer data on dose initiation and titration than there are with ACEIs. ELITE II used "low"-dose losartan, which was 50 mg/day. Val-HeFT used valsartan titrated from 40 mg b.i.d. to 160 mg/day. The Randomized Evaluation of Strategies for Left Ventricular Dysfunction (RESOLVED) pilot trial used candesartan at multiple doses of 4, 8 or 16 mg as monotherapy compared to 4 or 8 mg with the addition of enalapril 20 mg, compared to enalapril as monotherapy at 20 mg/day.[34] Most of the time, ARBs are begun after the patient has been on an ACEI for some time and is demonstrating intolerance. In these cases, there is no need to start the ARB at a very low "test" dose to see how the patient's blood pressure will tolerate the drug. One can then begin an ARB usually at a moderate dose (80 mg valsartan, 25–50 mg losartan).

Contraindications

These are similar to those for ACEIs and include: bilateral renal artery stenosis, serum creatinine greater than 3 mg/dL, potassium greater than 5.5 mmol/L, systolic blood pressure less than 80 mmHg, rash or angioedema.

Drug Interactions

As with ACEIs, overaggressive diuretic dosing can exacerbate the nephrotoxic and hypotensive effects of ARBs. Potassium retention with concurrent dosing of spironolactone is a concern. An interesting question involves the concurrent dosing of ACEIs, BBs and ARBs. Although the goal of therapy is to completely inhibit the RAAS and SNS, those patients in Val-HeFT trial who received all three agents trended not to do as well as those who received placebo instead of valsartan when added to standard therapy of ACEI and BB.[33]

Beta-Blockers

Initiation of BBs should begin once the acute exacerbation of HF has been stabilized (unless the episode is associated with an acute ischemic event with tachycardia and hypertension and therefore BBs are part of initial therapy). BBs should be started at very low doses and titrated up about every week as patients tolerate. They are the third "cornerstone" in HF therapy, added once the patient is on a stable oral diuretic dose and a moderate ACEI dose (approximately 10 mg lisinopril or the equivalent). One should not wait until the patient is at the high doses of ACEIs that were achieved in the major trials before adding on BBs. It should be noted that BBs were not part of the standard of care when those trials were run and therefore not a high percentage of the patients in these trials were on BBs. Given the overwhelming evidence of the benefit BBs in the treatment of HF,[35–41] physicians should not be prevented from giving BBs because a patient is relatively hypotensive due to too high a dose of an ACEI, ARB, or other antihypertensive agent. Even patients with class IV HF have been shown to benefit from BBs.[42] The question as to which BB to use is open to debate; those shown to reduce morbidity and mortality in randomized trials include carvedilol, metoprolol tartrate (short-acting), metoprolol succinate (sustained-release) and bisoprolol.[41] The results of the ongoing Carvedilol or Metoprolol European Trial (COMET) will be very important in answering this question. In the in-patient setting, BB therapy is often initiated with metoprolol tartrate 6.25–12.5 mg b.i.d. or carvedilol 3.125 mg b.i.d. Metoprolol succinate is now available in a 25-mg dose which is scored and can be given at a low starting dose (12.5 mg, which is equivalent to 6.25 mg b.i.d. of metoprolol tartrate). If possible, the dose of metoprolol tartrate should be titrated to the point where it can be changed over to an equivalent dose of metoprolol succinate, as dividing up the metoprolol tartrate tablets at such low doses as an outpatient is virtually impossible. Metoprolol tartrate 12.5 mg b.i.d. can be converted to succinate at 25 mg/day, and this is achieved by splitting the 50 mg tablet. Stable outpatients (New York Heart Association class II) can usually start with a dose of 25 mg of metoprolol succinate a day or carvedilol 3.125 mg b.i.d.. In the Metoprolol Controlled-release Randomized Intervention Trial (MERIT), the target dose was 200 mg of metoprolol succinate a day, titrated up over a period of 8 weeks, with the average dose being 159 mg/day;[40] for carvedilol, the target dose was 25 mg b.i.d., with the average daily dose being 47 mg/day.[37] In practice, patients may have a lot of difficulty achieving doses at those levels peaking at 50–100 mg of metoprolol succinate and carvedilol 12.5 mg b.i.d.. It should be noted that, at least in the carvedilol trials, there was an open-label run-in period, and those patients who could not tolerate low-dose carvedilol (6.25 mg b.i.d.) were excluded from the trial. This may explain why a higher percentage of patients achieved "target" doses of carvedilol in the trial compared to what is attained in some cases in general practice.[43] Contrary to the results from ATLAS, there is evidence for a significant "dose–response" with BB, at least carvedilol. The Multicenter Oral Carvedilol in Heart Failure Assessment (MOCHA) investigators documented an increase in EF and a decrease in cardiovascular hospitalizations and mortality with increasing doses from 6.25 to 25 mg b.i.d..[38]

Contraindications

Absolute contraindications include: resting heart rate (HR) below 60 beats/min, advanced heart block (in the absence of a pacemaker), severe reactive airways disease. Concern about masking diabetic reactions is a relative contraindication.[25]

Monitoring

Patients need weekly HR and blood pressure follow-up while their doses are being titrated, either in the office or by phone if patients have a home blood-pressure machine (which also often records the HR). Dose-limiting side effects include dizziness, lethargy, and fatigue. These symptoms are most often reported with carvedilol, perhaps due to the nonselective beta-blockade or the alpha-blockade.[43] It has been our experience that these symptoms are not necessarily a reflection of too rapid an upward titration, but can also occur after the patient has been at steady state for some time. They improve when patients are switched to a selective beta$_1$-antagonist such as metoprolol succinate. (This is a personal observation and may not reflect other physicians' experiences.) Patients with severe underlying lung disease may not tolerate the beta$_2$ effects of carvedilol and may also tolerate the selective agent better.

Drug Interactions

Patients already on digoxin may develop high-grade atrioventricular block, especially with underlying conduction system disease. Patients with glaucoma may need to switch from eye drops containing beta-blocker to nonbeta-blocking formulations to avoid excessive bradycardia, as there are often significant systemic effects from the beta-blocker in the eye drops. Patients with significant left ventricular dysfunction (left ventricular EF less than 40%) should not be on medications such as diltiazem and verapamil, and these medications should be discontinued prior to initiating BBs.

Diuretics

Loop diuretics such as furosemide, torsemide, and bumetanide are the mainstay of the therapy of most patients with congestive heart failure. Furosemide and torsemide have longer half-lives than bumetanide and therefore have the advantage of being dosed less frequently throughout the day. The bioavailability of furosemide is approximately 50%, and the oral dose is therefore twice what the intravenous dose was while the patient was hospitalized. Torsemide is completely absorbed in its oral form and there does not need to be any change in dosing level when intravenous administration is changed over to oral.[23] Given its better bioavailability, torsemide is an excellent choice for patients with right heart failure and increased bowel edema and subsequently reduced absorption. It should be noted that some studies have demonstrated that patients have fewer hospitalizations and less fatigue and that the overall cost of care is lower on torsemide—so perhaps, despite its higher pharmacy cost, its long-term use may actually result in savings and better outcomes.[23,44]

Initiation

Furosemide dosing generally starts at 20–40 mg/day, often in split dosing, as once the duration of action is complete, the nephron more avidly retains sodium and therefore there is a "rebound" effect. In patients with underlying renal insufficiency, these doses have to be adjusted upward. If furosemide is dosed b.i.d. in an outpatient setting, the patient should take the second dose in the mid- to late afternoon (approximately 3 p.m., to avoid too much nocturia). The half-life of torsemide is longer than furosemide and it can therefore be dosed once a day in most situations. The goal weight loss is 1–2 pounds a day in outpatients who have mild to moderate fluid retention.

Maintenance

Once patients have achieved a stable diuretic regimen, they need to know how to manage fluctuations in their fluid status, usually brought on by dietary indiscretions or, occasionally, other medications. Sliding-scale diuretic instructions should be reviewed with patients so that they can take an extra dose of a diuretic should they gain an extra 2–3 pounds over a 24–48-h period. As a precautionary measure, it is not unreasonable to have patients take an extra dose of diuretic after they have a high-sodium-load meal (Chinese food, ham, etc.).

Monitoring

Electrolytes, BUN and creatinine should be checked within 3–5 days of initiating or changing a diuretic or diuretic dose. Phone contact with the office, HF nurse coordinator, or Visiting Nurse Association (VNA) visit to check symptoms of lightheadedness, fatigue, and any orthostatic signs and symptoms is also important. Hypokalemia is less of an issue when patients are also on ACEIs and ARBs, but hyperkalemia and renal insufficiency are real concerns.

Drug Interactions

Overly aggressive diuretic dosing can result in prerenal azotemia and exacerbate the nephrotoxicity of ACEIs and ARBs. Non-HF medications—particularly the NSAIDs, which inhibit the natriuretic effect of diuretics—can limit the effectiveness of the diuretic.[25] As stated in the ACEI section, the newer COX-2 agents appear to be particularly potent in this regard. These agents can also cause renal failure, due to their own negative effects on renal function, resulting in electrolyte imbalance, renal failure and possible digoxin toxicity. NSAIDs are particularly troublesome, because so many of them are over-the-counter that patients do not necessarily consider them when they discuss their medication lists with the physician or the nurse.

Combination Diuretics

In patients who do not respond sufficiently to a single loop agent, many times adding a low-dose thiazide agent (commonly metolazone although any thiazide will work) is extremely effective in achieving a brisk diuresis.[23,25] In these instances, frequent electrolyte and renal function panels need to be checked (i.e., within 2 days of instituting combination therapy) as this combination can result in large potassium loss. A potential drawback to these regimens is that they are a little complicated for some patients, as metolazone needs to be taken approximately half an hour prior to taking the loop diuretic. This can be cumbersome, especially for patients on multiple medications. Metolazone can have adverse effects on glucose metabolism as well.

Spironolactone

Given the evidence produced in the Randomized Aldactone Evaluation Study (RALES), spironolactone is now the fourth cornerstone in the therapy for HF. The doses found to be effective were remarkably low, and its benefits were felt to be due to its cardioprotective effects from its blockade of aldosterone, as opposed to any true diuretic effect.[45]

Initiation

Dosing can begin at 12.5 mg/day, up to 50 mg/day, although the average dose in the trial was 26 mg/day.

Contraindications

Serum creatinine greater than 2.5 mg/dL and/or a serum potassium greater than 5.0 mmol/L were part of the exclusion criteria in the RALES trial and should serve as guidelines for the use of spironolactone.

Monitoring

Patients need electrolytes, BUN and creatinine monitored weekly while doses are being adjusted, especially if patients are on an ACEI or ARB, as this interaction can precipitate hyperkalemia.

Digoxin

Initiation

If patients are already on digoxin, they should stay on it, as withdrawing digoxin can result in increased hospitalizations and worsening symptoms. The major question remains, if patients are in normal sinus rhythm, and are not on digoxin, should it be added? Although there continues to be debate, the Digitalis Investigation Group (DIG) trial[21] did demonstrate reduced hospitalizations, although no mortality benefit. The benefits of digoxin are probably not so much in its inotropic properties but in its neurohumoral properties, which are manifested at a low dose (0.125 mg). Therefore, the proarrhythmic complications seen in the trials and in some practices may be a function of the higher dosing of digoxin (0.25 mg).[46,47] In the absence of the need for rate control for atrial fibrillation, therefore, digoxin can be started at 0.125–0.25 mg/day without a loading regimen for patients in sinus rhythm or atrial fibrillation with a well-controlled ventricular response.

Drug Interactions

Multiple drug interactions occur with digoxin, but in patients with abnormal ventricles, the only agents that are of clinical importance are amiodarone and spironolactone. Quinidine is rarely used for atrial fibrillation any more, and drugs such as verapamil, propafenone, and flecainide are not used in patients with significant systolic dysfunction.

Combination of Isosorbide Dinitrate and Hydralazine

This combination is indicated for those patients who are intolerant of ACEI/ARBs because of allergic reaction, renal failure, hyperkalemia or other contraindications (e.g., pregnancy).

Dosing

This is an extremely difficult regimen for patients to comply with, given the multidose schedule. Vasodilator Heart Failure Trial (V-HeFT) I and II used very high doses of isosorbide dinitrate (ISDN) and hydralazine—up to 160 mg/day of ISDN and 300 mg/day of hydralazine (average 136 mg ISDN and 270 mg hydralazine in V-HeFT I, and 100 mg ISDN and 199 mg hydralazine in V-HeFT II).[17,18] There is no ATLAS or MOCHA trial for this combination to compare low versus high dosing of these agents. Starting dose is 10 mg t.i.d. of ISDN and 10 t.i.d.–q.i.d. of hydralazine. Both are titrated upwards by 10 mg increments every couple of days to 20–30 mg t.i.d. of each. Doses are then held for a week at that level before they are increased further. Symptoms and blood pressure are then assessed, and doses can then be advanced. If the t.i.d. dosing is tolerated in terms of blood pressure, symptoms and compliance, a fourth dose of each can be added. Since there are no data on the use of extended-release nitrate preparations, their use is not recommended. The peak and trough effect of the shorter-acting ISDN, may in fact, make this regimen better tolerated, allowing some escape from the nitrate effect during the day.

Monitoring

If the patient complains of increasing fatigue and breathlessness, there is the possibility of hemolytic anemia, and a complete blood count should be checked. Erythrocyte sedimentation rate and antinuclear antibody (ANA) should be checked if the patient complains of myalgias, arthralgias, indigestion, or nausea to rule out hydralazine-induced lupus-like syndrome.

Drug Interactions

There are very few interactions with hydralazine. Hydralazine can reduce the liver's first-pass effect on BBs (propranolol and metoprolol) and therefore effectively increase the effects of these drugs, potentiating their mutual hypotensive effects. Also, food intake greatly affects hydralazine absorption, with absorption being much greater on an empty stomach. Therefore, patients should be instructed to take hydralazine consistently, whether it is with or without food, for a consistent effect.[48]

Calcium-Channel Blockers

There was initial interest in the use of amlodipine, especially in patients with nonischemic cardiomyopathy, due to the results of the Prospective Randomized Amlodipine Survival Evaluation I (PRAISE I) trial.[49] However, these findings have been called into question by the results of PRAISE II, where amlodipine was not shown to have any benefit.[50] Therefore, at this time there is no place for the use of calcium-channel blockers in the treatment of patients with systolic dysfunction.

Summary

The outpatient pharmacologic management of HF has become far more complex than it was in the digoxin and diuretic era. The focus has shifted from treating the *end* of the process, to treating the process *itself.* The target now is not the weakened muscle, but the forces at work which brought it to that state, namely the RAAS and SNS. As physicians taking care of these patients, we now have a number of agents at our disposal. ACEIs and ARBs are relatively recently developed agents (within the past decades) and are the new starting points. Beta-blockers, once considered heretical in the treatment of systolic dysfunction, are now the "standard of care". A forgotten diuretic, spironolactone, has been resurrected and has found a new role. Even digoxin, always thought to exert its therapeutic role as our only oral positive inotropic agent, now perhaps has a place in the neurohumoral armamentarium. We should take a cue from our colleagues in hematology/oncology and infectious disease, as rarely is a patient treated with a single chemotherapy agent, and many severe infections are treated with multiple antibiotics. Each chemotherapy agent and antibiotic is designed to interrupt the cell cycle at different stages. As cardiologists, we are dealing with a similar situation in HF. We have a syndrome which is driven by the interaction of multiple systems. Our *goal*, therefore, should be to use as many agents as possible, each directed at *multiple targets*, and titrating each up to doses that *individual* patients can tolerate. If the resting heart rate remains high and blood pressure allows, as long as there is no evidence of significant heart block, beta-blockers can be titrated. If, on the other hand, there is resting bradycardia or significant conduction system disease, ACE inhibitors can be titrated. We can, therefore, customize the guidelines designed for the population with congestive heart failure to the individual, and thereby significantly alter the natural history of this syndrome patient by patient.

References

1. Packer M. Do angiotensin-converting enzyme inhibitors prolong life in patients with heart failure treated in clinical practice? *J Am Coll Cardiol* 1996;28: 1323–1327.
2. Cohn JN. The prevention of heart failure: a new agenda. *N Engl J Med* 1992; 327:725–727.
3. Hobbs RE. Results of the ATLAS study: high or low doses of ACE inhibitors for heart failure? *Clev Clin J Med* 1998;65:539–542.
4. Packer M, Poole-Wilson PA, Armstrong PW, et al. Comparative effects of low and high doses of the angiotensin-converting enzyme inhibitor, lisinopril, on the morbidity and mortality of chronic heart failure. ATLAS Study Group. *Circulation* 1999;100:2312–2318.
5. The CONSENSUS Trial Study Group. Effects of enalapril on mortality in severe congestive heart failure: Results of the Cooperative North American Scandinavian Enalapril Survival Study. *N Engl J Med* 1987;316:1429–1435.
6. Pfeffer MA, Lamas GA, Vaughan DE, Parisi AF, Braunwald E. Effect of captopril on progressive ventricular dilatation after anterior myocardial infarction. *N Engl J Med* 1988;319:80–86.
7. Pfeffer MA, Braunwald E, Moye LA, et al. Effect of captopril on mortality and morbidity in patients with left ventricular dysfunction after myocardial infarction: Results of the Survival and Ventricular Enlargement Trial. *N Engl J Med* 1992;327:669–677.
8. SOLVD Investigators. Effects of enalapril on survival in patients with reduced left ventricular ejection fractions and congestive heart failure. *N Engl J Med* 1991:325:293–302.
9. SOLVD Investigators. Effects of enalapril on mortality and the development of heart failure in asymptomatic patients with reduced left ventricular ejection fraction. *N Engl J Med* 1992;327:685–691.
10. Shah MR, Granger CB, Bart BA, McMurray JJ, et al. Sex-related differences in the use and adverse effects of angiotensin-converting enzyme inhibitors in heart failure: the study of patients intolerant of converting enzyme inhibitors registry. *Am J Med* 2000;109:489–492.
11. Bart BA, Ertl G, Held P, et al. Contemporary management of patients with left ventricular systolic dysfunction: Results from the Study of Patients Intolerant of Converting Enzyme Inhibitors (SPICE) Registry. *Eur Heart J* 1999;20: 1182–1190.
12. Chin M, Wang J et al. Utilization and dosing of angiotensin-converting enzyme inhibitors for heart failure: Effect of physician specialty and patient characteristics. *J Gen Intern Med* 1997;12:563–566.
13. Echemann M, Zannad F, Briancon S, et al. Determinants of angiotensin-converting enzyme inhibitor prescription in severe heart failure with left ventricular systolic dysfunction: The EPICAL Study. *Am Heart J* 2000;139: 624–631.
14. Roe CM, Motheral BR, Teitelbaum F, Rich MW. Angiotensin-converting enzyme inhibitor compliance and dosing among patients with heart failure. *Am Heart J* 1999;138:818–825.

15. Stafford RS, Saglam D, Blumenthal D. National patterns of angiotensin-converting enzyme inhibitor use in congestive heart failure. *Arch Intern Med* 1997;157:2460–2464.
16. Rich MR, Luther P. Temporal trends in pharmacotherapy for congestive heart failure at an academic medical center: 1990–1995. *Am Heart J* 1998;135:367–372.
17. Cohn JN, Archibald DG, Ziesche S, et al. Effect of vasodilator therapy on mortality in chronic congestive heart failure: results of a Veterans Administration Cooperative Study. *N Engl J Med* 1986;314:1547–1552.
18. Cohn JN, Johnson G, Ziesche S, et al. A comparison of enalapril with hydralazine–isosorbide dinitrate in the treatment of chronic congestive heart failure. *N Engl J Med* 1991;325:303–310.
19. Ward RE, Gheorghiade M, Young JB, Uretsky B. Economic outcomes of withdrawal of digoxin therapy in adult patients with stable congestive heart failure. *J Am Coll Cardiol* 1995;26:93–101.
20. Packer M, Gheorghiade M, Young JB, et al. Withdrawal of digoxin from patients with chronic heart failure treated with angiotensin-converting enzyme inhibitors. RADIANCE Study. *N Engl J Med* 1993;329:1–7.
21. Digitalis Investigation Group. The effect of digoxin on mortality and morbidity in patients with heart failure. *N Engl J Med* 1997;336:525–533.
22. Cody RJ. Clinical trials of diuretic therapy in heart failure: research directions and clinical considerations. *J Am Coll Cardiol* 1993;22(suppl A):165A–171A.
23. Brater DC. Diuretic therapy in congestive heart failure. *Congest Heart Fail* 2000;6:197–201.
24. Elliott HL, Meredith PA. Clinical implications of the trough : peak ratio. *Blood Press Monit* 1996;1(suppl 1):S47–S51.
25. Consensus recommendations for the management of chronic heart failure. *Am J Cardiol* 1999;83(suppl 2A):1A–38A.
26. Weinfeld MS, Chertow GM, Stevenson LW. Aggravated renal dysfunction during intensive therapy for advanced chronic heart failure. *Am Heart J* 1999;138:285–290.
27. Teerlink JR, Massie BM. The interaction of ACE inhibitors in heart failure: torn between two lovers. *Am Heart J* 1999;138:193–197.
28. Hall Dd. The aspirin–angiotensin-converting enzyme inhibitor tradeoff: to halve and halve not. *J Am Coll Cardiol* 2000;35:637–639.
29. Latini R, Tognoni G, Maggioni AP, et al. Clinical effects of early angiotensin-converting enzyme inhibitor for acute myocardial infarction are similar in the presence and absence of aspirin: systematic overview of individual data from 96,712 randomized patients. Angiotensin-converting Enzyme Inhibitor Myocardial Infarction Collaborative Group. *J Am Coll Cardiol* 2000;35:1801–1807.
30. Leor J, Reicher-Reiss H. Aspirin and mortality in patients treated with angiotensin-converting enzyme inhibitors: A cohort study of 11,575 patients with coronary artery disease. *J Am Coll Cardiol* 1999;33:1920–1925.
31. Jamali AH, Tang WH, Khot UN, Fowler MB. The role of angiotensin receptor blockers in the management of chronic heart failure. *Arch Intern Med* 2001;161:667–672.
32. Pitt B, Poole-Wilson PA, Segal R, et al. Effect of losartan compared with captopril on mortality in patients with symptomatic heart failure: randomised trial. The Losartan Heart Failure Survival Study, ELITE II. *Lancet* 2000;355:1582–1587.

33. Cohn JN, Tognoni G, Val-HeFT Investigators. The effect of the angiotensin receptor blocker valsartan on morbidity and mortality in heart failure: the Valsartan Heart Failure Trial (Val-HeFT). Paper presented at the American Heart Association 73rd Scientific Session, November 2000, New Orleans.
34. Cohn JN. A strategy to reduce the mortality of heart failure. In: O'Connor C, ed. *Blocking Angiotensin II: The Goal for All CVD Treatment Strategies.* http://cardiology.medscape.com/CMECircle/cardiology/2000/CME01/pnt-CME01.html.
35. Eichhorn E. The paradox of β-adrenergic blockade for the management of congestive heart failure. *Am J Med* 1992;92:527–538.
36. Fisher ML, Gottlieb SS, Plotnick GD, et al. Beneficial effects of metoprolol in heart failure associated with coronary artery disease: a randomized trial. *J Am Coll Cardiol* 1994;23:943–950.
37. Packer M, Bristow M, Cohn JN, et al. The effect of carvedilol on morbidity and mortality in patients with chronic heart failure. *N Engl J Med* 1996;334:1349–1355.
38. Bristow M, Gilbert E, Abraham WT, et al. Carvedilol produces dose-related improvements in left ventricular function and survival in subjects with chronic heart failure. *Circulation* 1996;94:2807–2816.
39. Heidenreich PA, Lee TT, Massie BM. Effect of beta-blockade on mortality in patients with heart failure: a meta-analysis of randomized clinical trials. *J Am Coll Cardiol* 1997;30:27–34.
40. MERIT-HF Study Group. Effect of metoprolol CR/XL in chronic heart failure: Metoprolol CR/XL Randomised Intervention Trial in Congestive Heart Failure (MERIT-HF). *Lancet* 1999;353:2001–2007.
41. Smith AJ, Wehner JS, Manley HJ, Richardson AD, Beal J, Bryant PJ. Current role of β-adrenergic blockers in the treatment of chronic congestive heart failure. *Am J Health Syst Pharm* 2001;58:140–145.
42. Packer, M. COPERNICUS results. Paper presented at the 4th Annual Scientific Meeting of Heart Failure Society of America, Boca Raton, FL, 2000.
43. McMurray JJV. Major β-blocker mortality trials in chronic heart failure: a critical review. *Heart* 1999;82(suppl IV):IV14–IV22.
44. Murray MD, Forthofer MM, Bennett SJ, et al. Effectiveness of torsemide and furosemide in the treatment of CHF: results of a prospective, randomized trial [abstract]. *Circulation* 1999;100(suppl I):I-300.
45. Pitt B, Zannad F, Remme WJ, et al. The effect of spironolactone on morbidity and mortality in patients with severe heart failure. Randomized Aldactone Evaluation Study Investigators. *N Engl J Med* 1999;341:709–717.
46. Packer M. End of the oldest controversy in medicine: Are we ready to conclude the debate on digitalis? *N Engl J Med* 1997;336:575–576.
47. Slatton ML, Irani WN, Hall SA, et al. Does digoxin provide additional hemodynamic and autonomic benefit at higher doses in patients with mild to moderate heart failure and normal sinus rhythm? *J Am Coll Cardiol* 1997;29:1206–1213.
48. Hydralazine HCl Oral: Drug Interactions. Medscape DrugInfo with First Databank and ASHP.
49. Gattis WA, O'Connor CM. Effect of amlodipine on mode of death in advanced heart failure. *Cardiol Rev* 2001;18:13–19.
50. Borzak S. Subset analysis caveats. *Cardiol Rev* 2001;18:19–23.

Chapter 11

Continuum of Care: Prevention to End of Life

Salpy V. Pamboukian, MD, FACC and Nancy M. Albert, MSN, RN, CCNS, CCRN, CNA

Heart failure represents the culmination of a variety of cardiac diagnoses. The most common cause in the United States is coronary atherosclerosis, with hypertension following closely behind. Once heart failure develops, many aspects of its treatment, both pharmacologic and nonpharmacologic, are the same regardless of the underlying etiology.

Prevention of conditions that lead to heart failure has enormous potential to impact the cost of health care today. As a result, the area of preventative cardiology has burgeoned in the last decade. This chapter will summarize the major trials of preventative cardiology, including lipid lowering, hypertension treatment, hormone replacement therapy, diet, vitamin supplementation, and prevention of ischemic heart disease.

Once heart failure develops, the clinician must be able to prognosticate the condition in order to make decisions regarding further therapies, including cardiac transplantation or left ventricular assist device (LVAD). Many factors have been shown to predict a patient's survival, which will be reviewed.

Finally, once all therapeutic options have been exhausted, the physicians and nurses, along with other members of the health-care team, must formulate a plan for issues surrounding the end of life. This therapeutic plan is made in collaboration with the patient and his or her family.

From: Jessup M, McCauley KM (eds). *Heart Failure: Providing Optimal Care*. Elmsford, NY: Futura, an imprint of Blackwell Publishing; ©2003.

Prevention

Lipid-Lowering Therapy

A comprehensive body of evidence exists extolling the benefits of lipid-lowering therapy in both primary and secondary prevention of cardiovascular disease. The first major randomized, double-blind, placebo-controlled trial of lipid lowering was the 4S, or Scandinavian Simvastatin Survival Study. A total of 4444 patients, ranging in age from 35 to 70 years, with a history of myocardial infarction or angina and serum cholesterol 5.5–8.0 mmol/L were randomized to simvastatin 20–40 mg versus placebo. Premenopausal women, patients with myocardial infarction within 6 months, congestive heart failure or scheduled revascularization with coronary bypass or angioplasty were not included. After a median follow-up of 5.4 years, total cholesterol decreased by 25%, low-density lipoprotein (LDL) decreased by 35%, high-density lipoprotein (HDL) increased by 8% and triglycerides decreased by 10% in the simvastatin treated patients. Mortality was 12% in the placebo group versus 8% in the simvastatin group ($P = 0.0003$). The Kaplan–Meier 6-year probability of survival was 87.7% in the placebo group versus 91.3% in the simvastatin group. The relative risk of having a coronary event in the simvastatin group was 0.73 (CI 0.66–0.80, $P < 0.00001$).[1]

The benefit of cholesterol reduction in patients with coronary disease with average cholesterol levels was examined in the Cholesterol and Recurrent Events (CARE) study. Over 4000 patients ranging in age from 21 to 75 years old who had experienced a myocardial infarction in the preceding 3–20 months where randomized to pravastatin 40 mg/day or placebo. Total cholesterol in the study group was less than 240 mg/dL, with LDL levels of 115–174 mg/dL. Patients with symptomatic heart failure or left ventricular ejection fraction less than 25% were excluded. The majority of patients were Caucasian (93%) males (86%). Median follow-up was 5 years. The primary endpoint was fatal coronary event or nonfatal myocardial infarction. Pravastatin lowered LDL by 32%, producing a risk reduction in the primary endpoint of 24% (CI 9–36%, $P = 0.03$). The effect was more pronounced in women compared to men, with a risk reduction of 46% versus 20%, respectively. The reduction in coronary events was also greater in patients with higher pretreatment levels of LDL cholesterol. There were no significant reductions in overall mortality.[2]

The Long-term Intervention with Pravastatin in Ischemic Disease (LIPID) trial extended the results of these two previous trials. This study enrolled 9014 subjects aged 31–75 years who had a myocardial infarction in the previous 3–36 months. Of these, 1516 patients were female. For patients to qualify, the plasma cholesterol level at randomization was required to be between 155 and 271 mg/dL, with the fasting triglyceride level less than 445 mg/dL. Patients with a clinically significant medical or surgical event within the previous 3 months, cardiac failure, renal or hepatic disease, or using a lipid-lowering agent, were excluded. The primary outcome was death from coronary heart disease. Death from coronary disease occurred in 8.3% of patients in the placebo group versus 6.4% in the treatment arm, a relative risk reduction of 24% ($P < 0.001$). Overall mortality was 14.1% in the placebo group versus 11% in the pravastatin group, a relative risk reduction of 22% ($P < 0.001$). The incidence of all cardiovascular outcomes was lower in patients receiving pravastatin, including myocardial infarction (29% risk reduction, $P < 0.001$), stroke (19% risk reduction, $P < 0.001$), and coronary revascularization (20% risk reduction, $P < 0.001$).[3] This is a convincing body of evidence for lipid lowering in secondary prevention in patients with a wide range of cholesterol levels.

An equally robust body of evidence exists for lipid lowering in primary prevention. The West of Scotland Coronary Prevention Study (WOSCOPS) assessed whether pravastatin therapy (40 mg/day) versus placebo reduced the incidence of acute myocardial infarction and mortality from coronary heart disease in hypercholesterolemic men without a history of prior myocardial infarction. Over 6000 men aged 45–64 years with fasting LDL >252 mg/dL before diet, or >155 after diet, were eligible. Five percent had angina, and 78% were ex- or current smokers. Compared to baseline values, pravastatin reduced plasma total cholesterol levels by 20% and LDL cholesterol by 26%. Coronary events were reduced by 31% (CI 17–43%, $P < 0.001$) and death from all cardiovascular causes was reduced by 32% (CI 3–53%, $P = 0.033$).[4] Clearly, the population represented in WOSCOPS was moderate to high risk.

The primary preventative benefits have also been observed in patients with average serum cholesterol levels, women and older persons. The Air Force Coronary Atherosclerosis Prevention Study (AFCAPS/TexCAPS) compared lovastatin, 20 mg to 40 mg daily, to placebo for prevention of first acute major coronary event in men and women without clinically evident atherosclerosis and average cholesterol levels. The mean total cholesterol was 221 mg/dL, mean LDL was 150 mg/dL, and mean HDL was 36 mg/dL for men and 40 mg/dL for women. Lovastatin reduced the incidence of first acute major coronary event by 37% overall, 34% in men, 54% in women and 29% in the elderly. Patients in the lovastatin group also had a 33% reduction in procedures such as coronary bypass and angioplasty and a 34% reduction in hospitalization due to unstable angina.[5] The effects of cholesterol lowering on coronary atherosclerosis in normocholesterolemic patients have also been confirmed angiographically in the recent Simvastatin/Enalapril Coronary Atherosclerosis Trial (SCAT). In a 2–2 factorial design, 460 patients received simvastatin or placebo and enalapril or placebo and were evaluated by angiogram at baseline and at closeout, 3–5 years later, or when clinically indicated by symptoms. Baseline cholesterol levels were not significantly different between groups. Mean LDL was 3.39 mmol/L in the simvastatin-treated group at baseline, compared with 3.33 mmol/L in the placebo group. During the trial, LDL decreased by 30.5% in the simvastatin group ($P < 0.001$). Although no differences were observed between groups in all-cause mortality or cardiovascular events, simvastatin treated patients required less revascularization procedures (6% versus 12%, $P = 0.021$) and angioplasties (3% versus 9%, $P = 0.020$). Quantitative coronary angiography demonstrated that simvastatin-treated patients had less progression of coronary disease, as indicated by less decrease in mean and minimum diameter and less percent diameter stenosis over time. Enalapril had an angiographically neutral effect, but clinically, there was a significant decrease in the combined endpoint of death/myocardial infarction/stroke.[6]

Hypertension

Control of hypertension has the potential to impact tremendously on the prevalence of heart failure. Hypertension is defined as a systolic blood pressure of >140 mmHg over a diastolic blood pressure of >90 mmHg and can be classified into three stages according to severity[7] (Table 1). Diuretics and beta-blockers remain the drugs of choice in

Table 1

Classification of Blood Pressure for Adults Aged 18 Years and Older. Copyright American Medical Association © 1997. All rights reserved

	Blood Pressure, mmHg	
Category	Systolic	Diastolic
Optimal	<120 and	<80
Normal	<130 and	<85
High-normal	130–139 or	85–89
Hypertension		
Stage 1	140–159 or	90–99
Stage 2	160–179 or	100–109
Stage 3	≥180 or	≥110

From: JNC VI, *Archives of Internal Medicine*, 1997, with permission.

uncomplicated hypertension, as they are the only drugs which have been shown to reduce cardiovascular morbidity and mortality in prospective trials.[8–10] More recently, the recommendation for using beta-blocker as first-line therapy has been challenged in a meta-analysis of randomized trials which used diuretics and/or beta-blockers and reported morbidity and mortality outcomes in elderly patients with hypertension. Two-thirds of the patients on diuretics as monotherapy were well controlled, versus less than one-third of those treated with beta-blockers. Diuretic therapy was found to be superior to beta-blockers with regard to all endpoints and was effective in preventing cerebrovascular events, fatal stroke, coronary disease, cardiovascular mortality and all cause mortality.[11]

Thiazide diuretics remain the preferred drugs for the treatment of isolated hypertension in the elderly and have been demonstrated to reduce fatal and nonfatal heart failure by 50% as well as reduce left ventricular mass, a powerful predictor of cardiovascular mortality.[12,13]

Although the role of angiotensin-converting enzyme inhibitors in patients with heart failure is well defined, its role in the treatment of hypertension is less clearly established. The Captopril Prevention Project (CAPPP) trial compared captopril to conventional therapy with diuretics and beta-blockers. The primary endpoint was a composite of fatal and nonfatal myocardial infarction, stroke and other cardiovascular deaths. Over 5000 patients participated in each arm. There was no significant difference in the primary endpoint between the two groups, but the captopril group had a higher rate of fatal and nonfatal stroke (relative risk 1.25, CI 1.01–1.55, $P = 0.044$). This may have been due to a more frequent history of transient ischemic attack (TIA) or higher blood pressures at baseline and throughout the study in the captopril group. Angiotensin-converting enzyme (ACE) inhibitors have been shown to reduce death, myocardial infarction, and stroke in a broad range of high-risk patients who do not have low ejection fraction or heart failure. The Heart Outcomes Prevention Evaluation (HOPE) study randomized high-risk patients who had evidence of vascular disease or diabetes plus one other cardiovascular risk factor (hypertension, smoking, dyslipidemia, or microalbuminuria) without heart failure or low ejection fraction to ramipril or placebo for a mean of 5 years. Treatment with ramipril significantly reduced death from cardiovascular causes, myocardial infarction, revascularization procedures, heart failure, cardiac arrest, complications of diabetes, and death from any cause.[14] ACE inhibitors have also been found to be renoprotective in patients with type 1 diabetes mellitus with nephropathy.[15]

In general, antihypertensive therapy should be tailored to the individual based on the presence of comorbid conditions.

Diet

Much attention has been paid recently to the impact of diet and other lifestyle factors on the development of cardiovascular disease. The "Mediterranean diet" was recently evaluated in the Lyons Diet Heart Study. This diet, based on traditional Mediterranean diets rich in fish oils and certain vegetable oils containing α-linolenic acid, was shown to decrease cardiovascular mortality by 76% and new myocardial infarctions by 73% in individuals with a history of cardiovascular disease.[16] The Diet and Reinfarction Trial (DART) randomized over 2000 postmyocardial infarction patients to an increase in fatty fish intake (two to three portions per week), a reduction in dietary fat, or an increase in dietary fat. Although the risk of reinfarction did not differ, those advised to eat fatty fish had a significant 29% reduction in all-cause mortality.[17] The Dietary Approaches to Stop Hypertension (DASH) diet, rich in vegetables, low-fat dairy foods, and reduced saturated and total fat, significantly decreased systolic and diastolic blood pressures by 5.5 and 3 mmHg, respectively, compared to the control diet, based on the average American diet.

Several randomized trials of the effect of vitamin E supplementation on cardiovascular events have failed to demonstrate clear benefits.[18–20] More recently, the HOPE trial randomly assigned over 9500 high-risk patients to vitamin E 400 IU or placebo, with a mean follow-up of 4.5 years. Although there were no adverse events in the patients receiving vitamin E, there was no benefit with regards to all cause mortality, cardiovascular mortality, myocardial infarction or stroke.

There is long-standing debate as to whether dietary sodium is associated with the development of hypertension. Two meta-analyses of randomized trials did not find compelling evidence for sodium restriction in the normotensive population.[21,22] In those with hypertension, reduction of sodium intake modestly reduces blood pressure and it might be used as a supplementary treatment.[21] Larger decreases in blood pressure were observed in trials of older hypertensive individuals (mean age >45).[22]

Based on these and other data linking high dietary saturated fat intake and development of cardiovascular disease, the American Heart Association currently recommends a diet emphasizing vegetables, fruits, and whole grains and limiting fats, saturated fats, and refined carbohydrates.

Hormone Replacement Therapy

The issue of hormone replacement therapy (HRT) in postmenopausal females has recently garnered a lot of attention in both the popular and scientific media. Abundant epidemiological studies suggested a reduction of cardiovascular events with the use of HRT, but the first randomized, double-blind, placebo-controlled trial to examine the issue of HRT in secondary prevention was the Heart and Estrogen/ Progestin Replacement study (HERS). A total of 2763 postmenopausal women, younger than 80 years, with coronary disease were randomized to 0.625 mg of conjugated equine estrogens plus 2.5 mg of medroxyprogesterone acetate or placebo. Patients were followed for an average of 4.1 years. Overall, there were no significant differences between the groups in the primary outcome of nonfatal myocardial infarction and cardiovascular death, or in any of the secondary outcomes. Although there was a strong trend for reduction in the primary endpoint at years 4 and 5, with a 33% decrease in coronary heart disease, there was a disturbing 4.1% increase in cardiovascular events in the treatment group at 1 year compared to a 2.7% incidence in the placebo group.[23,24] Based on this study, the initiation of HRT for secondary prevention cannot be advocated, but may be continued in women already taking HRT who sustain a cardiovascular event.

Ischemic Heart Disease

Antiplatelet therapy with aspirin (80–325 mg) has been shown to decrease mortality in patients with coronary artery disease and lower risk of recurrent infarction, stroke and vascular death in the order of 25%.[25] No antiplatelet agent has been proven to be superior to aspirin, and it is standard treatment unless a clear contraindication exists.

Beta-blockers have been shown to lower mortality both early in the acute treatment of myocardial infarction and as secondary prevention after myocardial infarction. At least 29 randomized beta-blocker trials with over 28,970 patients have examined intravenous, followed by oral, beta-blocker therapy in acute myocardial infarction, demonstrating about a 13% relative reduction in the risk of mortality.[26] The Thrombolysis in Myocardial Ischemia (TIMI) IIB[27] trial studied the combination of beta-blocker therapy and thrombolysis with recombinant tissue plasminogen activator. Metoprolol was given either immediately, intravenously followed by orally, or deferred until day 6 and given only orally. Overall, there were no differences in mortality between the early and late regimens, nor was left ventricular function improved. However, there was a lower incidence of reinfarction and recurrent chest pain in the immediate intravenous group. This indicates that intravenous betablockade in the setting of early reperfusion may not enhance salvage of myocardium, but may confer benefit by means of anti-ischemic effect.[26]

Revascularization with coronary artery bypass surgery has been shown to be superior to medical therapy, with regard to mortality, in certain anatomical subgroups, including those with left main coronary stenosis, multivessel disease with decreased left ventricular function, and three-vessel disease, which includes the proximal left anterior descending artery.[28] Angioplasty has been compared to coronary bypass surgery in patients with multivessel disease with comparable mortality, expect in treated diabetics, whose 5-year survival has been shown to be significantly better after coronary artery bypass surgery,[29] and with the advent of stents, both clinical and angiographic outcomes are improved as compared with standard balloon angioplasty, including less need for subsequent intervention and lower re-stenosis rates.[30,31] Detection of viable myocardium using nuclear imaging, dobutamine echocardiography, and positron-emission tomography (PET) scanning also identifies a group of high-risk patients who may have mortality benefit from revascularization.[32–34] The mechanisms for improved survival may be related to improvement in left ventricular function, decreased ventricular remodeling, decreased propensity to arrhythmias, and likelihood of fatal ischemic events.[35]

Prognostic Factors in Patients with Advanced Heart Failure

Once heart failure develops, the patient must be risk-stratified in order to guide ongoing therapy, including potential cardiac transplantation and implantation of a ventricular assist device. Even if a patient is not a candidate for these more advanced therapies, determining a patient's prognosis is important in addressing issues related to end of life.

Etiology of Heart Failure

Many studies have demonstrated worse prognosis in patients with ischemic cardiomyopathy compared to those with dilated cardiomyopathy.[36–38] However, contradictory evidence exists. The Studies of Left Ventricular Dysfunction (SOLVD) and Vasodilator Heart Failure Trial (V-HeFT) II revealed no significant predictive value of coronary artery disease for mortality.[39,40] In the Cooperative North Scandinavian Enalapril Survival Study (CONSENSUS), overall mortality in patients with ischemic cardiomyopathy treated with standard medical therapy (diuretic, digoxin, ACE inhibitor) was much higher compared to those with other causes of heart failure.[41] Gradman and colleagues observed increased total mortality and occurrence of sudden death with nonischemic etiology by univariate analysis, although not all patients were classified by coronary angiography.[42]

Provocative Testing

Rather than looking at etiology alone, observing response to provocative testing may be a more meaningful predictor of mortality in both ischemic and nonischemic cardiomyopathy. Low-dose dobutamine responsiveness in idiopathic dilated cardiomyopathy has been found to correlate with maximal oxygen consumption, and by multivariate analysis, lower percentage change in end-systolic volume index was significantly associated with clinical deterioration and death.[43] In patients with ischemic cardiomyopathy, the demonstration of viable myocardium by dobutamine echocardiography or uptake of F-18 deoxyglucose on PET scanning has been shown to independently predict subsequent cardiovascular events.[44,45] Proposed mechanisms for this observation include increased propensity for malignant arrhythmias in ischemic segments, increased likelihood of subsequent myocardial infarction, and decline in ejection fraction and remodeling.[45]

Ventricular Function

Measurement of left ventricular ejection fraction by echocardiography may be inaccurate and has not been shown in a majority of analyses to predict prognosis.[46–48] Other echocardiographic parameters of systolic function which have been shown to correlate with prognosis include left ventricular fractional shortening,[49] left ventricular end-systolic[50] and end-diastolic dimensions,[51] mitral E point septal separation,[50] and wall motion index.[52]

In contrast, numerous studies have demonstrated that left ventricular ejection fraction determined by radionuclide ventriculography predicts mortality.[36,42,53] Data from the V-HeFT I and II trials demonstrated that change in left ventricular ejection fraction over time was a predictor of mortality, with a decline of greater than 5 units associated with the worst prognosis. Interestingly, patients taking the combination of hydralazine–isosorbide dinitrate (Isordil) had a significantly higher improvement in ejection fraction compared with those taking enalapril, even though survival was superior in the enalapril-treated group.[54]

Right ventricular dysfunction is also an independent risk factor for increased mortality,[55,56] and may indicate that the primary myocardial insult was large enough to include both ventricles, or that the severity of left ventricular dysfunction has resulted in secondary right ventricular dysfunction. In fact, in one multivariate analysis, right ventricular ejection fraction <35% at rest was the most potent predictor of death and was found to better predict overall and event-free survival than peak exercise oxygen consumption.[57]

Neurohormonal Factors

Neurohormonal compensatory mechanisms serve to maintain cardiac function and performance over the short term. However, over time, these mechanisms have deleterious effects. Hyponatremia, as a marker of renin–angiotensin system activation, independently predicts prognosis.[58] Increased circulating levels of various neurohormones have been shown to portend a poor prognosis including norepinephrine,[59,60] atrial natriuretic peptide,[61] brain natriuretic peptide,[62] and endothelin-1.[63]

One caveat is that the correlation between neurohormones and mortality is not always seen in patients receiving heart failure drug therapy. In the CONSENSUS trial, a positive correlation between mortality and levels of angiotensin II, aldosterone, norepinephrine, epinephrine and atrial natriuretic factor was observed in the placebo group, but not in the enalapril group.[64] Data from the V-HeFT II trial demonstrated increased plasma norepinephrine concentrations in the hydralazine–Isordil-treated group during the first year of follow-up,[60] despite the fact that this combination had been shown to decrease mortality up to 2 years compared with placebo in the V-HeFT I trial.[65] With the current standard drug regimens in heart failure, data regarding neuorhormonal levels should be cautiously interpreted.

Invasively Obtained Hemodynamics

Resting hemodynamic measurements have been found to correlate variably with prognosis. However, hemodynamic response to therapy may have more prognostic value. Pulmonary capillary wedge pressure obtained after medical optimization is more relevant than the pulmonary capillary wedge pressure during an acute decompensation. In one study, if pulmonary artery capillary wedge pressure could be lowered below 16 mmHg with vasodilator therapy while maintaining cardiac output and blood pressure, 1-year survival was 83%, versus 38% in those who did not respond ($P = 0.0001$).[66]

Exercise Performance

In chronic heart failure, cardiopulmonary exercise testing is used to as an objective means of defining functional capacity. A variety of cut-offs of peak Vo_2 have been proposed to indicate timing for cardiac transplantation, although generally a peak Vo_2 of less than 14 mL/kg/min is accepted as the threshold below which cardiac transplantation is considered. This is based on the study by Mancini and coworkers, which showed one and 2-year survival to be only 47% and 32% respectively in patients with a peak VO_2 ≤14 mL/kg/min not accepted for transplantation versus 1- and 2-year survival of 94% and 84% in those with peak VO_2 ≥14 mL/kg/min. Patients with a peak VO_2 of ≤ 14 mL/kg/min who were listed for transplantation had a 1-year survival of 70%.[67] Further refinement of this measurement with adjustment to lean body mass may increase the prognostic value of cardiopulmonary stress testing, especially in women and the obese, with a proposed cut-off of 19 mL/kg of lean body mass/min used for timing transplantation.[68] Peak VO_2 expressed as a percentage of predicted values for age and gender may also be a more meaningful measurement, particularly in women.[69]

Other parameters such as ventilatory response to exercise (minute ventilation/carbon dioxide production or V_E/VCO_2)[70,71] and heart rate response to exercise (chronotropic index)[70] have also been shown in multivariate analyses to independently predict increased mortality.

Arrhythmias

It has been suggested that atrial fibrillation is associated with increased mortality,[72] but data from the V-HeFT studies did not demonstrate atrial fibrillation to be associated with increased major morbidity or mortality in mild to moderate heart failure.[73] This has been confirmed by more recent reports.[74]

Although patients with heart failure are clearly at increased risk of sudden death, the presence of nonsustained ventricular tachycardia has been linked to worse prognosis in some,[75,76] but not all studies.[77,78] However, the recent Multicenter Automatic Defibrillator Implantation Trial (MADIT) and Multicenter Unsustained Tachycardia Trial (MUSTT) showed that in patients with coronary artery disease, left ventricular ejection fraction less that 40%, nonsustained ventricular tachycardia and inducible ventricular tachycardia on electrophysiological testing, therapy with implantable defibrillator reduced mortality significantly versus antiarrhythmic therapy.[79,80] In patients with nonischemic cardiomyopathy and nonsustained ventricular arrhythmias, the role of implantable defibrillator versus amiodarone is currently being investigated in the Sudden Cardiac Death in Heart Failure Trial (SCD-HeFT).

Other markers on the surface electrocardiogram, which may indicate increased risk of arrhythmic events or mortality, include QT and QRS dispersion[81] and T wave alternans during exercise stress.[82]

End-of-Life Care

Managing patients in end-of-life heart failure requires moving from the traditional paradigm of cure and substantial prolongation of life to a paradigm focusing on compassion, provision of comfort measures, restoration of functional capacity, and control or alleviation of symptoms to meet health needs. It is a comprehensive program of management of the patient's physical, psychological, sociocultural, and spiritual needs and values to promote an optimal quality of life. It is predicted that by 2050, seniors over the age of 65 will double and those over the age of 85 will quadruple. The graying of Americans, coupled with the knowledge that the incidence of heart failure continues to be rising, may help healthcare professionals increase their awareness of the benefits of palliation and hospice care when a patient's cardiac condition becomes advanced, suffering is obvious, and death appears imminent. The key dimensions of palliation—evaluation, explanation, management, monitoring and attention to detail—will be discussed. In addition, development of a heart failure-specific hospice/palliative care program will be discussed as a means to achieving the key dimensions of palliation.

Evaluation: Is End of Life Discernible in Advanced Heart Failure?

In determining if a patient is ready for end-of-life measures, the first step in the process is to assess the patient's overall condition and heart condition, to ensure that factors reflecting end of life are present. One method is to use the National Hospice Organization's medical guidelines to determine prognosis in heart disease (Table 2).[83] There are two issues with this guideline content. First, the Study to Understand Prognoses and Preferences for Outcomes and Risks of Treatments (SUPPORT) group found that the median predicted chance for survival for 2 months on the day before actual death in patients with advanced heart failure was 62%.[84] This SUPPORT result reflects the fact that patients with advanced heart failure may not appear ready for death compared with patients dying from other terminal diseases and that it may be very difficult to discern precursors to sudden cardiac death, which accounted for the large variation in predicted chance for 2-month survival and actual death. A second problem with these guidelines is that we now know the benefits of beta-blocker therapy in patients with systolic left ventricular dysfunction. In fact, the addition of beta-blockers in the treatment regimen has led to a 30–65% reduction in all-cause mortality in five individual trials and a 35–40% decrease in combined death and hospitalization; these improvements are more substantial than the addition of angiotensin-converting enzyme inhibitors (ACEIs) and other vasodilators.[85] Therefore, it is no longer acceptable to assume a patient is optimized on therapy unless beta-blockers are a part of the therapy regimen (unless contraindications are documented).

Table 2

National Hospice Organization Medical Guidelines for Determining Prognosis in Heart Disease

Must meet *all* of the following:

1 Recurrent congestive heart failure symptoms at rest (New York Heart Association functional class IV; ejection fraction less than 20% is supplemental evidence but not mandatory)

2 Persistent symptoms despite being optimally treated with vasodilators and diuretics
If not on vasodilators, a valid medical reason should be documented
Note: beta-blocker therapy is not included in optimal drug therapy

3 History of the following in patients who are optimally treated but continue to have refractory symptoms:

- Symptomatic ventricular tachycardia or supraventricular tachycardia resistant to drugs
- A cardiac arrest and subsequent resuscitation that occurs in any setting
- Unexplained syncope
- Cardiogenic brain embolism
- Concomitant human immunodeficiency virus infection

Evaluation refers to the process of determining probability and pattern recognition. As seen above in the SUPPORT study, it is difficult to tell when death is imminent in heart failure. It is possible to use investigative means (e.g., maximum oxygen consumption) to provide more information upon which the health-care provider can make a better determination, but it is not necessary to do so. In the *Épidémiologie de l'Insuffisance Cardiaque Avancée en Lorraine* (EPICAL) study, Alla and colleagues derived a score for prognostic prediction for patients with severe heart failure of ischemic or dilated cardiomyopathy etiology from readily available data.[86] The database tested 28 prognostic factors and developed a three-tiered survival classification for ischemic and dilated etiologies. Patients with ischemic cardiomyopathy were classified as having low survival (less than or equal to 25% 1-year survival rate) if three of the following four factors were present: serum sodium below 138 mmol/L, resting heart rate greater than 100 beats/min, serum creatinine greater than 180 µmol/L (2.0 mg/dL), and a history of prior decompensation. In patients with dilated cardiomyopathy, low survival was based on the presence of at least five of the following seven factors: serious comorbidity (e.g., cancer, cirrhosis, arteritis, cerebral vascular accident, and bronchopneumonopathy), heart failure diagnosis at least 3 months old, patient was institutionalized or dependent on assistance from relatives, serum sodium below 138 mmol/L, resting heart rate greater than 100 beats per minute, serum creatinine greater than 180 µmol/L, and age greater than 70 years. The stratification tool developed by Alla and colleagues can be used to make decisions about shifting care measures towards a quality-of-life focus as part of a patient-centered model of care.

Explanation

Once it is determined that prognosis is poor and that cardiac transplantation, assist device, or surgical options are not appropriate, the second key dimension of palliation begins. In the explanation phase, it is important to review each of the patient's recurring symptoms that one hopes to impact through palliative measures. This is done by providing a description of each symptom, determining its cause, determining possible mechanisms (devices or means) which may alter it (i.e., rest or sitting versus lying position), and assessing for nonphysical factors which may impact its incidence and prevalence. Dyspnea, pain, abdominal fullness/nausea/early meal satiety, palpitations and cough are frequently encountered symptoms that must be addressed.

Management

Whenever possible, correcting correctable causes of symptoms must be addressed first. Nondrug therapies should be attempted before turning to symptomatic drug treatment whenever possible. Managing symptoms to enhance comfort requires a balancing of the art and science of care management. If the patient experiences breathlessness from consuming high sodium foods, the caregiver must find a solution that allows for comfortable food ingestion but also controls or eliminates periods of dyspnea. This requires frequent reassessment of signs and symptoms of volume overload, including subclinical signs such as a new or worsening S_3 gallop, a positive abdominojugular reflux test, slow weight gain, or an elevated jugular venous pressure in the absence of edema or respiratory crackles. Health-care providers must make the connection between the patient's recurring symptoms causing distress and diet and/or fluid indiscretion so that an adequate management plan can be designed and implemented.

The cause of worsening symptoms might be nonadherence to medication, which could be due to a variety of factors. If economic factors are prevalent, social work consultation might aide in providing a solution to the high cost of the multitude of medications heart failure patients must take. It is also prudent to reassess the patient's current medications, including over-the-counter therapies, to assure that the patient is not taking medications (such as nonsteroidal anti-inflammatory agents, nasal decongestants, sodium-based antacids, or herbal therapies known to cause diuretic intolerance or sodium and water retention—ginseng, gingko) which augment deleterious symptoms.

It is also important to assess for signs of end-organ hypoperfusion, which may indicate that the patient's condition has advanced to a more terminal state. At this stage, the patient may require an increase in diuretic dose and initiation of antianxiety medications to relieve symptoms. In addition, if pain becomes more prevalent, broad-spectrum analgesia should be incorporated into the treatment plan. Generally, the World Health Organization's three-step analgesia ladder should be used as a guide to relieving pain.[87] This stepped approach starts with a nonopioid (Tylenol) plus an adjuvant (corticosteroid for appetite stimulation and anti-inflammatory action, antidepressant, antispasmodic, or muscle relaxant—benzodiazepines—as needed), then stepping up to a weak opioid plus a nonopioid and adjuvant, then finally stepping up toward a strong opioid plus nonopioid and adjunct to provide relief. When narcotics are ordered, a bowel management program with laxatives must also be prescribed to overcome hypersegmentation in the colon. Morphine is the drug of choice when opioids are needed, since it provides the most versatility; it is available in sustained-release, immediate-release, oral solution and rectal suppositories.[88] Other implications associated with new or worsening end-organ hypoperfusion are that the patient and family must be prepared for death (if this process has not already begun) and that patients must be able to retain as much control and autonomy as possible. Health-care providers must offer choices to the patient and promote autonomy through education and compliance monitoring/counseling.

If we assume the patient is being correctly treated with core heart failure medications (ACEI or vasodilator replacements if ACEI is contraindicated, beta-blockers, diuretics, spironolactone and digoxin) at doses recommended by national consensus guidelines,[85,89] then palliative therapies should not focus on the addition of new heart failure drug therapies. Instead, emphasis should be placed on psychological support related to fear, anxiety, pain and depression and palliative medications and lifestyle changes to optimize function.

Management issues and controversies in end-of-life heart failure management include decisions related to implanted cardioverter–defibrillators and the use of intravenous inotropes. There is no consensus related to a patient's request for cardioverter–defibrillator device inactivation. If a patient is having multiple shocks per day from intractable arrhythmias, and this leads to complaints of pain, fear, and increased anxiety, an electrophysiology cardiologist should be consulted to determine options related to device settings. In some situations, the device is deactivated, or if the battery life is diminished due to multiple shocks, the cardiologist and patient may agree not to replace the battery.

There are clearly written consensus guidelines available to direct use of intravenous inotropes, dobutamine and milrinone, during end-of-life heart failure management.[89] Intermittent "pulse" therapy is not recommended, even in advanced heart failure. Continuous intravenous inotrope infusion through a central catheter (Hickman catheter) may provide comfort, increase functional capacity, and improve quality of life in advanced heart failure even though there is a trade off of proarrhythmia and increased mortality with long-term use. The initiation of these agents in end-of-life care may prevent hospital readmission for decompensation due to a recurring hypoperfusion state. It may allow the patient to have additional quality time at home with family. Key discussions that must be carried out prior to hospital discharge between the primary health-care provider and patient/family include drug up-titration if hypoperfusion occurs or worsens and the need for electrocardiogram (ECG) monitoring on a routine basis or in the presence of signs of ventricular tachycardia, such as palpitations and syncope. If the inotrope agent is truly being used to increase comfort through symptom relief, and the patient and family understand the risks and benefits of this therapy as a palliative measure, then it should not be up-titrated and ECG monitoring should not be necessary.

Monitoring and Attention to Details

These two final key dimensions of palliation are essential elements that promote a trusting physician or health-care professional–patient relationship and satisfying communication. There is no substitute for effective communication as a foundation to quality end-of-life care. The health-care team must be willing to take the time to ask the right questions and listen to the patient and family.

Effective Communication

Health-care providers must incorporate specific themes of conversation (Table 3) and respond to patients in ways that help them feel that their fears, ideas, feelings, and expectations are understood.[90] Specific components of effective communication that lead to improved care include understanding cultural differences among patients; listening to patient preferences in relation to themselves, their families, their lives and their hopes and futures; reassuring patients that you will stay actively involved in their care; addressing the patient's emotional and spiritual needs; and delivering messages in person, in a clear, straightforward manner using understandable terminology, in a quiet and comfortable setting, and in a way that reinforces the patient's sense of control.[91]

Table 3

Topics in End-of-life Heart Failure Conversations

- Unfavorable prognosis and treatment failure
- Physical and emotional symptoms
- Maintenance of autonomy and functional capacity
- Treatment choices and family responses
- Aggressive care near death
- Advance care planning
- Concerns about one's ability to cope
- Family burden (financial and emotional challenges)
- Life goals and other life-closure issues
- Anticipatory mourning
- Survivor bereavement
- The meaning of illness and the suffering it creates

The SUPPORT and Hospitalized Elderly Longitudinal Project (HELP) studies addressed characteristics of patients dying from heart failure who were seriously ill and over 80 years of age.[92] Lynn and colleagues found that over 75% of patients were conscious and 60% were able to communicate. Severe dyspnea was common (65%), and 43% had severe pain, but less than 20% had severe confusion. In the last 3 days of life, 12% of patients with heart failure received feeding tubes, 12% were placed on a ventilator, 15% had cardiopulmonary resuscitation, and 42% of patients received at least one of the three treatments. In addition, in the last 3 days before death, family members reported that nearly 50% of patients preferred comfort measures and that they perceived that care was not in accord with patient preferences approximately 12% of the time.[92] When reviewing SUPPORT data, Levenson and coworkers found that over 60% of patients with heart failure preferred comfort care and 47% preferred "do not resuscitate" status in the last 1 month to 3 days before death.[93] During this same time period of 1 month to 3 days before death, nearly 70% of patients would rather die than spend all of their remaining time on a ventilator, nearly 60% felt the same regarding feeding tube placement, but only 32% of patients would rather die than spend their remaining days in a nursing home.[93]

Health-care professionals must not assume that end-of-life heart failure patients are mentally impaired and unable to make decisions concerning their future. The SUPPORT and HELP findings above provide credence for actions to be taken to overcome patient barriers (concealing the extent of their feelings and fears, cultural prohibitions, overestimating cure), medical care system barriers (busy schedules, taking responsibility, no compensation for psychosocial conversations), and physicians or other professional care provider barriers (fear of causing pain or delivering bad news, lack of knowledge of advance directives, viewing death as the enemy, medicolegal concerns, feeling threatened by discussions, anticipating disagreement with patient/family). Utilization of a patient-centered care approach will augment mutual participation relationships, enhance interpersonal communication skills, and assist with the need to understand the meaning of illness for the patient.

Advance Directives

One aspect of attending to details is to incorporate advance planning into your practice. Once the diagnosis of heart failure has been made and the patient exhibits ongoing signs of poor prognosis, decisions regarding medical management wishes and what is not wanted can be made in advance. Types of advance directives include a living will, durable power of attorney for health care by naming a health-care proxy and any document or chart notation that states the patient's wishes for specific aspects of care, such as resuscitation and ventilator management, in a clear manner. The use of advance directives can serve as a blueprint for treatment decisions and can also be used to initiate and promote discussion between physician and patient so that a mutual understanding develops.[94] Well-written, specifically stated or disease-specific advance directives can ultimately reduce patient, family, and physician stress. In addition, family members derive comfort in knowing they are augmenting decisions that their loved ones desired.

Hospice Care and Resuscitation Preferences

Since heart failure is a condition that we know to be progressive and often leading to functional disability, a well-written advance directive should include palliative measures related to identification of caregivers and location of care. Hospice care offers patients more than just a facility or service prior to death. It is a "philosophy about the significance of death and dying within the context of human existence and a powerful movement to return that experience to its proper place in human affairs."[95] In hospice care, hope can flourish through comfort and knowing comfort will be secured through whatever means necessary to relieve pain and control symptoms. In addition, other essential elements of hospice care are inclusion of the family or significant other as a unit of care; empowerment and encouragement of the patient and family in daily care; multidisciplinary team services as needed (social workers, chaplain, therapists, bereavement counselors); spiritual care, especially when questions of reconciliation and meaning at the end of life become prominent; and long-term support of family and friends beyond the patient's death.[95]

Issues that the heart failure team must overcome when working with the hospice care team are ensuring that hospice care members understand heart failure pathophysiology, medical management (including the use of continuous intravenous inotrope therapy as a palliative care measure), the importance of lifestyle modifications in daily care, and prognostic signs and symptoms. Most hospice care teams are very knowledgeable regarding care of patients with cancer and neurologic problems, but very uninformed of routine care and disease progression of heart failure. Education of hospice team members is crucial if they are to truly offer the kind of services they promote. One mechanism to ensure optimal care is to design a physician order sheet specifically for the care of patients with end-of-life heart failure. It should include specific treatment approaches for dyspnea, pain, cough, fluid overload, and anxiety that are consistent with heart failure management themes. Physician-initiated, nurse-mediated care algorithms could promote comfort and possibly prevent avoidable deterioration in condition (i.e., aggressive diuretic therapy with a 3–5-pound weight gain). Nurses who manage heart failure patients in a hospice care program need to understand the interrelationship between diet, fluids, and symptoms so that they are not promoting comfort foods and fluids at the cost of hastening suffering (dyspnea) and death. Proper use of inotrope therapies, vital signs, laboratory, and testing procedures can also be enhanced through preprinted physician order sheets and nurse-mediated algorithms. A heart failure-specific hospice program should have a physician champion who is a cardiologist, or someone who understands care management strategies in heart failure and can educate and promote optimal care by all team members.

Formal palliative and hospice care programs are especially beneficial if they can prevent repeated hospitalizations that are associated with a progressively declining quality of life in heart failure. Another benefit of palliative and hospice care is the attention to resuscitation preferences. In severe congestive heart failure, results from the SUPPORT project, which prospectively studied resuscitation preferences in patients who were admitted with exacerbation of severe heart failure, found that only 23% of patients stated that they did not want to be resuscitated. Physician perception differed from the patient's wishes in 24% of all cases.[96] Cardiopulmonary resuscitation (CPR) futility is not only considerable with regard to poor patient survival, it also is associated with substantial costs and places a large burden on our health-care system. It is important to specifically discuss the patient's CPR desires before they become critically ill and require hospitalization and then again after hospital discharge, since the SUPPORT project found that many patients who chose not to be resuscitated when hospitalized changed their minds within 2 months of discharge.[96] In the heart failure patient population, it is difficult to predict patient wishes and patient wishes are likely to change as their condition waxes and wanes. Hospice programs may mandate that patients are assigned a "do not resuscitate" status before they enter or on entry into their program; this may ultimately alleviate anxiety and worry associated with resuscitation preferences for both the patient and family.

Conclusion

The burden that heart failure places on the patient and his or her family, the health-care system, and society is tremendous. With the aging population, unfortunately, this burden is only growing with time. The most effective way of dealing with the future burden of heart failure is to prevent it altogether. Clinicians have to be aggressive in treating underlying heart failure-producing conditions. This is not always easy to do. It may be difficult to convince an asymptomatic patient with hypertension or hypercholesterolemia of the necessity of drug therapy. But this is the challenge that lies ahead.

Once heart failure develops, a variety of factors help determine prognosis. Therapeutic options such as ventricular assist device (VAD) and cardiac transplantation are only offered once the patient's risk of death from heart failure is felt to be worse than the risks associated with VADs and the complications associated with cardiac transplantation, such as long-term immunosuppression. Even if the patient is not deemed to be a candidate for these types of interventions, the clinician and the patient both need to be aware of the long-term prognosis so that a plan of care may be formulated.

Issues surrounding end-of-life care are often neglected until late in the course of heart failure. A significant proportion of patients succumb to sudden death, making it difficult to truly predict when end of life is near. However, a large number do die of progressive pump failure, requiring a shift in the treatment paradigm from therapy focused on cure to treatment focused on comfort.

Caring for heart failure patients truly represents a continuum encompassing those who are asymptomatic, across the varying degree of symptoms to those facing the specter of imminent death. Although challenging, it is this spectrum that makes treating patients with heart failure both intellectually and emotionally rewarding.

References

1. Scandinavian Simvastatin Survival Study Group. Randomized trial of cholesterol lowering in 4444 patients with coronary heart disease. *Lancet* 1994;344:1383–1389.
2. Sacks FM, Pfeffer MA, Moye LA, et al. The effect of pravastatin on coronary

events after myocardial infarction in patients with average cholesterol levels. *N Engl J Med* 1996;335:1001–1009.
3. LIPID Study Group. Prevention of cardiovascular events and death with pravastatin in patients with coronary heart disease and broad range of initial cholesterol levels. *N Engl J Med* 1998;339:1349–1357.
4. Shepard J, Cobbe SM, Ford I, et al. Prevention of coronary heart disease with pravastatin in men with hypercholesterolemia. *N Engl J Med* 1995;333:1301–1307.
5. Downs JR, Clearfield M, Weis S, et al. Primary prevention of acute coronary events with lovastatin in men and women with average cholesterol levels. *JAMA* 1998;279:1615–1622.
6. Teo KK, Burton JR, Buller CE, et al. Long-term effects of cholesterol lowering and angiotensin-converting enzyme inhibition on coronary atherosclerosis. The Simvastatin/Enalapril Coronary Atherosclerosis Trial (SCAT). *Circulation* 2000;102:1748–1754.
7. Joint National Committee on Prevention, Detection, Evaluation and Treatment of High Blood Pressure. The sixth report of the Joint National Committee on Prevention, Detection, Evaluation and Treatment of High Blood Pressure. *Arch Intern Med* 1997;157:2413–2446.
8. SHEP Cooperative Research Group. Prevention of stroke by antihypertensive drug treatment in older persons with isolated systolic hypertension: Final results of the Systolic Hypertension in the Elderly Program (SHEP). *JAMA* 1991;265:3255–3264.
9. Daholf B, Lindholm LH, Hansson L, et al. Morbidity and mortality in the Swedish Trial in Old Patients with Hypertension (STOP-Hypertension). *Lancet* 1991;338:1281–1285.
10. MRC Working Party. Medical Research Council trial of treatment of hypertension in older adults: principal results. *BMJ* 1992;304:405–412.
11. Messerli FH, Grossman E, Goldbourt U. Are β-blockers efficacious as first-line therapy for hypertension in the elderly? A systematic review. *JAMA* 1998;279:1903–1907.
12. SHEP Cooperative Research Group: Prevention of heart failure by antihypertensive drug treatment in older persons with isolated systolic hypertension. *JAMA* 1997;278:212–216.
13. Ofili EO, Cohen JD, St. Vrain JA, et al. Effect of treatment of isolated systolic hypertension on left ventricular mass. *JAMA* 1998;279:778–780.
14. The Heart Outcomes Prevention Evaluation Study Investigators. Effects of an angiotensin-converting-enzyme inhibitor, ramipril, on cardiovascular events in high risk patients. *N Engl J Med* 2000;342:145–153.
15. Lewis EJ, Hunsicker LG, Bain RP, Rhode RD. The effect of angiotensin-converting enzyme inhibition on diabetic nephropathy. *N Engl J Med* 1993; 329:1456–1462.
16. de Lorgeril M, Renaud S, Mamelle N, et al. Mediterranean alpha-linolenic acid-rich diet in secondary prevention of coronary heart disease. *Lancet* 1994;343:1454–1459.
17. Burr ML, Gilbert JF, Holliday RM, et al. Effects of changes in fat, fish and fiber intakes on death and myocardial reinfarction: diet and reinfarction trial (DART). *Lancet* 1989;ii:757–761.
18. Stephens NG, Parsons A, Schofield PM, et al. Randomized control trial of vitamin E in patients with coronary disease: Cambridge Heart Antioxidant Study. *Lancet* 1996;347:781–786.
19. Rapola JM, Virtamo J, Ripatti S, et al. Randomized trial of α-tocopherol and β-

carotene supplements on incidence of major coronary events in men with previous myocardial infarction. *Lancet* 1997;349:1715–1720.

20. GISSI-Prevenzione Investigators (Gruppo Italiano per lo Studio della Sopravvivenza nell'Infarto Miocardico). Dietary supplementation with n-3 polyunsaturated fatty acids and vitamin E after myocardial infarction: results of the GISSI-Prevenzione trial. *Lancet* 1999;354:447–455.
21. Graudal NA, Gallpe AM, Gared P. Effects of sodium restriction on blood pressure, renin, aldosterone, catecholamines, cholesterols, and triglyceride: A meta-analysis. *JAMA* 1998;279:1383–1391.
22. Midgley JP, Matthew AG, Greenwood CMT, et al. Effect of reduced dietary sodium on blood pressure: A meta-analysis of randomized controlled trials. *JAMA* 1996;275:1590–1597.
23. Hulley S, Grady D, Bush T, et al. Randomized trial of estrogen plus progestin for secondary prevention of coronary heart disease in postmenopausal women. *JAMA* 1998;280:605–613.
24. Foody J. Preventive cardiology. *Curr Opin Cardiol* 1999;14:382–391.
25. Antiplatelet Trialists' Collaboration. Collaborative overview of randomised trials of antiplatelet therapy, 1: Prevention of death, myocardial infarction, and stroke by prolonged antiplatelet therapy in various categories of patients. *BMJ* 1994;308:81–106.
26. Braunwald E, Zipes DP, Libby P, eds. *Heart Disease: A Textbook of Cardiovascular Medicine*. Philadelphia: Saunders, 2001:1168.
27. Roberts R, Rogers WJ, Mueller HS, et al. Immediate versus deferred betablockade following thrombolytic therapy in patients with acute myocardial infarction: Results of the Thrombolysis in Myocardial Infarction (TIMI) II-B study. *Circulation* 1991;83:422–437.
28. Yusef S, Zucker D, Peduzzi P, et al. Effect of coronary artery bypass grafts on survival: Overview of 10-year results from randomised trials by the Coronary Artery Bypass Graft Surgery Trialists collaboration. *Lancet* 1994;344: 563–570.
29. The Bypass Angioplasty Revascularization Investigation (BARI) Investigators. Comparison of coronary bypass surgery with angioplasty in patients with multivessel disease. *N Engl J Med* 1996:335:217–225.
30. Serruys PW, de Jaegere P, Kiemeneij F, et al. A comparison of balloon-expandable-stent implantation with balloon angioplasty in patients with coronary artery disease. *N Engl J Med* 1994;331:489–495.
31. Versaci F, Gaspardone A, Tomai F, et al. A comparison of coronary-artery stenting with angioplasty for isolated stenosis of the proximal left anterior descending coronary artery. *N Engl J Med* 1997;336:817–822.
32. Bax JJ, Poldermans D, Elhendy A, et al. Improvement of left ventricular ejection fraction, heart failure symptoms and prognosis after revascularization in patients with chronic coronary artery disease and viable myocardium detected by dobutamine stress echocardiography. *J Am Coll Cardiol* 1999; 34:163–169.
33. Bax JJ, Wijns W, Cornel JH, Visser FC, Boersma E, Fioretti PM. Accuracy of currently available techniques for prediction of functional recovery after revascularization in patients with left ventricular dysfunction due to chronic coronary artery disease: Comparison of pooled data. *J Am Coll Cardiol* 1997; 30:1451–1460.
34. Gioia G, Powers J, Heo J, Iskandrian AS. Prognostic value of rest-redistribution tomographic thallium-201 imaging in ischemic cardiomyopathy. *Am J Cardiol* 1995;75:759–762.

35. Braunwald E, Zipes DP, Libby P, eds. *Heart Disease: A Textbook of Cardiovascular Medicine.* Philadelphia: Saunders, 2001:1317.
36. Adams KF, Dunlap SH, Sueta CA, et al. Relation between gender, etiology and survival in patients with symptomatic heart failure. *J Am Coll Cardiol* 1996;28:1781–1788.
37. Franciosa JA, Wilen M, Ziesche S, Cohn JN. Survival in men with severe chronic left ventricular failure due to either coronary heart disease or idiopathic dilated cardiomyopathy. *Am J Cardiol* 1983;51:831–836.
38. Bart BA, Shaw LK, McCants CB, et al. Clinical determinants of mortality in patients with angiographically diagnosed ischemic or nonischemic cardiomyopathy. *J Am Coll Cardiol* 1997;30:1002–1008.
39. Yusuf S. Effect of enalapril on survival in patients with reduced left ventricular ejection fractions and congestive heart failure. *N Engl J Med* 1991;325:293–302.
40. Johnson G, Carson P, Francis GS, et al. Influence of prerandomization (baseline) variables on mortality and on the reduction of mortality by enalapril. Veterans Affairs Cooperative Study on Vasodilator Therapy of Heart Failure (V-HeFT II). *Circulation* 1993;87(suppl VI):VI32–VI39.
41. Swedberg K, Kjekshus J. Effects of enalapril on mortality in severe congestive heart failure: Results of the Cooperative North Scandinavian Enalapril Survival Study (CONSENSUS). *Am J Cardiol* 1988;62:60A–66A.
42. Gradman A, Deedwania P, Cody R, et al. Predictors of total mortality and sudden death in mild to moderate heart failure. *J Am Coll Cardiol* 1989;14: 564–570.
43. Scruntinio D, Napoli V, Passantino A, et al. Low-dose dobutamine responsiveness in idiopathic dilated cardiomyopathy: relation to exercise capacity and clinical outcome. *Eur Heart J* 2000;21: 927–934.
44. Williams MJ, Odabashian J, Lauer MS, et al. Prognostic value of dobutamine echocardiography in patients with left ventricular dysfunction. *J Am Coll Cardiol* 1996;27:132–139.
45. Kamthorn SL, Marwick TH, Cook SA, et al. Prognosis of patients with left ventricular dysfunction, with and without viable myocardium after myocardial infarction. *Circulation* 1994;90:2687–2694.
46. Pozzoli M, Traversi E, Cioffi G, et al. Loading manipulations improve the prognostic value of Doppler evaluation of mitral flow in patients with chronic heart failure. *Circulation* 1996;95:1222–1230.
47. Saxon LA, Stevenson WG, Middlekauff JR, et al. Predicting death from progressive heart failure secondary to ischemic or idiopathic dilated cardiomyopathy. *Am J Cardiol* 1993;72:62–65.
48. Morley D, Brozena SC. Assessing risk by hemodynamic profile in patients awaiting cardiac transplantation. *Am J Cardiol* 1994;73:379–383.
49. Dargie HJ, Cleland JGF, Leckie BJ, et al. Relation of arrhythmias and electrolyte abnormalities to survival in patients with severe chronic heart failure. *Circulation* 1987;75:IV98–IV107.
50. Wong M, Johnson G, Shabetai R, et al. Echocardiographic variables as prognostic indicators and therapeutic monitors in chronic congestive hart failure: Veterans Affairs Cooperative Studies V-HeFT I and II. *Circulation* 1993;87:V 165–170.
51. Lee TH, Hamilton MA, Stevenson LW, et al. Impact of left ventricular cavity size on survival in advance heart failure. *Am J Cardiol* 1993;72:672–676.
52. Madsen BK, Videbaek R, Stokholm H, et al. Prognostic value of echocardio-

graphy in 190 patients with chronic congestive heart failure. *Cardiology* 1996; 87:250–256.
53. Keogh AM, Baron DW, Hickie JB. Prognostic guides in patients with idiopathic or ischemic cardiomyopathy assessed for cardiac transplantation. *Am J Cardiol* 1990;65:903–908.
54. Cintron G, Johnson G, Francis G, et al. Prognostic significance of serial changes in left ventricular ejection fraction in patients with congestive heart failure. *Circulation* 1993;87(suppl VI):VI17–VI23.
55. Ghio S, Gavazzi A, Campana C, et al. Independent and additive prognostic value of right ventricular systolic function and pulmonary artery pressure in patients with congestive heart failure. *J Am Coll Cardiol* 2001;37:183–188.
56. Polak JF, Holman L, Wynne J, et al. Right ventricular ejection fraction: an indicator of increase mortality in patients with congestive heart failure associated with coronary artery disease. *J Am Coll Cardiol* 1983;2:217–224.
57. DiSalvo TG, Mathier M, Semigran MJ, Dec GW. Preserved right ventricular ejection fraction predicts exercise capacity and survival in advanced heart failure. *J Am Coll Cardiol* 1995;25:1143–1153.
58. Lee WH, Packer M. Prognostic importance of serum sodium concentration and its modification by converting-enzyme inhibition in patients with severe chronic heart failure. *Circulation* 1986;73:257–267.
59. Cohn JN, Levine B, Olivari MT, et al. Plasma norepinephrine as a guide to prognosis in patients with chronic congestive heart failure. *N Engl J Med* 1984;311:819–823.
60. Francis GS, Cohn JN, Johnson G, et al. Plasma norepinephrine, plasma renin activity, and congestive heart failure: Relations to survival and the effects of therapy in V-HeFT II. *Circulation* 1993;87(suppl VI):VI40–VI48.
61. Gottlieb SS, Kukin ML, Ahern D, Packer M. Prognostic importance of atrial natriuretic peptide in patients with chronic heart failure. *J Am Coll Cardiol* 1989;13:1534–1539.
62. Yu CM, Sanderson JE. Plasma brain natriuretic peptide: An independent predictor of cardiovascular mortality in acute heart failure. *Eur J Heart Fail* 1999; 1:59–65.
63. Pousset F, Isnard R, Lechat P, et al. Plasma endothelin-1 is a strong prognostic marker in chronic heart failure. *Eur Heart J* 1997;18:254–258.
64. Swedberg K, Eneroth P, Kjekshus J, et al. Hormones regulating cardiovascular function in patients with severe congestive heart failure and their relationship to mortality. *Circulation* 1990;82:1730–1736.
65. Cohn JN, Archibald DG, Ziesche S, et al. Effect of vasodilator therapy on mortality in chronic congestive heart failure: Results of a Veterans Administration Cooperative Study. *N Engl J Med* 1986;314:1547–1552.
66. Stevenson LW, Tillisch JH, Hamilton M, et al. Importance of hemodynamic response to therapy in predicting survival with ejection fraction ≤20% secondary to ischemic or nonischemic cardiomyopathy. *Am J Cardiol* 1990;66: 1348–1354.
67. Mancini DM, Eisen H, Kussmaul W, et al. Value of peak exercise oxygen consumption for optimal timing of cardiac transplantation in ambulatory patients with heart failure. *Circulation* 1991;83:778–786.
68. Osman AF, Mehra MR, Lavie CJ, et al. The incremental prognostic importance of body fat adjusted peak oxygen consumption in chronic heart failure. *J Am Coll Cardiol* 2000;36:2126–2131.
69. Richards DR, Mehra MR, Ventura HO, et al. Usefulness of peak oxygen consumption in prediction outcome of heart failure in women versus men. *Am J Cardiol* 1997;80:1236–1238.

70. Francis DP, Shmim W, Davies LC, et al. Cardiopulmonary exercise testing for prognosis in chronic heart failure: Continuous and independent prognostic value form V_E/V_{CO_2} and peak V_{O_2}. *Eur Heart J* 2000;21:154–161.
71. Robbins M, Francis G, Pashkow FJ, et al. Ventilatory and heart rate responses to exercise: Better predictors of heart failure mortality than peak oxygen consumption. *Circulation* 1999;100:2411–2417.
72. Middlekauf HR, Stevenson WG, Stevenson LW. Prognostic significance of atrial fibrillation in advanced heart failure. *Circulation* 1991;84:40–48.
73. Carson PE, Johnson GR, Dunkman B, et al. The influence of atrial fibrillation on prognosis in mild to moderate heart failure. The V-HeFT studies. *Circulation* 1993;87(suppl VI):VI102–VI110.
74. Mahoney P, Kimmel S, DeNofrio D, et al. Prognostic significance of atrial fibrillation in patients at a tertiary medical center referred for heart transplantation because of severe heart failure. *Am J Cardiol* 1999;83:1544–1547.
75. Reese DB, Silverman ME, Gold MR, Gottlieb SS. Prognostic importance of the length of ventricular tachycardia in patients with nonischaemic congestive heart failure. *Am Heart J* 1995;130:489–493.
76. De Maria R, Gavazzi A, Caroli A, et al. Ventricular arrhythmias in dilated cardiomyopathy as an independent prognostic hallmark. *Am J Cardiol* 1992;69: 1451–1457.
77. Wilson JR, Schwartz JS, St. John Sutton M, et al. Prognosis in severe heart failure: relation to hemodynamic measurements and ventricular ectopic activity. *J Am Coll Cardiol* 1983:403–410.
78. Teerlink JR, Jalaluddin M, Ander S, et al. Ambulatory ventricular arrhythmias in patients with heart failure do not specifically predict an increase risk of sudden death. *Circulation* 2000;101:40–46.
79. Buxton AE, Lee KL, Fisher JD, et al. A randomized study of the prevention of sudden death in patients with coronary artery disease. *N Engl J Med* 1999;341: 1882–1890.
80. Moss AJ, Hall WJ, Cannom DS, et al. Improved survival with an implanted defibrillator in patients with coronary artery disease at high risk for ventricular arrhythmia. *N Engl J Med* 1996;335:1933–1940.
81. Anasasiou-Nana MI, Nanas JN, Karagounis LA, et al. Relation of dispersion of QRS and QT in patients with advanced congestive heart failure due to cardiac and sudden death mortality. *Am J Cardiol* 2000;85:1212–1217.
82. Klingenheben T, Zabel M, D'Agostino RB, et al. Predictive value of T-wave alternans for arrhythmic events in patients with congestive heart failure. *Lancet* 2000;356:651–652.
83. National Hospice Organization. *Hospice Care: A Physician's Guide.* Arlington, VA: National Hospice Organization, 1998:43–44.
84. Lynn J, Harrell F, Cohn F, Wagner D, Connors AF. Prognoses of seriously ill hospitalized patients on the days before death: implications for patient care and public policy. *New Horiz* 1997;5:56–61.
85. American College of Cardiology/American Heart Association Task Force. ACC/AHA guidelines for the evaluation and management of chronic heart failure in the adult: executive summary. *J Am Coll Cardiol* 2001;38:2101–2113.
86. Alla F, Briancon S, Juilliere Y, et al. Differential clinical prognostic classifications in dilated and ischemic advanced heart failure: The EPICAL study. *Am Heart J* 2000;139:895–904.
87. World Health Organization. *Cancer Pain Relief.* Geneva: World Health Organization, 1997.
88. Bruera E, Bylock I. End-of-life care: Management of pain and discomfort. *Patient Care* 2000;34(21):38–40, 49–50, 52, 55–56, 59–62, 65, 69–71.

89. Heart Failure Society of America. HFSA guidelines for management of patients with heart failure caused by left ventricular systolic dysfunction: Pharmacological approaches. *J Card Fail* 1999;5:357–382.
90. Larson DG, Tobin DR. End-of-life conversations: Evolving practice and theory. *JAMA* 2000;284:1573–1578.
91. Buckman R, Byock I, Fry VL. End-of-life care: Talking with patients and families. *Patient Care* 2000;34(21):16–18, 20, 29, 33–36.
92. Lynn J, Teno JM, Phillips RS, et al. Perceptions of family members of the dying experience of older and seriously ill patients. *Ann Intern Med* 1997;126:97–106.
93. Levenson JW, McCarthy EP, Lynn J, et al. The last six months of life for patients with congestive heart failure. *J Am Geriatr Soc* 2000;48:S101–S109.
94. Emanuel E, Goold SD, Hammes BJ, et al. End-of-life care: A detailed examination of advance directives. *Patient Care* 2000;34(21):92–94, 97–98, 101–102, 105–108.
95. Caloras D, Coloney M, Kangas CA, et al. End-of-life care: The virtues of hospice. *Patient Care* 2000;34(21):72–74, 76–78, 80–81, 85–91.
96. Krumholz HM, Phillips RS, Hamel MB, et al. Resuscitation preferences among patients with severe congestive heart failure: Results from the SUPPORT Project. *Circulation* 1998;98:648–655.

Chapter 12

Surgical Management of Heart Failure

David Zeltsman, MD and Michael A. Acker, MD

Cardiac failure remains the leading cause of death in the United States, affecting more than 5 million people, with greater than 700,000 deaths annually. Approximately a third of heart failure patients are in New York Heart Association (NYHA) class III/IV. The cost of caring for these patients is growing and approaches $50 billion per year.

Traditionally, heart failure has been thought secondary to impaired left ventricular pump performance. According to this view, systolic dysfunction is secondary to contractile failure. Recently, a new view of heart failure has been developed where systolic dysfunction is thought secondary to a structural increase in ventricular chamber volume. Instead of contractile failure leading to chamber dilatation, chamber dilatation occurs as an early response that results in decreased wall motion that is mandated to generate a normal stroke volume from a larger end-diastolic volume. *Remodeling* is the term used to refer to the pathologic change in chamber length and shape not related to a preload-mandated increase in sarcomere length. As the heart remodels and dilates, the radius of curvature increases, increasing wall tension, leading to increased myocardial oxygen consumption, decreased subendocardial blood flow, impaired energetics and increased arrhythmias. Overall, poor prognosis directly correlates with the degree of remodeling.[1]

According to this view, remodeling, not contractile failure, is the key to the severity of depression of ejection fraction and poor prognosis. The process has also been shown to be reversible. Current therapies that improve mortality, such as angiotensin-converting enzyme inhibitors and new-generation beta-blockers, can inhibit progressive chamber remodeling and improve survival. In these studies, beta-blockers and

From: Jessup M, McCauley KM (eds). *Heart Failure: Providing Optimal Care*. Elmsford, NY: Futura, an imprint of Blackwell Publishing; ©2003.

angiotensin-converting enzyme (ACE) inhibitors consistently improved left ventricular function and long-term outcomes and significantly decreased all-cause hospitalization rate and mortality. Further data suggest that survival benefits attributed to ACE inhibitors and beta-blockers can be attributed to the reversed remodeling properties of these drug groups.[2–12]

Nevertheless, despite the significant advances in the pharmacological support of failing heart, the results remain far from perfect. The mortality continues to be high and hospitalization costly. There is a growing understanding that old—as well as new and evolving—surgical therapies, which in the past were contraindicated for the failing heart, can be used successfully to impact on the process of ventricular remodeling and improve cardiac function.

Cardiac transplantation remains the gold standard of surgical therapies for advanced and end-stage heart failure. However, the Achilles heel of heart transplantation is the persistent and worsening shortage of organ donors. Only approximately 2000 heart transplants are done each year in the United States. Although 4296 patients were on the United Network for Organ Sharing (UNOS) national patient waiting list as of April 2001, only 49% will proceed to heart transplantation.[13–15] Despite its success, transplantation is epidemiologically trivial. It will remain a very limited option that trades one disease for another and can only be applied to a small number of patients who potentially could benefit. Therefore, an aggressive search must be made for alternative surgical management of end-stage heart disease.

The most frequently reported indication for heart transplantation in the United States is coronary artery disease, accounting for 44.6% of the patients.[13] Surgical revascularization for patients with ejection fractions less than 20%, to recruit hibernating myocardium, is becoming commonplace.[16] These patients are generally more sick, with more perioperative risk factors and, though having increased hospital mortality of approximately 4%–6%,[17] they enjoy 90% and 64% survival at 1 and 5 years, respectively.[17] Patients with ischemic cardiomyopathy, evidence of viable myocardium, and presence of bypassable vessels can be revascularized with permissible risk, achieving 88% perioperative survival, with 72% of the patients alive at 1 year. These results are reproducible and have been reported by different authors.[18–21]

Mitral valve repair for both primary and secondary severe mitral regurgitation in dilated cardiomyopathic ventricles with ejection fraction less than 30% is being actively pursued. Mitral insufficiency is an important complication of dilative cardiomyopathy resulting from enlargement of the mitral annular ventricular apparatus, with ensuing loss of valve leaflet coaptation.[22–24] As the annular dilation progresses, centrally located functional regurgitant jet develops, despite structural preservation of chordal and papillary muscle complex.[24] Ischemic mitral regurgitation appears to be more complex and is multifactorial, resulting from deformational changes in the ventricular geometry, annular dilatation, and papillary muscle dysfunction. Often, the posterior leaflet becomes functionally restricted as a result of ventricular enlargement. In patients with significant (>2+) secondary mitral regurgitation, mitral valve repair should be considered in NYHA class III/IV patients with dilated cardiomyopathies. Bolling and coworkers have demonstrated operative mortality <5%, with significant improvement in NYHA class symptoms, as well as good survival rates at 1 and 2 years.[23,24] The annuloplasty is performed with a complete ring and undersizing the mitral annulus and offers effective correction of mitral regurgitation in heart failure patients. The procedure is well tolerated, and the elimination of mitral regurgitation contributes to reversed remodeling, with restoration of elliptical left ventricular contour and decreased sphericity.[24] If mitral valve repair is not possible, it is essential that mitral valve replacement be performed with retention of the subchordal attachments. Preservation of both the anterior and posterior chorded attachments to the papillary muscles helps to maintain normal ventricular geometry and function following mitral valve replacement.[25–28]

The concept of surgically reversing the remodeling process—partial left ventriculectomy—for patients with class IV idiopathic dilated cardiomyopathies was introduced by Batista in 1996. He described an operation in which normal muscle between the anterior and posterior papillary muscles is resected along with mitral valve repair/replacement, to restore the ventricle to a more normal volume–mass–diameter relationship. The reduction in ventricular diameter, according to Laplace's law, results in decreased ventricular wall tension and thus improved systolic performance.[29,30] Although many patients improved markedly, perioperative mortality was high (>20%) in many reports. In the largest and best-controlled series, from the Cleveland Clinic, perioperative mortality was only 3.2%, but 16% required left ventricular assist devices following the procedure. Many patients improved to allow removal from the transplant list, but freedom from death, need for left ventricular assist device (LVAD), need for transplant, or return to class IV heart failure symptoms amounted to 50% and 37% at 1 and 2 years. After initial success, many patients would redilate.[31,32] Overall enthusiasm for the procedure has waned. Selection criteria need to improve before the role of partial left ventriculectomy for end-stage heart failure patients can be determined.

Direct surgical restoration of left ventricular geometry, with reduction in left ventricular size, has evolved over the last few years from partial left ventriculectomy to a modification of the Dor procedure for left ventricular aneurysm,[33] known as endoventricular circular patch plasty or surgical ventricular restoration (SVR). This procedure is considered for patients with ischemic cardiomyopathies with status post large anterior wall myocardial infarctions resulting in dilated spherical left ventricles associated with an area of anterior akinesia or dyskinesia. An endoventricular Dacron patch is used to exclude akinetic or dyskinetic portions of the anterior wall and septum, to restore a more normal size and shape to the left ventricle. This then results in more normal ventricular geometry (an elliptical instead of a spherical ventricle) and improved systolic performance. A recent report on the results of this procedure in 586 patients, combined usually with coronary artery bypass grafting, reported an overall mortality of 7.7%. The left ventricular and systolic volume index decreased from 98 ± 95 to 64 ± 40 mL/m^2, while left ventricular ejection function improved from 29.5% to 40% postoperatively.[34–36] Carefully controlled studies need to be performed to determine if decreased ventricular size results in diastolic compromise, if the increase in ejection fraction in smaller ventricles translates to an increase stroke volume, and whether further remodeling occurring after the operation limits its overall long-term success.[36] A National Institutes of Health-sponsored multicentered randomized trial is planned for patients with heart failure and coronary artery disease amenable to surgical revascularization. In patients with reported left ventricular dysfunction, surgical ventricular restoration (SVR) and surgical revascularization will be randomized to either surgical revascularization alone or to surgical revascularization and SVR, to determine its impact on cardiac function and overall survival.

Recently, new girdling devices to limit or to reverse ventricular remodeling have been evaluated. Lessons learned from the clinical experience with dynamic cardiomyoplasty revealed that much of its benefit was derived from the girdling effect of the muscle wrap, and not from an increase in stroke volume as originally conceived. The prosthetic external constraint CardioCor (Acorn Cardiovascular, Inc.) is currently under active clinical investigation, based on the belief that heart failure is primarily the result of ongoing ventricular remodeling. Preclinical evaluation in canine models of chronic dilated cardiomyopathy and heart failure have demonstrated a halting or reversal of ventricular remodeling and preservation or improved cardiac function. In addition, improved myocyte contraction and relaxation, enhance inotropic response, as well as altered gene expression, have been demonstrated.[37–42] In over 60 patients who have had the Acorn jacket placed in Europe, no evidence of coronary or ventricular constriction has been seen for up to 2 years.[43] Currently, a randomized, prospective, multicenter phase-2 Food and Drug Administration (FDA) study is underway in patients with NYHA class III heart failure comparing the efficacy of the Acorn jacket in dilated left ventricles with and without mitral insufficiency. Recently, in a chronic animal model of heart failure following acute myocardial infarction, placement of the Acorn jacket following the infarction prevented further ventricular remodeling in comparison with control animals at 2 months. Further ventricular dilatation was halted, infarct size was decreased, and systolic function was improved. In this model, the Acorn jacket was effective in preventing the progression of heart failure due to acute myocardial infarction.[44,45] In the future, this device or something similar may be used prophylactically in patients with large myocardial infarctions, to prevent subsequent remodeling and heart failure.

Mechanical ventricular assistance as a bridge to transplantation is an established therapy. A 70% success to transplantation after implantation of a left ventricular assist device can be expected. The TCI HeartMate is the most successful device, with the lowest incidence of stroke, despite patients being managed on only one aspirin daily. Patients can be sent home to wait for a suitable heart to become available. These devices allow patients in cardiogenic shock, from a variety of causes, not only to live but to be mobile and rehabilitated prior to their transplant. The expert use of a variety of different ventricular assist devices for left, right, and biventricular support is mandatory for any cardiac transplant center today.[46–49]

Recently, there have been a number of published reports of prolonged (weeks to months) left ventricular assist device support used as a bridge to recovery. Muller and colleagues report a number of patients with dilated cardiomyopathy improving after weeks to months of left ventricular unloading.[50] Others feel that this approach in patients with chronic heart failure is very unpredictable and rarely successful.[51] In patients presenting with fulminant acute myocarditis, however, such support has been particularly successful, resulting in full cardiac recovery in many cases.[52,53]

The success of the TCI HeartMate as a bridge to transplantation has led to its consideration as a permanent or destination device. This is currently being studied in class IV patients who are not transplant candidates in a multicenter, prospective, randomized study (the Randomized Evaluation of Mechanical Assistance in the Treatment of Congestive Heart Failure, REMATCH).[54] Although this study is still ongoing, the Achilles heel of this and other present-day devices may turn out to be a high incidence of infection—in the drive line, exit site, pump pocket, or true endocarditis. Until this complication is drastically reduced, these devices cannot be considered for permanent placement.

A new generation of assist devices will soon be entering initial phase 1 and 2 studies. Axial flow pumps (HeartMate II, DeBakey, Jarvik) have been developed that are tiny compared to present general pulsatile pumps, while still capable of up to 10 L of flow. The LionHeart (Arrow International), currently undergoing phase-1 FDA evaluation, is a destination device that is a totally intracorporeal left ventricular assist device powered by transcutaneous energy transmission, with no drive line crossing the skin. Within the very near future, total artificial hearts (Abiocor, Abiomed) will also be entering clinical trials.[55,56]

In summary, an aggressive approach to surgical revascularization, correction of mitral insufficiency, or reversal of left ventricular remodeling by new girdling devices, or directly by the Dor procedure in end-stage heart failure, should be considered in any patient who has exhausted current pharmacologic therapy. The development and clinical use of a new generation of totally intracorporeal assist devices, permanently implanted in patients with end-stage heart failure who are not transplant candidates—overcoming present-day problems of thromboembolism, infection, and large size—will be a clinical reality within the near future.

References

1. Cohn JN. Structural basis for heart failure. *Circulation* 1995;91:2504–2507.
2. Pfeffer MA, Braunwald E, Moye LA, et al. Effect of captopril on mortality and morbidity in patients with left ventricular dysfunction after myocardial infarction: Results of the survival and ventricular enlargement trial. The SAVE Investigators. *N Engl J Med* 1992;327:669–677.
3. The Acute Infarction Ramipril Efficacy (AIRE) Study Investigators. Effects of ramipril on mortality and morbidity of survivors of acute myocardial infarction with clinical evidence of heart failure. *Lancet* 1993;342:821–828.
4. Kober L, Torp-Pedersen C, Carlsen JE, et al. A clinical trial of the angiotensin-converting enzyme inhibitor trandolapril in patients with left ventricular dysfunction after myocardial infarction. Trandolapril Cardiac Evaluation (TRACE) Study Group. *N Engl J Med* 1995;21;333:1670–1681.
5. CIBIS Investigators and Committee. A randomized trial of beta-blockade in heart failure: the Cardiac Insufficiency Bisoprolol Study (CIBIS). *Circulation* 1994;94:1765–1773.
6. CIBIS II Investigators and Committees. The Cardiac Insufficiency Bisoprolol Study (CIBIS II): a randomized trial. *Lancet* 1999;353:9–13.
7. MERIT-HF Study Group. Effects of metoprolol CR/XL in chronic heart failure: metoprolol CR/XL randomized trial in congestive heart failure. *Lancet* 1999;353:2001–2007.
8. Packer M, Bristow MR, Cohn JN, et al. The effect of carvedilol on morbidity and mortality in patients with chronic heart failure. U.S. Carvedilol Heart Failure Study Group. *N Engl J Med* 1996;334:1349–1355.
9. Yancy CW, Fowler MB, Colucci WS, et al. Race and the response to adrenergic blockade with carvedilol in patients with chronic heart failure. U.S. Carvedilol Heart Failure Study Group. *N Engl J Med* 2001;344:1358–1365.
10. Aikawa Y, Rohde L, Plehn J, et al. Regional wall stress predicts ventricular remodeling after anteroseptal myocardial infarction in the Healing and Early Afterload Reducing Trial (HEART): an echocardiography-based structural analysis. *Am Heart J* 2001;141:234–242.
11. Konstam MA, Kronenberg MW, et al. Effects of the angiotensin-converting enzyme inhibitor enalapril on the long-term progression of left ventricular

dilatation in patients with asymptomatic systolic dysfunction. SOLVD (Studies of Left Ventricular Dysfunction) Investigators. *Circulation* 1993;88:2277–2283.

12. Australia/New Zealand Heart Failure Research Collaborative Group. Randomized, placebo-controlled trial of carvedilol in patients with congestive heart failure due to ischemic heart disease. *Lancet* 1997;349:375–380.
13. Keck BM, Bennett LE, Rosendale J, Daily OP, Novick RJ, Hosenpud JD. Worldwide thoracic organ transplantation: A report from the UNOS/ISHLT International Registry for Thoracic Organ Transplantation. *Clin Transpl* 1999: 35–49.
14. U.S. Scientific Registry of Transplant Recipients and the Organ Procurement and Transplantation Network. 2000 Annual Report: Transplant Data 1989–2000. Rockville, MD/Richmond, VA: HHS/HRSA/OSP/DOT and UNOS (http://www.unos.org/Data/anrpt_main.htm).
15. Transplant Patient Data Source (May 11, 2001). Richmond, VA: United Network for Organ Sharing (http://www.patients.unos.org/data.htm).
16. Pagano D, Bonser RS, Camici PG. Myocardial revascularization for the treatment of postischemic heart failure. *Curr Opin Cardiol* 1999;14:506–509.
17. Trachiotis GD, Weintraub WS, Johnston TS, Jones EL, Guyton RA, Craver JM. Coronary artery bypass grafting in patients with advanced left ventricular dysfunction. *Ann Thorac Surg* 1998;66:1632–1639.
18. Dreyfus GD, Duboc D, Blasco A, et al. Myocardial viability assessment in ischemic cardiomyopathy: benefits of coronary revascularization. *Ann Thorac Surg* 1994;57:1402–1407.
19. Tjan TD, Kondruweit M, Scheld HH, et al. The bad ventricle: Revascularization versus transplantation. *Thorac Cardiovasc Surg* 2000;48:9–14.
20. Lansman SL, Cohen M, Galla JD, et al. Coronary bypass with ejection fraction of 0.20 or less using centigrade cardioplegia: long-term follow-up. *Ann Thorac Surg* 1993;56:480–485.
21. Kaul TK, Agnihotri AK, Fields BL, Riggins LS, Wyatt DA, Jones CR. Coronary artery bypass grafting in patients with an ejection fraction of twenty percent or less. *J Thorac Cardiovasc Surg* 1996;111:1001–1012.
22. Hendren WG, Nemec JJ, Lytle BW, et al. Mitral valve repair for ischemic mitral insufficiency. *Ann Thorac Surg* 1991;52:1246–1251.
23. Bolling SF, Pagani FD, Deeb GM, Bach DS. Intermediate-term outcome of mitral reconstruction in cardiomyopathy. *J Thorac Cardiovasc Surg* 1998;115:381–386.
24. Smolens IA, Pagani FD, Bolling SF. Mitral valve repair in heart failure. *Eur J Heart Fail* 2000;2:365–371.
25. Sintek CF, Pfeffer TA, Kochamba G, Fletcher A, Khonsari S. Preservation of normal left ventricular geometry during mitral valve replacement. *J Heart Valve Dis* 1995;4:471–475.
26. Sarris GE, Cahill PD, Hansen DE, Derby GC, Miller DC. Restoration of left ventricular systolic performance after reattachment of the mitral chordae tendineae: The importance of valvular–ventricular interaction. *J Thorac Cardiovasc Surg* 1988;95:969–979.
27. Natsuaki M, Itoh T, Tomita S, et al. Importance of preserving the mitral subvalvular apparatus in mitral valve replacement. *Ann Thorac Surg* 1996;61: 585–590.
28. Komeda M, David TE, Rao V, Sun Z, Weisel RD, Burns RJ. Late hemodynamic effects of the preserved papillary muscles during mitral valve replacement. *Circulation* 1994;90:II190–194.
29. Batista RJ, Santos JL, Takeshita N, Bocchino L, Lima PN, Cunha MA. Partial

left ventriculectomy to improve left ventricular function in end-stage heart disease. *J Card Surg* 1996;11:96–97.

30. Batista RJ, Verde J, Nery P, et al. Partial left ventriculectomy to treat end-stage heart disease. *Ann Thorac Surg* 1997;64:634–638.
31. McCarthy JF, McCarthy PM, Starling RC, et al. Partial left ventriculectomy and mitral valve repair for end-stage congestive heart failure. *Eur J Cardiothorac Surg* 1998;13:337–343.
32. Etoch SW, Koenig SC, Laureano MA, Cerrito P, Gray LA, Dowling RD. Results after partial left ventriculectomy versus heart transplantation for idiopathic cardiomyopathy. *J Thorac Cardiovasc Surg* 1999;117:952–959.
33. Dor V, Saab M, Coste P, Kornaszewska M, Montiglio F. Left ventricular aneurysm: a new surgical approach. *Thorac Cardiovasc Surg* 1989;37:11–19.
34. Athanasuleas CL, Stanley AW Jr, Buckberg GD, Dor V, DiDonato M, Blackstone EH. Surgical anterior ventricular endocardial restoration (SAVER) in the dilated remodeled ventricle after anterior myocardial infarction. RESTORE group. Reconstructive Endoventricular Surgery, returning Torsion Original Radius Elliptical Shape to the LV. *J Am Coll Cardiol* 2001;37:1199–1209.
35. Dor V, Sabatier M, Di Donato M, Montiglio F, Toso A, Maioli M. Efficacy of endoventricular patch plasty in large postinfarction akinetic scar and severe left ventricular dysfunction: comparison with a series of large dyskinetic scars. *J Thorac Cardiovasc Surg* 1998;116:50–59.
36. Di Donato M, Sabatier M, Dor V, et al. Effects of the Dor procedure on left ventricular dimension and shape and geometric correlates of mitral regurgitation one year after surgery. *J Thorac Cardiovasc Surg* 2001;121:91–96.
37. Sabbah HN, Sharov VG, Chaudhry PA, Suzuki G, Todor A, Morita H. Chronic therapy with the Acorn Cardiac Support Device in dogs with chronic heart failure: three and six months hemodynamic, histologic and ultrastructural findings [abstract]. *J Heart Lung Transplant* 2001;20:189.
38. Sabbah HN, Gupta RC, Sharov VG, et al. Prevention of progressive left ventricular dilation with the Acorn Cardiac Support Device down regulates stretch-response proteins and improves sarcoplasmic reticulum recycling in dogs with chronic heart failure [abstract]. *J Am Coll Cardiol* 2001;37(suppl A):474A.
39. Saavedra F, Tunin R, Mishima T, et al. Reverse remodeling and enhanced adrenergic reserve from a passive external ventricular support in experimental dilated heart failure [abstract]. *Circulation* 2000;102(suppl):501.
40. Sabbah HN, Gupta RC, Sharov VG, et al. Prevention of progressive left ventricular dilation with the Acorn Cardiac Support Device (CSD) down regulates stretch-mediated p21ras, attenuates myocyte hypertrophy and improves sarcoplasmic reticulum calcium cycling in dogs with heart failure [abstract]. *Circulation* 2000;102(suppl): 683.
41. Chaudry PA, Mishima T, Sharov VG, et al. Passive epicardial containment prevents ventricular remodeling in heart failure. *Ann Thor Surg* 2000;70: 1275–1280.
42. Gupta RC, Sharov VG, Mishra S, Todor A, Sabbah HN. Chronic therapy with the Acorn Cardiac Support Device (CSD) attenuates cardiomyocyte apoptosis in dogs with heart failure [abstract]. *J Am Coll Cardiol* 2001; 37(suppl A):478A.
43. Kleber FX, Sonntag S, Krebs H, Stantke K, Konertz W. Follow-up on passive cardiomyoplasty in congestive heart failure: influence on the Acorn Cardiac

Support Device on left ventricular function [abstract]. *J Am Coll Cardiol* 2001;37(suppl A):143A.

44. Pilla JJ, Brockman DJ, Blom AS, et al. Prevention of dilatation using the Acorn cardiac support devise (CSD) results in reversed remodeling and improvement of function [poster]. American Heart Association, Scientific Session 2001, Anaheim, CA, November 2001.
45. Pilla JJ, Blom AS, Brockman DJ, et al. Ventricular constraint using the Acorn cardiac support device (CSD) limits infarct expansion [poster]. American Heart Association, Scientific Session 2001, Anaheim, CA, November 2001.
46. Goldstein DJ, Oz MC. Mechanical support for postcardiotomy cardiogenic shock. *Semin Thorac Cardiovasc Surg* 2000;12:220–228.
47. McCarthy PM, Portner PM, Tobler HG, Starnes VA, Ramasamy N, Oyer PE. Clinical experience with the Novacor ventricular assist system: Bridge to transplantation and the transition to permanent application. *J Thorac Cardiovasc Surg* 1991;102:578–586.
48. Levin HR, Chen JM, Oz MC, et al. Potential of left ventricular assist devices as outpatient therapy while awaiting transplantation. *Ann Thorac Surg* 1994;58: 1515–1520.
49. Sun BC, Catanese KA, Spanier TB, et al. 100 long-term implantable left ventricular assist devices: the Columbia Presbyterian interim experience. *Ann Thorac Surg* 1999;68:688–694.
50. Muller J, Wallukat G, Weng YG, et al. Weaning from mechanical cardiac support in patients with idiopathic dilated cardiomyopathy. *Circulation* 1997;15: 96:542–549.
51. Mancini DM, Beniaminovitz A, Levin H, et al. Low incidence of myocardial recovery after left ventricular assist device implantation in patients with chronic heart failure. *Circulation* 1998;98:2383–2389.
52. McCarthy RE, Boehmer JP, Hruban RH, et al. Long-term outcome of fulminant myocarditis as compared with acute (nonfulminant) myocarditis, *N Engl J Med* 2000;342:690–695.
53. Acker MA. Mechanical circulatory support for patients with acute/fulminant myocarditis. *Ann Thorac Surg* 2001;71(3 suppl):S73–76; discussion S82–85.
54. Rose EA, Moskowitz AJ, Packer M, et al. The REMATCH trial: rationale, design, and end points. Randomized Evaluation of Mechanical Assistance for the Treatment of Congestive Heart Failure. *Ann Thorac Surg* 1999;67:723–730.
55. Mann DL, Willerson JT. Left ventricular assist devices and the failing heart: A bridge to recovery, a permanent assist device, or a bridge too far? *Circulation* 1998;98:2367–2369.
56. Frazier OH. Future directions of cardiac assistance. *Semin Thorac Cardiovasc Surg* 2000;12:220–228.

Chapter 13

The Management of Heart Failure's Electrical Complications: Device Therapy

John M. Fontaine, MD

Introduction

Approximately 4.8 million individuals in the United States suffer from congestive heart failure and it is estimated that 500,000 new cases are diagnosed annually. Cardiac mortality is directly related to New York Heart Association (NYHA) functional classification and may be due to progression of heart failure or sudden death due to ventricular tachyarrhythmias, bradyarrhythmia, or asystole. In order to significantly impact survival in patients with heart failure, one must address the electrical or arrhythmia complications of this disease. These complications include frequent and complex ventricular ectopy, including unsustained ventricular tachycardia, sustained ventricular tachycardia/fibrillation, and atrial fibrillation. In this chapter, a discussion of current management strategies for evaluating and treating the electrical complications of heart failure is presented. Evidence from randomized clinical trials is presented in support of these treatment strategies. Current recommendations for primary and secondary prevention of sudden cardiac death are discussed. A discussion of resynchronization or biventricular pacing therapy for congestive heart failure, patient selection, hemodynamic benefits and results of early clinical trials are presented first.

Although recent pharmacological treatments with angiotensin-converting enzyme (ACE) inhibitors, beta-blockers and spironolactone have been shown to reduce morbidity and mortality in patients with NYHA class II–IV heart failure and improve quality of life, prognosis is

From: Jessup M, McCauley KM (eds). *Heart Failure: Providing Optimal Care.* Elmsford, NY: Futura, an imprint of Blackwell Publishing; ©2003.

still poor despite these advances.[1–3] Moreover, cardiac mortality in these patients is significantly higher in those who have a prolonged QRS duration (>120 ms).[4] The prevalence of an interventricular conduction delay in patients with chronic heart failure has been estimated to be between 27% and 53%.[5] An intraventricular or interventricular conduction delay (IVCD) will manifest itself as a left bundle branch block (LBBB) in up to 60% of patients with congestive heart failure. These conduction abnormalities result in ventricular dyssynchrony and abnormalities in ventricular activation, with subsequent reduction in ventricular filling and relaxation time. To a lesser extent, these patients also may have prolonged atrioventricular (AV) conduction time, which may result in diastolic mitral regurgitation and decreased forward flow. Recently, multisite biventricular pacing has been proposed as a new therapeutic modality which produces cardiac resynchronization, thus augmenting stroke volume and improving left ventricular filling and relaxation time.

In this section, a discussion of the clinical manifestations of an intraventricular conduction delay in patients with chronic heart failure, the mechanism by which biventricular pacing improves cardiac performance, and preliminary trial results demonstrating the efficacy of this treatment modality are presented.

Clinical Manifestations of Intraventricular and Interventricular Conduction Delay

An intraventricular or interventricular conduction delay (IVCD) in patients with congestive heart failure has deleterious effects on systolic function and left ventricular filling and relaxation time. A QRS duration of >120 ms in these patients adversely effects mortality and often may induce or exacerbate mitral regurgitation. In a study by Xiao and colleagues, the presence of an LBBB was associated with an increase of over 80% in left ventricular preejection contraction time and a 60% decrease in left ventricular relaxation time. In addition, a negative correlation between the QRS duration and left ventricular dP/dt results. The wider the QRS duration, the lower is left ventricular contractility.[6] In the same study, evaluation of left ventricular diastolic function revealed that left ventricular filling time was significantly reduced in patients with dilated cardiomyopathy and an LBBB. Ventricular dyssynchrony is often seen in patients with a normal QRS duration and congestive heart failure, but the magnitude of this dyssynchrony is greatest in patients with an IVCD. Presence of an IVCD, particularly an LBBB, is associated with septal dyskinesis or paradoxical wall motion, presystolic or diastolic mitral regurgitation due to early papillary muscle activation, reduced diastolic filling time and reduced dP/dt.

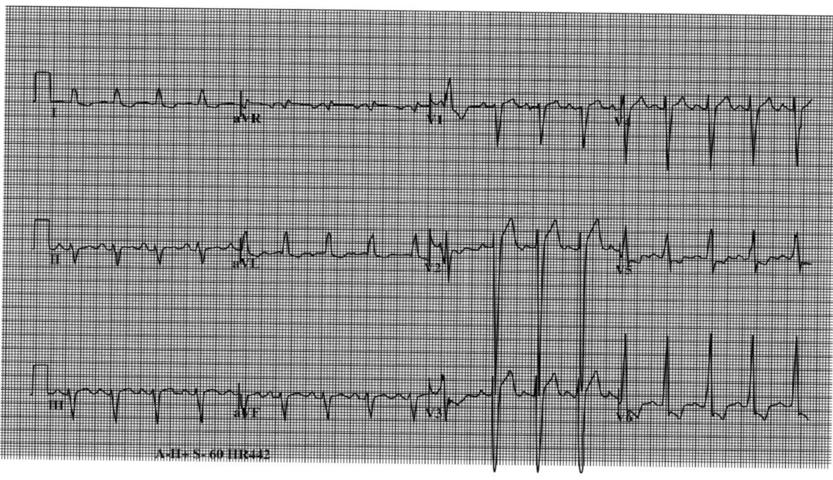

Figure 1. This 12-lead electrocardiogram (ECG) demonstrates a typical left bundle branch block (LBBB) pattern with a QRS duration of 150 ms. This patient has chronic congestive heart failure, an left ventricular ejection fraction (LVEF) of 15%, and is a candidate for resynchronization therapy.

In the Vesnarinone Study (VEST), 3654 patients with NYHA class II–IV were evaluated and cardiac mortality assessed based on the QRS duration noted on the surface ECG.[4] The QRS duration, in addition to age, serum creatinine, left ventricular ejection fraction (LVEF), and resting heart rate were found to be independent predictors of mortality. A fivefold increase in the relative risk for cardiac mortality was noted in the group of patients with the widest QRS duration when compared with those with the narrowest.

Figure 1 demonstrates a 12-lead electrocardiogram (ECG) obtained from a patient with a dilated cardiomyopathy, chronic heart failure, and an LVEF of 15%. He has an IVCD that is of an LBBB pattern.

Cardiac Resynchronization

Multisite biventricular pacing, also referred to as biventricular pacing or cardiac resynchronization therapy, has been proposed as a new modality by which simultaneous right and left ventricular electrical stimulation can be used to reduce the ventricular dyssynchrony noted in chronic heart failure patients with an IVCD. The rationale for providing this therapy is based on the high prevalence (27–53%) of an IVCD and documented ventricular systolic and diastolic dysfunction in these patients. Several preliminary studies have shown that permanent biventricular pacing results in immediate hemodynamic benefits and improved symptoms, exercise time, and distance walked during a 6-minute walk test.[7–10]

Cazeau and colleagues recently published results from the Multisite Stimulation and Cardiomyopathy (MUSTIC) trial.[11] In this study, 67 patients with a mean age of 63 years and NYHA class III heart failure, who were on stable pharmacologic therapy, underwent biventricular pacing therapy. This study had a randomized, single-blind, crossover design that evaluated the effects of biventricular pacing or ventricular (inactive) pacing, at a rate of 40 beats/min, on predefined endpoints. The primary endpoint was the distance walked during a 6-minute walk test, and the secondary endpoint was the quality of life, based on the Minnesota Living with Heart Failure Questionnaire. Left ventricular pacing was achieved through a lead placed in the coronary sinus (the customary approach nowadays) and positioned laterally, midway between the base and the apex of the left ventricle. In this trial, 48 patients completed both phases of the study. The results show that there was a 23% increase in distance walked (399 ± 100 meters versus 326 ± 134 meters; $P < 0.001$). The quality-of-life score improved by 32% ($P < 0.001$), peak oxygen uptake increased by 8% ($P < 0.03$), and hospitalizations were reduced by 66% ($P < 0.05$). Although blinded, the biventricular pacing mode was preferred by 85% of patients ($P < 0.001$). The authors concluded that biventricular pacing is technically complex, but feasible, and results in improved exercise tolerance and quality of life in chronic heart failure patients with an IVCD.

Recently, data from a separate study, the Myocardial Infarction Risk Recognition and Conversion of Life-threatening Events into Survival (MIRACLE) trial, evaluated the effects of biventricular pacing in a single-blind, randomized, crossover study of 266 patients with chronic congestive heart failure and a QRS duration >150 ms.[12] Forty-four centers in the United States and Canada were involved in this trial. There were 134 patients randomized to cardiac resynchronization therapy, whereas 132 patients were in the control group. The mean age of the patient population was 65 years; 90% were in NYHA class III and 10% were in class IV. The mean LVEF was 21%. A 93% implant success rate was achieved. The endpoints in this trial were quality of life, NYHA classification, and 6-minute walk test response. The results demonstrated a 65% improvement in NYHA class to either category I or II in the resynchronization therapy group, whereas a 30% improvement was noted in the control group. A significant difference was noted in peak oxygen consumption, total exercise time (with a 100-s improvement in exercise duration), LVEF (improved by 6% in the resynchronization group), and left ventricular end-diastolic dimension (decreased by 0.5 cm in the resynchronization group).

Patient Selection/Methodology of Resynchronization Therapy

The treatment goals in providing cardiac resynchronization therapy are:

- To improve global ventricular synchrony
- To organize ventricular activation, thus improving LVEF
- To improve cardiac efficiency by augmenting oxygen consumption
- To reduce NYHA classification
- To improve symptoms, exercise tolerance and the patient's sense of well-being

In order to achieve these goals, proper selection of patients for cardiac resynchronization therapy is needed. At the moment, it appears that patients with a prolonged QRS duration of >150 ms and an LBBB pattern clearly benefit from this therapy. However, questions remain whether patients with a right bundle branch block or a QRS duration between 120 and 150 ms benefit. Some benefit in patients with minimal QRS prolongation has been seen in uncontrolled trials. Controlled trials are needed in order to confirm these results. Multisite biventricular pacing has been shown to be beneficial in patients with atrial fibrillation. In patients with normal AV conduction who undergo biventricular pacing, the VDD pacing mode should be carefully programmed in order to maximize biventricular stimulation and minimize fusion beats, which may result as a consequence of normal AV conduction.[13]

Technical considerations in biventricular pacing have been related to the ability to achieve stable lead position for left ventricular stimulation. Initially, a thoracotomy approach was utilized, but because of increased morbidity and mortality in these high-risk patients, left ventricular sites were subsequently accessed through the coronary sinus, and this became the more widely accepted approach. Figure 2 demonstrates a coronary sinus venogram obtained following insertion of the right ventricular lead, but before insertion of the left ventricular pacing lead. A coronary sinus venogram is necessary to delineate the coronary venous anatomy and should be performed prior to coronary sinus lead placement. In Fig. 2, this venogram illustrates the presence of a large posterior ventricular branch with its lateral tributaries. The development of suitable coronary sinus leads that can be utilized for left ventricular stimulation, in addition to new delivery systems (i.e., guiding catheters and sheaths) that can be used to expeditiously position the left ventricular lead in the coronary sinus, has facilitated resynchronization therapy. A

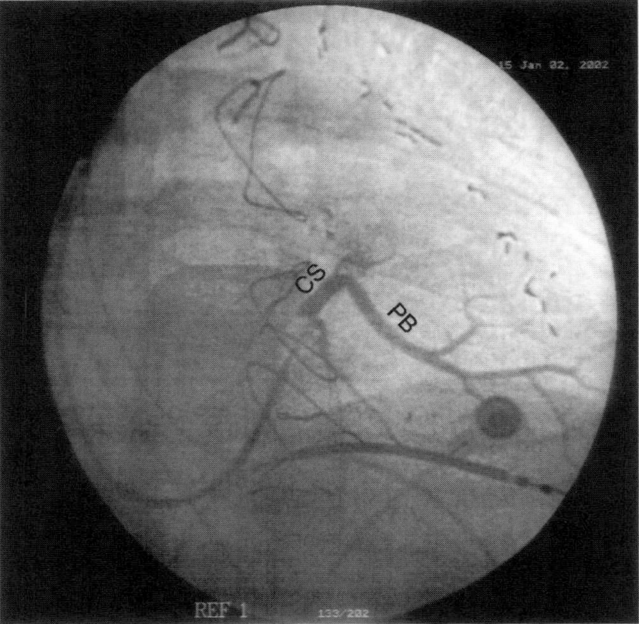

Figure 2. This image illustrates a coronary sinus venogram obtained in the right anterior oblique projection. The main coronary sinus (CS) along with a large posterior branch (PB) and its lateral tributaries are demonstrated. A right ventricular lead positioned in the apex is evident.

chest radiograph of the biventricular pacing system is shown in Fig. 3. A posteroanterior and lateral chest film illustrates significant cardiomegaly in a patient with congestive heart failure, an IVCD, and permanent atrial fibrillation. In the lateral film, it is evident that the left ventricular lead is positioned in the posterolateral base of the left ventricle and widely separated from the right ventricular apical lead. This is generally considered an ideal location for the left ventricular (LV) lead.

Blanc and coworkers reported that left ventricular pacing alone, rather than biventricular pacing, resulted in benefits in cardiac resynchronization similar to those afforded by multisite biventricular pacing.[14] These results will have to be confirmed by subsequent controlled clinical trials. The question remains whether left ventricular pacing alone would be preferred in patients with atrioventricular conduction abnormalities. Another concern that has not been fully evaluated is the issue regarding the site where the left ventricle should be paced. Access to left ventricular sites is limited based on the coronary venous anatomy. Most investigators have positioned the left ventricular lead in a lateral branch

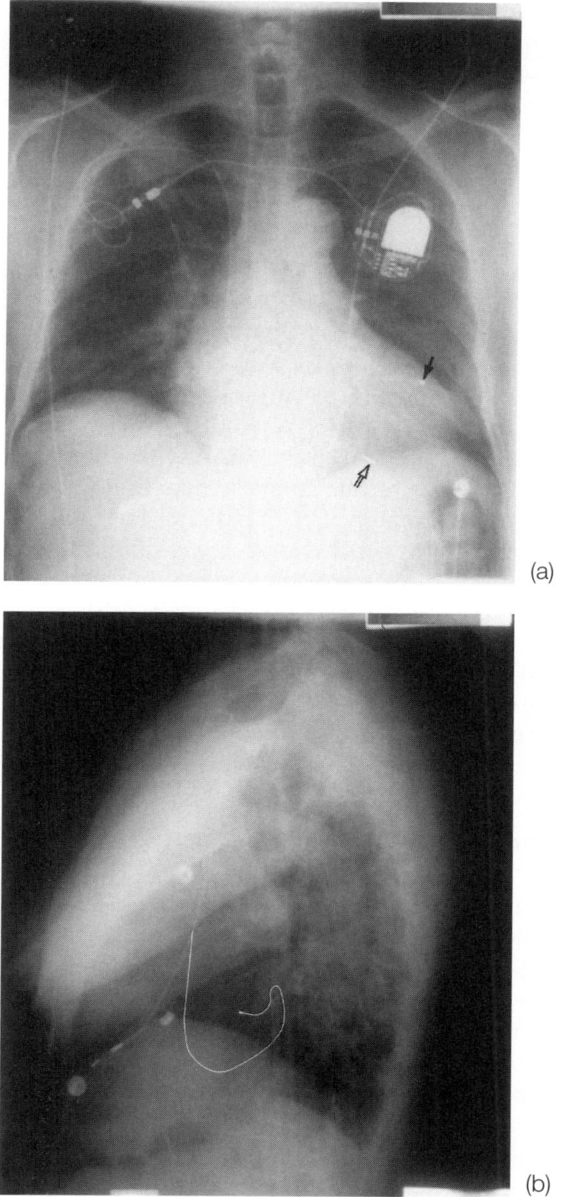

Figure 3. (a) This anterior posterior chest radiograph illustrates the biventricular pacing system. The downward-pointing arrow illustrates the left ventricular pacing electrode located along the epicardial surface of the posterolateral left ventricle. The right ventricular lead is positioned at the apex (upward-pointing arrow). (b) The lateral film illustrates a left ventricular pacing lead that courses through the main coronary sinus and lies in its posterolateral branch.

of the coronary sinus, midway between the apex and base. Whether one site or multiple sites in the left ventricle need to be paced in order to maximally reduce ventricular dyssynchrony also needs to be evaluated. The determination of the most appropriate site for left ventricular pacing that would be associated with the greatest degree of narrowing of the paced QRS complex for the best hemodynamic benefit also needs to be assessed.

Conclusion

Multisite biventricular pacing has been shown to be beneficial in improving cardiac hemodynamics, exercise tolerance, ejection fraction, NYHA classification, oxygen consumption and quality of life in randomized controlled trials. These trials have clearly shown short-term benefits in hemodynamic parameters and clinical symptoms in heart failure patients with an IVCD. Cardiac resynchronization therapy is technically achievable in approximately 90% of patients, but the selection of the appropriate patient for biventricular pacing is still undergoing evaluation. In addition, appropriate methods of assessing patients regarding the specific site for pacing, the degree of ventricular dyssynchrony and the reduction in dyssynchrony associated with cardiac resynchronization therapy need to be defined. Finally, it is clear that functional benefit and quality of life improvement are documented in a number of studies; however, further investigations regarding the impact on morbidity, mortality and cost-effectiveness will have to be carried out.

Electrical Complications of Heart Failure

Heart failure is diagnosed in approximately 500,000 cases annually. The prevalence increases with advancing age. The prevalence of heart failure correlates well with the increased prevalence of coronary artery disease in the population over the age of 65.[15–17]

Arrhythmia complications in patients with heart failure include ventricular tachycardia, ventricular fibrillation, atrial fibrillation, and bradyarrhythmias, including AV block and sinus node dysfunction. Patients with ischemic cardiomyopathy are more likely to have ventricular tachycardia occurring as a result of a reentry mechanism than patients with nonischemic cardiomyopathy. Other mechanisms, such as triggered activity or stretch-induced chloride channel activation—particularly in the dilated heart or in patients with atrioventricular valvular dysfunction—contribute to ventricular arrhythmias seen in heart failure patients.[18,19]

Mortality in patients with heart failure may be due to progression of heart failure, ventricular tachyarrhythmias, and bradyarrhythmias.

These deaths may be sudden or nonsudden and are often difficult to classify. Current classification of the cause of death in patients with left ventricular dysfunction utilizes a modification of the Hinkle–Thaler criteria, whereby the presence of circulatory failure before death is considered death due to heart failure, whereas death occurring without prior evidence of circulatory collapse is considered an arrhythmic death.[20] Based on these criteria, approximately one-half of all deaths in heart failure patients are thought to be sudden or a consequence of ventricular tachyarrhythmias, whereas the remaining deaths are thought to be due to other cardiac or noncardiac causes.[21,22] Classification of the causes of death is often difficult and imprecise, despite the use of the Hinkle–Thaler criteria. With the advent of the stored electrogram in patients with an implantable cardioverter defibrillator (ICD), a better understanding of the cause of death in patients who seemingly die suddenly was obtained.[23,24] Electrogram data from patients dying suddenly failed to show any significant arrhythmia in the few hours preceding their death, whereas clinical data would suggest that these deaths may have been arrhythmic. In the absence of such electrogram data from the ICD, these patients would have been classified as having experienced an arrhythmic death.

Patients with congestive heart failure are susceptible to ventricular tachyarrhythmias, and several studies have suggested that the prevalence of these arrhythmias ranges from 40% to 70%.[22,23,25] In the subsequent section of this chapter, a discussion of the management of the various subgroups of patients with left ventricular systolic dysfunction and various arrhythmia qualifiers will be provided. This discussion will be based on results from recent randomized clinical trials that evaluated the treatment strategies for these patients and will provide direction for the clinician in the management of these patients.

Primary Prevention of Cardiovascular Mortality and Sudden Cardiac Death in Patients with Left Ventricular Dysfunction

Patients with chronic congestive heart failure are known to die from progression of their disease. The Studies of Left Ventricular Dysfunction (SOLVD) was a randomized, double-blind, placebo-controlled, multicenter trial that evaluated outcomes in 2569 adult patients with chronic heart failure.[26] In that study, treatment with the ACE inhibitor enalapril was compared with placebo (standard therapy) for its effect on overall cardiovascular mortality and progression of heart failure. The placebo group demonstrated a 40% and 36% overall and cardiovascular mortality rate, respectively, over a mean follow-up period of 41 months in comparison with the treatment group (35% and 31%, respectively), both representing a significant (16% and 18%) reduction in overall and cardiovascular mortality. In the prevention trial, retrospective analysis of 4228 asymptomatic patients with left ventricular dysfunction followed over a mean period of 34 months demonstrated a 22% versus 14% mortality in black and white patients, respectively. These data demonstrated an increase in mortality due to the progression of heart failure in both symptomatic and asymptomatic patients with left ventricular systolic dysfunction. Other studies have since confirmed these data and support the use of ACE inhibitors as part of the treatment regimen in the primary prevention of cardiovascular mortality in patients with left ventricular systolic dysfunction.

Numerous studies have shown that patients with congestive heart failure and ventricular arrhythmias are at a higher risk for fatal cardiovascular events.[27–30] Patients with frequent and complex asymptomatic ventricular arrhythmias on Holter monitoring have been shown to demonstrate an annual mortality rate of approximately 15%; one-half of these deaths are sudden and presumably related to cardiac arrhythmias. Thus, asymptomatic ventricular arrhythmias in patients with congestive heart failure are associated with increased risk of overall mortality and sudden death. In a recent study, the Congestive Heart Failure Survival Trial of Antiarrhythmic Therapy (CHF-STAT), the impact of amiodarone on survival in patients with congestive heart failure and asymptomatic ventricular arrhythmias was evaluated.[25] CHF-STAT was a randomized double-blind placebo controlled multicenter study performed in 28 Veterans Hospital centers in the United States. This trial evaluated 674 patients with symptoms of congestive heart failure, LVEF of 40% or less, and 10 or more premature ventricular contractions (PVCs) per hour on ambulatory ECG monitoring. Patients were excluded if they had a history of symptomatic ventricular arrhythmia, sudden cardiac death or cardiac arrest, sustained ventricular tachycardia, uncontrolled thyroid disease, need for antiarrhythmic therapy, medical illness that was likely to be fatal within 3 years, or symptomatic hypotension. All patients in the study received vasodilator therapy, digoxin, and diuretic as needed. Three hundred and thirty-six patients were randomized to receive amiodarone, whereas 338 patients received placebo. The primary endpoint was overall mortality. The results of this study showed that there was no significant difference in overall mortality between the two treatment groups. The 2-year actuarial survival rate was 69% for the amiodarone group and 71% for the placebo group. After 2 years, the sudden death rate was 15% in the amiodarone group and 19% in the placebo group. This difference was not significant. However, a trend was noted toward a reduction in overall mortality among the patients with nonischemic cardiomyopathy who received amiodarone. Amiodarone was found to be beneficial in suppressing ventricular arrhythmias and increasing

LVEF by 42% ($P < 0.001$). Clinical characteristics of the patients in this study revealed that coronary artery disease was present in 72% of patients in the amiodarone group and 71% of those in the placebo group. In addition, 77% of patients in the amiodarone group had one or more episodes of ventricular tachycardia on ambulatory ECG, whereas 85% of these patients had similar arrhythmias in the placebo group. At randomization, the mean LVEF in the amiodarone and placebo group was 24.9 ± 8 and 25.7 ± 8%, respectively. Although the impact of amiodarone on ventricular arrhythmia suppression did not result in a decrease in overall mortality, a trend towards a beneficial effect in patients with nonischemic cardiomyopathy was noted. Further studies will be needed in this subgroup of patients to determine the benefits of empiric amiodarone therapy in patients with asymptomatic left ventricular dysfunction. Results of an earlier trial by the *Grupo de Estudio de la Sobrevida en la Insuficiencia Cardiaca en Argentina* (GESICA) suggested that empiric amiodarone therapy would be beneficial in reducing cardiovascular mortality in patients with left ventricular dysfunction and clinical evidence of heart failure.[31] The predominance of patients with coronary artery disease in CHF-STAT as compared to the GESICA trial, and the lack of blinding therapy in GESICA, may be reasons for discrepant results between the two trials.

To further risk-stratify patients with reduced left ventricular systolic function post myocardial infarction, several studies evaluated patients with asymptomatic unsustained ventricular tachycardia via electrophysiology study and guided antiarrhythmia therapy based on the results of programmed ventricular stimulation.[32–34] The Multicenter Automatic Defibrillator Implantation Trial (MADIT) was one such trial, undertaken to assess survival in this subgroup of patients.[32] This trial, which began in December of 1990, was performed in 30 centers in the United States and two in Europe, and sought to evaluate all-cause mortality in patients with asymptomatic unsustained ventricular tachycardia (three or more beats at a rate ≥120 pulses/min) with an LVEF of <36%, who had inducible and nonsuppressible ventricular tachyarrhythmias during electrophysiology study. The reasons for exclusion from enrollment were: a previous history of a cardiac arrest, ventricular tachycardia resulting in syncope that was not associated with an acute infarction, symptomatic hypotension, myocardial infarction within 3 weeks of enrollment, coronary artery bypass grafting within 2 months, or coronary angioplasty within 3 months of enrollment. One hundred and ninety-six patients were enrolled, with 95 patients randomized to the implantable defibrillator group and 101 to conventional therapy, and the patients were followed over a mean follow-up period of 27 months. Approximately two-thirds of patients enrolled in this study had class II or III congestive heart failure. There was no significant difference between the

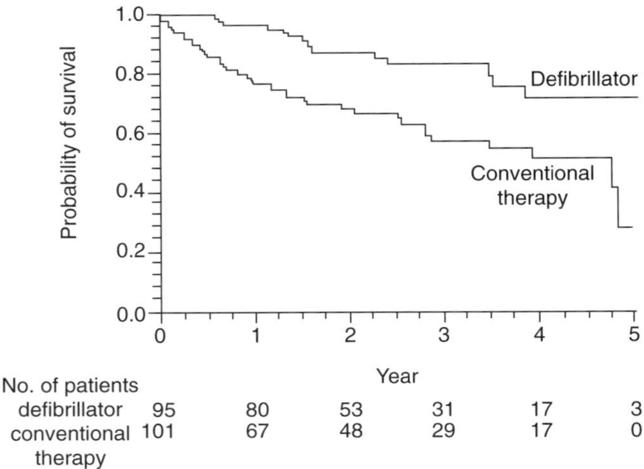

Figure 4. Kaplan–Meier survival curves of the probability of survival according to treatment strategy. The difference in survival was significant ($P = 0.009$). Reproduced with permission.

mean LVEF in the conventional treatment group (25%) and that in the amiodarone group (27%). This study was designed to have an 85% power to detect a 46% reduction in mortality in the defibrillator treatment group, as compared with the anticipated 2-year mortality rate of 30% among patients randomized to conventional therapy. Using a triangular sequential design, this study was terminated prematurely in March of 1996 in favor of the defibrillator treatment group. There were 15 deaths in the defibrillator group, whereas there were 39 deaths noted in the conventional treatment group (hazard ratio for overall mortality 0.46, 95% confidence interval 0.26–0.82, $P = 0.009$). The difference in survival between the two treatment groups is illustrated in Fig. 4. The use of beta-blockers and antiarrhythmia medications provided no benefit in survival in comparison with the defibrillator group. The 2-year mortality rate in the conventional group was 37% and similar to the anticipated pretrial estimate. These results were also comparable to the 2-year mortality rate observed in CHF-STAT study.[25] The patients in the CHF-STAT trial had a slightly higher ejection fraction for entry (≤40%), more had mild to moderate congestive heart failure and a more benign ventricular ectopy requirement for entry in the study (>10 PVCs per hour on ambulatory ECG). These results support the use of the implantable defibrillator in high-risk patients with coronary heart disease and left ventricular dysfunction who have asymptomatic spontaneous unsustained ventricular tachycardia with inducible and nonsuppressible ventricular arrhythmias during electrophysiology study. To provide effective screening of patients who fall into this subgroup studied in the MADIT, and to avoid selection bias, it would have been valuable to know the number of patients screened in that trial in order to identify eligible patients. The benefits of ICD therapy in this subgroup of patients were clearly shown. Electrophysiology testing was proven effective in risk stratification for primary prevention of sudden cardiac death in this patient population. Clinicians may be encouraged to refer patients such as those studied in MADIT for electrophysiology study.

In another recent trial, the value of electrophysiology study and ICD therapy as a primary prevention tool and treatment strategy, respectively, was evaluated in the postinfarction patient with reduced LVEF and unsustained ventricular tachycardia.[33] The Multicenter Unsustained Tachycardia Trial (MUSTT) was initiated in 1989 to test the hypothesis that antiarrhythmia therapy guided by electrophysiology study would reduce the risk of sudden death and cardiac arrest among patients with coronary artery disease, left ventricular dysfunction, and unsustained ventricular tachycardia. This trial involved 85 centers in the United States and Canada and enrolled patients with coronary artery disease, prior infarction who were at least 4 days post infarct with LVEF ≤40%, and asymptomatic unsustained ventricular tachycardia of three beats or more at a rate at or above 100 beats/min. Antiarrhythmia drug therapy in this study was randomly assigned, but not randomized. Patients in this study who had inducible ventricular tachyarrhythmias were randomized to electrophysiology-guided therapy or no antiarrhythmic therapy. Implantation of a defibrillator could be recommended after one unsuccessful drug test. A valuable component of this study was the use of a registry for patients who declined defibrillator therapy and received no antiarrhythmic drug therapy and for patients who were noninducible during electrophysiology study. The primary endpoint was cardiac arrest and death from arrhythmia, whereas the secondary endpoint included all-cause mortality, cardiac death, and spontaneous sustained ventricular tachyarrhythmias. As in the MADIT trial, death was categorized utilizing a modified Hinkle–Thaler classification. This study was initially designed to include 900 patients with inducible sustained ventricular tachyarrhythmias and to have an 80% and 90% power to detect event rates of 15% and 20%, respectively. At termination of enrollment in 1996, only 704 patients were enrolled and followed over a mean period of 39 months. There was no significant difference in the mean LVEF between the group of patients assigned to no therapy (29%) versus those who received electrophysiology-guided therapy (30%). Two-thirds of all patients had a history of New York Heart Association class II or III congestive heart failure, whereas none were in class IV. Based on

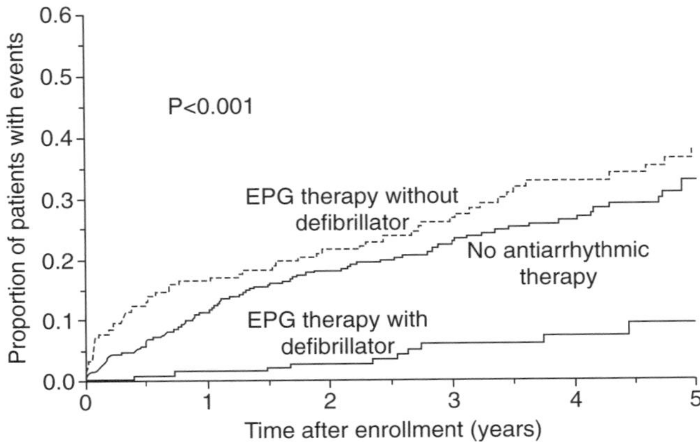

Figure 5. Kaplan–Meier estimates of the rates of cardiac arrest or arrhythmic death according to treatment with and without the implantable defibrillator (EPG, electrophysiology guided). Those patients who were assigned to no antiarrhythmic therapy were also compared to the defibrillator group. Reproduced with permission.

Kaplan–Meier survival analysis, the incidence of cardiac arrest or death from an arrhythmia was 25% among those receiving electrophysiology-guided therapy and 32% among those assigned to no therapy (relative risk 0.73; 95% confidence interval, 0.53–0.99), thus illustrating a significant reduction in risk of 27%. The overall mortality was 42% and 48%, respectively. The risk of a cardiac arrest or death from an arrhythmia among the patients who received defibrillator treatment was significantly lower than among the patients discharged without receiving defibrillator therapy (relative risk 0.24; 95% confidence interval, 0.13–0.45; $P < 0.001$) (Fig. 5). The survival curve for overall mortality based on treatment with or without a defibrillator is shown in Fig. 6. The authors concluded that electrophysiology-guided antiarrhythmia therapy with implantable defibrillators, but not with antiarrhythmic drugs, was associated with a reduced risk of sudden death in high-risk patients with coronary artery disease. In this trial, the use of beta-blockers was more frequent among patients assigned to receive no antiarrhythmia therapy. Forty percent of all patients were discharged receiving beta-blocker therapy.

In MUSTT, the use of electrophysiology study and ICD therapy in risk stratifying and managing patients at risk for arrhythmic death was found to be highly beneficial. The lack of benefit from antiarrhythmic drug therapy may occur as a result of the electrophysiology criteria used to define efficacy of therapy, or perhaps a changed cardiac substrate that occurred following the initial electrophysiology study. These data support the role of defibrillator therapy in this subgroup of patients; how-

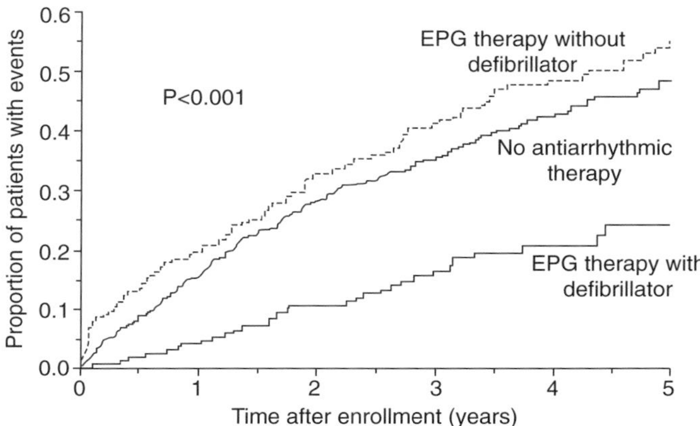

Figure 6. Kaplan–Meier estimates of the rates of overall mortality in patients treated with a defibrillator are compared with those patients receiving antiarrhythmic therapy without a defibrillator and those receiving no antiarrhythmic therapy. All comparisons showed a significant difference between groups (EPG, electrophysiology guided). Reproduced with permission.

ever, despite the proven value of the initial electrophysiology study, it is unclear whether repeat electrophysiology testing would be beneficial in identifying high-risk patients among those who were initially noninducible.

In MUSTT, the outcomes of 1397 patients in the registry who had no inducible ventricular tachyarrhythmias were compared to those with inducible ventricular tachyarrhythmias who were randomly assigned to receive no antiarrhythmic therapy. The prognostic value of electrophysiology study would thus be evaluated with this approach.[34] The mean LVEF in the registry patients was identical (29%) to those patients randomized to receive no antiarrhythmic therapy. In each group, 63% of patients had either class II or III congestive heart failure. The 2-year and 5-year rates for cardiac arrest or arrhythmic deaths were 12% and 24%, respectively, among patients in the registry, as compared with 18% and 32% among patients who were inducible, but received no antiarrhythmic therapy ($P = 0.005$). Thirty-five percent of registry patients were receiving beta-blocker therapy, as compared with 51% of patients assigned to the group with no antiarrhythmic therapy ($P = 0.001$), whereas 72% and 77% of patients in the registry who were inducible and on no antiarrhythmic therapy, respectively, were taking ACE inhibitors. The investigators concluded that patients with coronary artery disease, left ventricular dysfunction, asymptomatic unsustained ventricular tachycardia in whom sustained ventricular tachyarrhythmias could not be induced during electrophysiology study have a significantly lower risk of sudden death

Table 1

Clinical Characteristics of Patients with Left Ventricular Dysfunction in Primary and Secondary Prevention Studies of Sudden Cardiac Death and Overall Cardiac Mortality

		New York Heart Association				
Study	Mean EF %	Class I	Class II	Class III	Class IV	Arrhythmia type
CHF-STAT	25	8 (1.2%)	358 (55%)	279 (43%)		AF: 103 (15%) all had >10 VPC/h NSVT: 762 placebo, 337 amiodarone
MADIT	26	35%	65%		None	All had NSVT
MUSTT	30	37%	39%	24%	None	All had NSVT
AVID	32	48%		7, 12%	None	Sustained VT, VF; AF in 21% of ICD group, 26% of control group

AF, atrial fibrillation; AVID, Antiarrhythmics Versus Implantable Defibrillator trial; CHF-STAT, Congestive Heart Failure Survival Trial of Antiarrhythmic Therapy; EF, ejection fraction; ICD, implantable cardioverter defibrillator; MADIT, Multicenter Automatic Defibrillator Implantation Trial; MUSTT, Multicenter Unsustained Tachycardia Trial; NSVT, nonsustained ventricular tachycardia; VF, ventricular fibrillation; VPC, ventricular premature contraction; VT, ventricular tachycardia.

or cardiac arrest and lower mortality than similar patients with inducible sustained ventricular tachyarrhythmias. It is evident from these data that patients with heart failure have the electrical substrate and increased risk for sudden cardiac death that can be predicted by electrophysiology study. It is also evident that patients with complex ventricular arrhythmias and left ventricular dysfunction often have clinical evidence of class II and III congestive heart failure and are also at risk for cardiac death from progression of heart failure. Table 1 shows the relationship between heart failure and arrhythmia substrate in recent trials.

Implantable Cardioverter Defibrillator Use in Secondary Prevention

Recent publication of the Antiarrhythmics Versus Implantable Defibrillator (AVID) trial results demonstrated the efficacy of the defibrillator in the treatment of patients with sustained ventricular tachycardia or

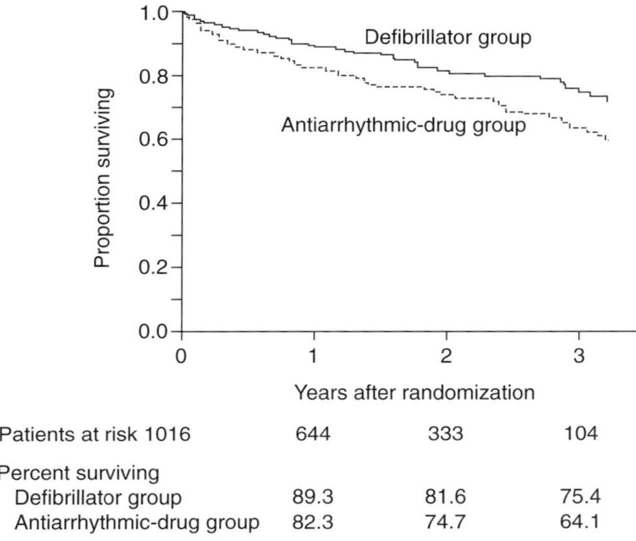

Figure 7. Overall survival in the Antiarrhythmics Versus Implantable Defibrillator (AVID) trial in the defibrillation treated group and in the group receiving antiarrhythmic drug treatment. Survival was significantly better in the defibrillation-treated group than in the antiarrhythmic drug-treated group ($P < 0.02$). Reproduced with permission.

those resuscitated from a cardiac arrest.[35] In this study, 1016 patients who were resuscitated from ventricular fibrillation or hemodynamically unstable sustained ventricular tachycardia, were randomized to receive defibrillator therapy or antiarrhythmic drug therapy with amiodarone. In that study, approximately 3% of patients were discharged on therapy with sotalol. Sixty percent of patients in AVID had evidence of congestive heart failure, 45% had ventricular fibrillation, and 55% had sustained ventricular tachycardia. Five hundred and seven patients were randomly assigned to treatment with the defibrillator, whereas 509 patients received antiarrhythmic drug therapy. The primary endpoint was overall mortality. The study found that overall survival was greater with implantable defibrillator therapy (89.3%) as compared with antiarrhythmic drug therapy (82.3%) at 1 year, 81.6 versus 74.7 at 2 years, and 75.4 versus 64.1 at 3 years ($P < 0.02$) (Fig. 7). This study was among the first multicenter studies that clearly showed the value of ICD therapy as a secondary prevention treatment strategy in patients resuscitated from fatal or near-fatal ventricular fibrillation, sustained ventricular tachycardia with syncope, or sustained ventricular tachycardia with an ejection fraction of <40%. The ICD was found to be superior to antiarrhythmic drug therapy for increasing overall survival.

Sudden Cardiac Death in Heart Failure

Although primary prevention modalities are available utilizing antiarrhythmic therapy guided by electrophysiology study for risk stratification of patients with poor left ventricular function and complex ventricular arrhythmias, this approach does not identify all patients who are at risk for sudden cardiac death. The Sudden Cardiac Death in Heart Failure Trial (SCD-HeFT) will serve as a primary prevention trial to assess the benefit of ICD therapy or amiodarone in patients with heart failure.[36] Heart failure patients enrolled in this trial will not require an arrhythmia qualifier. This study is expected to have a significant impact on the management of patients with heart failure, due to the number of patients with heart failure and potential for increasing the cost of care of these patients should a defibrillator be required for sudden cardiac death prophylaxis. The results of this study will not be known for a few years.

Atrial Fibrillation in Heart Failure Patients

Congestive heart failure is a serious condition that is often associated with the occurrence of complex ventricular as well as supraventricular arrhythmias. Among the most serious supraventricular arrhythmias is atrial fibrillation. Atrial fibrillation is common in patients with heart failure, ranging from 15% to 30% of these patients, and can impair exercise tolerance and hemodynamic performance and result in thromboembolic complications. Patients with heart failure are at greater risk for experiencing proarrhythmia complications of antiarrhythmic drug therapy, particularly if class I drugs are utilized.[37]

The Atrial Fibrillation Follow-up Investigation of Rhythm Management (AFFIRM) trial was undertaken to evaluate the benefits of maintaining sinus rhythm or providing rate control only, in the management of the patients with paroxysmal and persistent atrial fibrillation.[38] Patients were randomized to rate control versus cardioversion and rhythm control with amiodarone. The difference in total mortality between the two groups was assessed. The study has been completed, and no significant difference in mortality was observed between the rate or rhythm control strategies. One can speculate that perhaps only a subgroup of patients with heart failure would greatly benefit from maintaining sinus rhythm, whereas the overall number of patients with atrial fibrillation and preserved left ventricular function may not derive additional benefits pertaining to the maintenance of sinus rhythm.

In treating atrial fibrillation and attempting to regain sinus rhythm, one must weigh the benefits of antiarrhythmic drug therapy, as well as its adverse effects, versus the benefits of improved cardiac hemodynamics and amelioration of symptoms. Heart failure patients are likely to be treated with amiodarone or other class III arrhythmic agents such as dofetilide or sotalol. Alternative modalities available in the treatment of atrial fibrillation entail rate control with AV blocking drugs and anticoagulation, AV junctional ablation with subsequent rate control and anticoagulation, and radiofrequency-energy ablation of pulmonary vein foci of origin of atrial fibrillation. In a recent study, the Danish Investigations of Arrhythmia and Mortality on Dofetilide in Congestive Heart Failure (DIAMOND-CHF), the effects of dofetilide on survival and morbidity when used in patients with reduced left ventricular function and congestive heart failure were assessed.[39] This double-blind, randomized study in 1518 patients with symptomatic heart failure with severe left ventricular dysfunction demonstrated that dofetilide was effective in converting atrial fibrillation to sinus rhythm and preventing its recurrence. It was also associated with reduced hospitalizations for worsening heart failure and had no adverse effect on mortality.

Summary

In this chapter, the use of biventricular pacing as electrical therapy for congestive heart failure was discussed and evidence demonstrating its efficacy, beneficial effects on morbidity, and its ability to improve cardiac hemodynamics and exercise tolerance was demonstrated. Randomized clinical trials have clearly documented these benefits. Approval of these devices by the Food and Drug Administration (FDA) has been provided. The Medtronic InSync device (model no. 8140) and the Contak-CD (Guidant Corporation) recently received FDA approval for clinical use in the United States. Other manufacturers will soon complete their trials and also seek approval of their devices.

Randomized clinical trials such as the MADIT and MUSTT also have clearly shown the utility of electrophysiology study as a risk stratification tool and the ICD for primary prevention of sudden cardiac death in patients with left ventricular systolic dysfunction and heart failure. The AVID trial also demonstrated the overall and sudden death survival benefit of the ICD as the preferred secondary prevention treatment strategy. The results of the SCD-HeFT Trial will not be available for several years; thus, the role of the ICD versus antiarrhythmic drug therapy (mainly amiodarone) in the larger subgroup of patients with clinical heart failure without any ventricular arrhythmia will for now remain unanswered.

Atrial fibrillation remains the most significant supraventricular arrhythmia requiring therapy, particularly in patients with congestive heart failure, due to its prevalence in that patient population, impact on morbidity and mortality, and propensity to accelerate the progression of heart failure if inadequately treated. Although the results of the AFFIRM trial showed no difference in mortality between the two treatment strategies, it appears that patients with heart failure are more likely to require the maintenance of sinus rhythm and anticoagulation rather than rate control of atrial fibrillation plus anticoagulation with warfarin as the better treatment strategy. Further studies in this subgroup of patients with heart failure and persistent atrial fibrillation will be required in order to better assess the management strategy for these patients.

References

1. Consensus Trial Study Group. Effects of enalapril on mortality in severe congestive heart failure: Results of the north Scandinavian enalapril survival study. *N Engl J Med* 1987;316:1429–1435.
2. Bristow M. Beta-adrenergic receptor blockade in chronic heart failure. *Circulation* 2000;101:558–569.
3. The Randomized Aldactone Evaluation Study Investigators. The effect of spironolactone on morbidity and mortality in patients with severe heart failure. *N Engl J Med* 1999;341:709–717.
4. Venkateshawar K, Gottipaty K, Krelis P, et al. The resting electrocardiogram provides a sensitive and inexpensive marker of prognosis in patients with chronic congestive heart failure [abstract]. *J Am Coll Cardiol* 1999;33:145A.
5. Aaronson K, Schwartz S, Chen T, et al. Development and prospective validation of a clinical index to predict survival in ambulatory patients referred for cardiac transplant. *Circulation* 1997;95:2660–2667.
6. Xiao H, Roy C, Fujimoto S, et al. Natural history of abnormal conduction and its relation to prognosis in patients with dilated cardiomyopathy. *Int J Cardiol* 1996;53:163–170.
7. Cazeau S, Ritter P, Bakdach S, et al. Four chamber pacing in dilated cardiomyopathy. *Pacing Clin Electrophysiol* 1994;17:1974–1979.
8. Daubert JC, Cazeau S, Leclercq C. Do we have reasons to be enthusiastic about pacing to treat advanced heart failure? *Eur J Heart Fail* 1999;1:281–287.
9. Gras D, Mabo P, Tang T, et al. Multisite pacing as a supplemental treatment of congestive heart failure: Preliminary results of the Medtronic Inc. InSync Study. *Pacing Clin Electrophysiol* 1998;21:2249–55.
10. Alonso C, Leclercq C, Victor F, et al. Electrocardiographic predictive factors of long-term clinical improvement with multisite biventricular pacing in advanced heart failure. *Am J Cardiol* 1999;84:1417–1421.
11. Cazeau S, Leclercq C, Lavergne T, et al. Effects of multisite biventricular pacing in patients with heart failure and intraventricular conduction delay. *N Engl J Med* 2001;344:873–880.
12. Miracle Trial paper presented at the 50th Annual Scientific Session of the American College of Cardiology, Late Breaking Sessions, March 18–21, 2001, Orlando, Florida.
13. Kass DA, Chen CH, Curry C, et al. Improved left ventricular mechanics from acute VDD pacing in patients with dilated cardiomyopathy and ventricular conduction delay. *Circulation* 1999;99:1567–1573.
14. Blanc JJ, Etienne Y, Gilard M, et al. Evaluation of different ventricular pacing sites in patients with severe heart failure. *Circulation* 1997;96:3273–3277.

15. Massie BM, Shah NB: Evolving trends in the epidemiologic factors of heart failure. *Am Heart J* 1997;133:703–712.
16. Rodelheffer RJ, Jacobsen SJ, Gersh BJ, et al. The incidence and prevalence of congestive heart failure in Rochester, Minnesota. *Mayo Clin Proc* 1993;68: 1143–1150.
17. Gheorghiade M, Bonow RO: Chronic heart failure in the United States: A manifestation of coronary artery disease. *Circulation* 1998;7:282–289.
18. Pogwizd SM, Corr B. The contribution of nonreentrant mechanisms of malignant ventricular arrhythmias. *Basic Res Cardiol* 1992;87:115–129.
19. Franz MR, Cima R, Wang D. Electrophysiological effects of myocardial stretch and mechanical determinants for stretch activated arrhythmias. *Circulation* 1992;86:968–978.
20. Hinkle LE, Thaler HT. Clinical classification of cardiac deaths. *Circulation* 1982;65:457–464.
21. Uretsky BF, Sheahan RG. Primary prevention of sudden death in heart failure: Will the solution be shocking? *J Am Coll Cardiol* 1997;30:1589–1597.
22. The Defibrillator Study Group. Actuarial risk of sudden death while awaiting cardiac transplantation in patients with atherosclerotic heart disease. *Am J Cardiol* 1991;68:545–546.
23. Pratt CM, Greenway PS, Schoenfeld MH, et al. Exploration of the precision of classifying sudden cardiac death. *Circulation* 1996;93:519–524.
24. Epstein AE, Carlson MD, Fogoros RN, et al. Classification of death in antiarrhythmia trials. *J Am Coll Cardiol* 1996;27:433–442.
25. Singh SN, Fletcher RD, Fisher SG. Amiodarone in patients with congestive heart failure. *N Engl J Med* 1995;333:77–82.
26. SOLVD Investigators. Effect of enalapril on mortality and the development of heart failure in asymptomatic patients with reduced left ventricular ejection fraction. *N Engl J Med* 1992;327:669–677.
27. Holmes J, Kubo SH, Cody RJ, Kligfield P. Arrhythmias in ischemic and nonischemic dilated cardiomyopathy: prediction of mortality by ambulatory electrocardiography. *Am J Cardiol* 1985;55:146–151.
28. Meinertz TE, Hofmann T, Kasper W, et al. Significance of ventricular arrhythmias in idiopathic dilated cardiomyopathy. *Am J Cardiol* 1984;53:902–907.
29. von Olshausen K, Schafer A, Mehmel HC, Schwarz F, Senges J, Kubler W. Ventricular arrhythmias in idiopathic dilated cardiomyopathy. *Br Heart J* 1984;51:195–201.
30. Unverferth DV, Magorien RD, Moeschberger ML, Baker PB, Fetters JK, Leier CV. Factors influencing one-year mortality of dilated cardiomyopathy. *Am J Cardiol* 1984;54:147–152.
31. Doval HC, Nul DR, Grancelli HO, Perrone SV, Bortman GR, Curiel R. Randomised trial of low-dose amiodarone in severe congestive heart failure. Grupo de Estudio de la Sobrevida en la Insuficiencia Cardiaca en Argentina (GESICA). *Lancet* 1994;344:493–498.
32. Moss AJ, Hall JW, Cannom DS, et al. Improved survival with an implanted defibrillator in patients with coronary disease at high risk for ventricular arrhythmia. *N Engl J Med* 1996;335:1933–1940.
33. Buxton AE, Lee KL, Fisher JD, et al. A randomized study of the prevention of sudden death in patients with coronary artery disease. *N Engl J Med* 1999; 341:1882–1890.
34. Buxton AE, Lee KJ, DiCarlo L, et al. Electrophysiologic testing to identify patients with coronary artery disease who are at risk for sudden death. *N Engl J Med* 2000;342:1937–1945.

35. The Antiarrhythmics Versus Implantable Defibrillators (AVID) Investigators. A comparison of antiarrhythmic drug therapy with implantable defibrillators in patients resuscitated from near-fatal ventricular arrhythmias. *N Engl J Med* 1997;337:1556–1583.
36. Bardy GH. The Sudden Cardiac Death-Heart Failure Trial (SCD-HeFT). In: Woosley RL, Singh SN, eds. *Arrhythmia Treatment and Therapy*. New York: Dekker, 2000:323–342.
37. Flaker GC, Blackshear JL, McBride R, et al. Antiarrrhythmic drug therapy and cardiac mortality in atrial fibrillation (AFFIRM). *J Am Coll Cardiol* 1992;20:527–532.
38. Waldo AL. Management of atrial fibrillation: the need for AFFIRMative action. AFFIRM investigators. Atrial Fibrillation Follow-up Investigation of Rhythm Management. *Am J Cardiol* 1999;84:698–700.
39. Torp-Pedersen C, Moller M, Bloch-Thomsen PE, et al. Dofetilide in patients with congestive heart failure and left ventricular dysfunction. *N Engl J Med* 1999;341:857–865.

Chapter 14

Moving Ahead with Heart Failure: What Does the Future Hold?

James B. Young, MD

Over the past two decades, our understanding of the pathophysiology of heart failure has expanded substantially.[1–4] This insight has driven development and application of new drugs and devices for treatment of this challenging condition. Despite this fact, heart failure remains epidemic and patients suffer greatly with the problem. The morbidity and mortality of heart failure remain high. Indeed, recent studies of patients hospitalized for decompensated congestive heart failure indicate that the 6-month mortality and/or hospitalization rate is 20–30%. This observation, along with the profound suffering advanced congestive heart failure causes, pushes clinicians and investigators to develop even better approaches to diagnose, prevent, and treat the syndrome of heart failure. Perhaps it is important to first review the evolution of heart failure therapies as they relate to knowledge gained over the past several decades.

Evolution of Heart Failure Therapies

Table 1 summarizes how expanding insight into the pathophysiology and clinical characteristics of heart failure gained has impacted therapeutic strategies.[1] The syndrome of heart failure was most often linked to a dropsical condition with generalized edema caused by fluid retention. Obviously, treatments focused on removal of this abnormal fluid buildup. Of course, many dropsical conditions were not caused by heart failure (hepatic cirrhosis and myxedema, for example). After making the link between dropsical conditions and myocardial and circulatory

From: Jessup M, McCauley KM (eds). *Heart Failure: Providing Optimal Care.* Elmsford, NY: Futura, an imprint of Blackwell Publishing; ©2003.

Table 1

Evolution of Heart Failure Therapies

Clinical insights	Therapies
• Observation of a "dropsical", fluid-retaining condition	• Primitive diuretics • Lymphatic drains • Cavity taps • Foxglove tea
• Heart failure due to central pump inadequacy	• Cardiac glycosides • Other inotropes • Heart transplant • VAD/TAH
• Heart failure precipitated by "decompensated" LVH	• Antihypertensives • Valve repair
• Heart failure due to circulatory dysfunction	• Vasodilators
• Heart failure is an endocrinopathy	• ACEIs • ARBs • Beta-blockers • Aldosterone antagonism
• Heart failure is a fever	• Cytokine modulation

ACEI, angiotensin-converting enzyme inhibitor; ARB, angiotensin-receptor blocker; LVH, left ventricular hypertrophy; TAH, total artificial heart; VAD, ventricular assist device.

failure, primitive approaches included prescription of herbal diuretics, lymphatic and thoracic or abdominal cavity drainage, and even a primitive inotrope, as found in foxglove tea. Understanding that a central pump insufficiency was the prime defect in heart failure directed attention to the use of more sophisticated cardiac glycoside (inotropic) preparations and pursuit of alternative inotropic therapies. Obviously, cardiac transplantation and use of mechanical circulatory assist devices or total artificial hearts for end-stage heart failure are attractive, because these approaches more definitively address this primary problem. Understanding that ventricular hypertrophy was a cause of cardiac decompensation directed clinicians toward treating hypertension and valvular heart disease to prevent development of pathologic myocardial hypertrophy. We now know that treating these difficulties early is extraordinarily important if we wish to interdict heart failure at its inception. More recently, attention has been paid to the circulatory dysfunction of heart failure (in addition to the central pump inadequacy), and this has led to use of drugs having beneficial effects other than as a diuretic or inotrope. Indeed, the prescription of vasodilators for heart failure was a direct outgrowth of this. Clarification of the endocrinopathy and inflammatory nature of heart failure has supported the use of neurohormonal blocking agents and anti-inflammatory maneuvers to ameliorate the syndrome.

Even the definition of heart failure has changed.[1,4,5] The contemporary definition of heart failure is complicated. Heart failure is best understood as a milieu of cardiac pump dysfunction (either systolic or diastolic or varying combinations), myocardial remodeling (ventricular hypertrophy, chamber dilation, interstitial fibrosis), hormonal, cytokine, and neuroregulatory perturbation, all of which cause subsequent circulatory inadequacy. Structural heart lesions may precipitate or be a component of the syndrome, as may arrhythmias. Heart failure is no longer simply characterized as a dropsical state or inadequate cardiac output to meet the body's metabolic needs.

Also important has been the understanding that many different diseases can cause myocardial injury with subsequent acute or chronic myocardial dysfunction which leads to heart failure. Prevention of this primary injury has become paramount to successful interdiction of the syndrome. Future directions in heart failure diagnosis will undoubtedly focus upon even earlier identification of patients at risk for heart failure. Indeed, the recently published American College of Cardiology/ American Heart Association guidelines for heart failure diagnosis and management have created four distinct categorizations of patients either having, or at risk for developing, heart failure:[5]

- Stage A includes individuals with diseases placing them at high risk for having heart failure but without structural heart disease or symptoms of heart failure at the time of presentation. These are patients with hypertension, coronary heart disease, diabetes mellitus, individuals exposed to cardiotoxins such as alcohol or anthracyclines, or those with a history of familial cardiomyopathy.
- Stage B patients are those with structural heart disease but no traditional symptoms of heart failure. They are individuals who have had prior myocardial infarction, have known systolic or diastolic left ventricular dysfunction, or have asymptomatic valvular heart disease.
- Stage C patients are those with known structural heart disease and prior or current symptoms of heart failure. The symptoms might include short-windedness, fatigue, and reduced exercise tolerance or, perhaps, arrhythmias.
- Stage D patients are those with refractory heart failure who require specialized interventions to ameliorate symptoms. They are patients who have marked symptoms at rest despite maximal medical therapy (that is, those who are recurrently hospitalized or cannot be safely discharged from the hospital without specialized intervention).

This new categorization of heart failure will, undoubtedly, evolve even further.

Current Areas of Investigation in Heart Failure Therapeutics

Table 2 lists both general and specific areas where progress in heart failure is to be anticipated. New medications, including inotropic compounds, such as levosimendan, pimobendan, and enoximone, are currently being studied. These agents as a group are both calcium-sensitizing drugs and phosphodiesterase inhibitors.[6,7] Traditional neuro-

Table 2

Evolution of Heart Failure Therapies – General Areas of Progress

New medications
Inotropes (levosimendan, pimobendan, enoximone)
Neurohormonal antagonists (ARBs, endothelin antagonists, aldosterone antagonists, beta-blockers)
Diuretics (AVP antagonists)
Natriuretic peptides (BNP, NEP, ACEI)
Cytokine antagonists (P54 enzyme inhibitor)

New operations
Infarct "exclusion"
Elimination of valvular regurgitation
Atrial fibrillation operations
Remodeling surgery (Acorn, MyoSplint)
Cell transplants

Mechanical circulatory sustenance
New VADs (continuous versus pulsatile flow)
New TAHs
Alternative short-term support (ECMO, therapeutic shunts)

Electrophysiologic approaches
AICD
Biventricular pacing

Diagnostics
New definition of heart failure
Better echocardiography
BNP levels

ACEI, angiotensin-converting enzyme inhibitor; AICD, automatic implantable cardioverter defibrillator; ARB, angiotensin-receptor blocker; AVP, arginine vasopressin antagonist; BNP, B-natriuretic peptide; ECMO, extracorporeal membrane oxygenation; NEP, neutral endopeptidase inhibitor; TAH, total artificial heart; VAD, ventricular assist device.

hormonal antagonists, such as the angiotensin-receptor blocking drugs and aldosterone antagonists, as well as beta-blockers, are receiving new attention by focusing on heart failure patients not previously studied in clinical trials.[8–16] An evolving classification and development of neurohormonal antagonists includes the endothelin-blocking agents, such as bosentan and tezosentan.[17,18] Achieving effective diuresis with substantive safety has been difficult with currently available diuretics, and some arginine vasopressin antagonists are currently being developed and are in clinical trials.[1,2,4] Perhaps these drugs will be better and safer diuretics, alone or in combination with currently available agents. Natriuretic peptides have been studied as therapeutic agents and B-type natriuretic peptide (nesiritide) is now available for intravenous infusion in decompensated congestive heart failure patients.[19] The neutral endopeptidase/angiotensin-converting enzyme inhibitor omapatrilat conceptually provides unique advantages in heart failure patients.[20,21] Cytokine antagonists and immune-modulating systems are also still being evaluated.[22] Interestingly, a variety of new surgical procedures for advanced heart failure are emerging and being explored. Infarct exclusion operations with surgical removal of myocardial infarction scar and, sometimes, repair of mitral and/or tricuspid valve insufficiency provide effective surgical remodeling in heart failure.[23] In appropriately selected patients, this appears highly effective in attenuating symptoms and forestalling further detrimental remodeling. Also, elimination of valvular regurgitation in severely dilated hearts is gaining favor. A variety of operations for atrial fibrillation, a vexatious problem in the setting of heart failure, are now available. Other forms of remodeling surgery utilizing devices which constrain the heart (the Acorn cardiac support device) or reshape the left ventricle (the MyoSplint cardiac skewer) are currently being evaluated in clinical trials. Autologous and heterologous cell transplantation holds promise. Mechanical circulatory support devices, including new ventricular assist devices and new total artificial heart systems, continue to excite ill patients and heart failure treatment specialists.[24,25] Other alternative short-term support devices with improved extracorporeal membrane oxygenation system and devices to create therapeutic shunts may have promise. Electrophysiologic approaches to patients with heart failure include more widespread use of automated internal cardioverter defibrillating devices and biventricular cardiac resynchronization pacemakers.[26–28] Also important is the fact that new diagnostic procedures—including new definitions of heart failure, as already outlined, better echocardiographic techniques (including tissue Doppler characterization of failing hearts), and more routine use of neurohormonal levels such as B-natriuretic peptide quantification—are emerging.[5,29,30] The specifics of some of these advances are worth exploring.

Mechanical Circulatory Support

The long-term use of a left ventricular assist device for advanced end-stage heart failure in patients who are not candidates for cardiac transplantation has recently been reported.[24,25] The Randomized Evaluation of Mechanical Assistance for the Treatment of Congestive Heart Failure (REMATCH) trial randomly assigned 129 patients with end-stage heart failure who were ineligible for cardiac transplantation to receive either the HeartMate left ventricular assist device (68 patients) or continuation of "optimal" medical management (61 patients). Patients all had New York Heart Association (NYHA) class 4 heart failure. The primary reason for not being a heart transplant candidate was usually older age. The mean age of the study cohort was about 67 years, with approximately 80% being males. The majority had ischemic heart disease, and the mean left ventricular ejection fraction was approximately 17%. Around 70% of the patients were receiving continuous infusion of intravenous inotropic agents at the time of randomization. Kaplan–Meier survival analysis showed a reduction of 48% in the risk of death from any cause in the group that received left ventricular assist devices compared to the medical therapy group (relative risk 0.52; 95% confidence interval, 0.34–0.78; $P = 0.001$). The survival rate at 1 year was 52% in the device group and 25% in the medical therapy group ($P = 0.002$), and the rates at 2 years were 23% and 8% for each group, respectively ($P = 0.09$). The frequency of serious adverse events, however, in the device group was 2.3 times that in the medical therapy group (95% confidence interval, 1.86–2.95), with most problems relating to infection, bleeding, stroke, or device malfunction. Some aspects of quality of life were significantly improved at 1 year in the device group. Further study of the data suggested that it was the patients who were on continuous intravenous inotropic support who received all of the mortality benefit. No effect on survival was noted when patients not on inotropic support were compared to the left ventricular assist device group.

Bothersome was the morbidity, but nonetheless, this was the first clinical trial to demonstrate that "destination" therapy with left ventricular assist devices could achieve significantly improved outcomes compared to more rudimentary medical therapeutics. Perhaps encouraging is the fact that continuous-flow left ventricular assist devices such as the MicroMed, Jarvik 2000, and HeartMate II appear to be simpler units, with improved mechanical reliability and decreased infection rates. These devices are currently in trials to serve as a "bridge to heart transplantation," but soon will enter "destination" therapy studies.

Another approach to mechanical circulatory sustenance is the total artificial heart. The AbioCor system is an extremely sophisticated total cardiac prosthesis which is completely implantable. Energy sources are transmitted through the chest with a transcutaneous energy transmission system, and the device controller is completely implanted. The obvious advantage of this device is that no external penetrating communication exists. The absence of skin rents means that, hopefully, the incidence of device-related infection will drop to zero. In the seven recent implants, however, the majority of patients have either died or suffered significant morbidity with cerebrovascular events. Whether or not total artificial heart systems or ventricular assist devices will eventually predominate as destination therapy in treatment of end-stage heart failure is unclear, but many believe that left ventricular assist devices have the advantage.

Defibrillator Therapies

Sudden cardiac death has always been a vexing problem in patients with left ventricular systolic dysfunction. Troubling is the fact that many stable, compensated congestive heart failure patients with reasonable peripheral organ function would drop dead without warning. Several studies have suggested that routine antiarrhythmic prescription in these at-risk patient populations was not wise. On the other hand, several relatively small trials evaluated use of implantable defibrillators to attenuate mortality in these patients (with or without concomitant antiarrhythmic medications). The final results of the Multicenter Automatic Defibrillator Implantation Trial-II (MADIT-II) have been presented and confirm a survival benefit from implantable cardioverter defibrillators (ICDs) in patients with a history of myocardial infarction and left ventricular dysfunction manifest as an ejection fraction of 30% or less.[27] Previous results from the first MADIT and the Multicenter Unsustained Tachycardia Trial (MUSTT) had shown a benefit from ICD implantation in patients with heart disease, reduced ventricular function, unsustained ventricular arrhythmia, and inducible ventricular tachycardia at the time of electrophysiologic testing. These were relatively small trials. In the MADIT-I and MUSTT trials, patients underwent electrophysiologic testing to determine their risk of arrhythmia. MADIT-II, however, did not use this strategy. MADIT-II included 1232 patients from 71 United States and five European centers, and patients were randomized to receive either an ICD or continue on conventional medical therapy. Randomization was done in a 3:2 ratio, with 742 patients assigned to receive an ICD. Interestingly, the trial was halted early by the data safety and monitoring committee because of overwhelming efficacy noted in the ICD arm. During an average follow-up of 20 months, the mortality rate in the ICD group was only 14% compared to about 20% in the conventional therapy group—a 31% reduction in the risk of death, with highly significant P values. It is relevant to point out that the major impact the ICD had was on the diminution of sudden cardiac deaths. There was no impact, as might be expected, on deaths due to progressive heart failure, and hospitalization rates were not different between the two groups. This suggests that ICD implantation in heart failure patients meeting MADIT-II entry criteria will save lives but not interdict the progressive nature and pathophysiology of the heart failure syndrome. Coupling defibrillator technology to other heart failure treatment approaches designed to interdict disease progression is, obviously, important. The use of cardiac resynchronization therapy with biventricular pacing strategies could be the answer.

Biventricular Pacing to Achieve Cardiac Resynchronization

Cardiac dyssynergy is noted in about 30–50% of heart failure patients. It is marked by interventricular conduction defects and wide QRS complexes.[26,28] It is associated with higher morbidity and mortality. Small studies have demonstrated that cardiac resynchronization therapy with biventricular pacing can narrow the QRS complex, improve coordination of left ventricular contraction, improve diastolic filling parameters, and decrease mitral regurgitation. Two large clinical trials, the Myocardial Infarction Risk Recognition and Conversion of Life-threatening Events into Survival (MIRACLE) trial and the MIRACLE-ICD trial (both employing Medtronic devices), studied NYHA class 3 and 4 patients with symptomatic congestive heart failure despite optimal medication management.[26,28] The MIRACLE trial focused on patients without a pacemaker or ICD indication, whereas the MIRACLE-ICD trial studied patients with an ICD indication. These studies required prolonged QRS intervals (greater than 130 ms) for entry. Both clinical trials demonstrated significant and substantial effects on patients' symptoms, quality of life, maximal exercise times, maximal oxygen consumption and, at 6 months, physiologic improvement in cardiac pump performance that could be interpreted as beneficial reverse remodeling. Left ventricular volumes were decreased, diastolic filling times normalized, ejection fraction increased, and valvular regurgitation was lessened in many patients. Also important was the fact that in the MIRACLE-ICD trial, having a biventricular pacing system in place did not appear to be proarrhythmic and did not interfere with normal ICD function. Similar findings with the Guidant CONTAK-CD device have also been reported. This unit was recently approved by the Food and Drug Administration for use in New York Heart Association class III and IV congestive heart failure patients on reasonable medication therapies but still significantly symptomatic and having an ICD indication with a wide QRS complex.

The MIRACLE, MIRACLE-ICD, CONTAK-CD, and MADIT-II trials had quite broad implications with respect to the pool of patients who have ICD indications and symptomatic heart failure.[28] These patients appear to benefit from cardiac resynchronization therapy coupled to an ICD device. Resynchronization therapy appears to beneficially alter the pathophysiology of heart failure by interdicting detrimental ventricular remodeling, and the ICD seems to attenuate sudden cardiac death syndrome in these patients. Ongoing studies, such as the Comparison of Medical Therapy, Pacing and Defibrillation in Chronic Heart Failure (COMPANION) trial and Sudden Cardiac Death in Heart Failure Trial (SCD-HeFT), will give us more insight into proper patient selection and risk–benefit calculations for device implantation.[28]

New Applications of Older Pharmacologic Agents

The use of angiotensin-receptor blocking drugs in heart failure has been attractive, in view of the fact that angiotensin-converting enzyme (ACE) inhibitors have been so effective. Angiotensin-receptor blocking drugs may be better tolerated. On the other hand, angiotensin-receptor blocking agents do not activate the cyclooxygenase system as do angiotensin-converting enzyme inhibitors. Furthermore, angiotensin I levels are higher in patients receiving angiotensin-receptor blockers than in those on converting enzyme inhibitors. The recently published large-scale randomized trial of the angiotensin-receptor blocking agent valsartan in heart failure (Valsartan–Heart Failure Trial, Val-HeFT) produced interesting results and provided more insight into this important issue.[11] In that study, a total of 5010 patients with heart failure (NYHA class II–IV) were randomly assigned to receive 160 mg of valsartan or placebo twice daily. The primary efficacy analysis was mortality, with a second primary endpoint being the combined mortality and morbidity (defined as the incidence of cardiac arrest with resuscitation, hospitalization for heart failure, or receipt of intravenous inotropic or vasodilator therapy for at least four hours). Overall, mortality was similar in the two groups. However, the incidence of the combined endpoint was 13.2% less with valsartan than with placebo (relative risk 0.87; 97.5% confidence interval, 0.77–0.97; $P = 0.009$), predominantly because of a lower number of patients hospitalized for heart failure in the valsartan group ($P < 0.001$). Treatment with valsartan also resulted in significant improvements in NYHA class, ejection fraction, signs and symptoms of heart failure, and quality of life as compared with placebo. In a post-hoc analysis of the combined endpoint of mortality and morbidity, in subgroups defined according to baseline treatment with angiotensin-converting enzyme inhibitors or beta-blockers, valsartan had a favorable effect in patients receiving neither or one of these types of drugs. There was, however, an adverse effect in patients receiving both types of drug, although this point estimate observation was not statistically significant. Valsartan significantly reduces the combined endpoint of mortality and morbidity and improves clinical signs and symptoms in patients with heart failure when added to prescribed therapy. However, the post-hoc observation of an adverse effect on mortality and morbidity in the subgroup receiving valsartan, an angiotensin-converting enzyme inhibitor, and a beta-blocker raises concern about the potential safety of this specific combination. The ongoing Candesartan in Heart Failure Assessment in Reduction of Mortality (CHARM) trial, which is evaluating the angiotensin-receptor blocking agent candesartan in a wide spectrum of heart failure patients, will hopefully resolve some of these issues.

Perhaps of some additional relevance are recent studies evaluating angiotensin-receptor blocking agents in diabetics at risk of renal disease progression. Although these were not heart failure trials *per se*, some important insights into best-management practices for diabetics at risk of developing heart failure are presented. In the Reduction of Endpoints in Noninsulin-dependent Diabetes Mellitus with Angiotensin II Antagonist Losartan (RENAAL) study, patients were randomized to receiver either losartan or placebo in addition to standard therapies.[8–10] Both of these hypertensive diabetic groups continued to receive conventional blood-pressure medications, with 751 patients randomized to losartan 50 or 100 mg and 762 patients to placebo. The primary endpoint of the study was a composite measure consisting of time to the first occurrence of either doubling the serum creatinine, development of end-stage renal disease, or death. Results demonstrated that patients taking losartan had a significant reduction in the risk of renal disease progression by 16% ($P = 0.024$). About 44% of patients in the losartan group reached the primary composite endpoint, compared to 47% of patients in the placebo group. It was demonstrated that the renal protective effect of losartan was largely independent of its blood pressure-lowering effects. This study also examined the effects of treatment on cardiovascular events using a composite of heart attack, stroke, revascularization, hospitalization for unstable angina, hospitalization for heart failure, and cardiovascular death. There were similar effects in both treatment and control groups for this composite. When each of these events were analyzed, however, hospitalization for heart failure was significantly reduced in the losartan group (32% reduction, $P = 0.005$; 12% versus 17% for losartan and placebo). As has been noted in other studies of angiotensin-receptor blockers, losartan was generally well tolerated.

Irbesartan has also been demonstrated to slow progression of diabetic nephropathy and should be also looked at in the context of the losartan observations. Perhaps these beneficial effects are class-specific rather than drug-specific. Irbesartan has been studied recently, and it significantly slowed the development of diabetic nephropathy in hypertensive patients with type 2 diabetes and microalbuminuria.[9] The Irbesartan Microalbuminuria Type 2 Diabetes Mellitus in Hypertensive Patients (IRMA II) trial was a 2-year randomized international study focused on hypertension management. Specifically, this trial demonstrated that irbesartan significantly reduced progression from microalbuminuria to overt diabetic nephropathy by up to 70% ($P = 0.0004$), depending on the dose. The number of patients reaching the clinical endpoint of overt albuminuria was also significantly decreased with irbesartan in a dose-dependent manner in comparison with the control group (5.2% versus 15%, respectively; $P = 0.0004$). The percentage of patients with a reduction in microalbuminuria to normal levels was also increased with irbesartan therapy (33% versus 20%; $P = 0.006$). Like trials with losartan, the fact that blood pressure was controlled to nearly the same degree in the irbesartan and control groups suggests that some of the irbesartan benefit was independent of blood pressure reduction. This study, coupled with observations made in the previously reviewed trials, has great promise when one considers the prevalence of diabetes and renal insufficiency in heart failure.

These studies should also be viewed in light of the recently reported Losartan Intervention For Endpoint Reduction in Hypertension (LIFE) trial, which evaluated losartan in hypertensive patients without heart failure but with, sometimes, diabetes.[12,13] This trial evaluated cardiovascular morbidity and mortality in a double-blinded randomized parallel group study of over 9000 patients aged 55–80 years with essential hypertension. Participants were assigned to either daily losartan-based or atenolol-based antihypertensive treatment for at least 4 years, and until slightly over 1000 patients had a primary cardiovascular event (death, myocardial infarction, or stroke). Blood pressure fell by about 30 and 17 mmHg in the losartan and atenolol groups, respectively. The primary composite endpoint occurred in 508 losartan patients (about 24 per 1000 patient-years) and 588 atenolol patients (about 28 per 1000 patient years; relative risk 0.87; 95% confidence interval, 0.77–0.98; $P = 0.021$). There were 204 deaths from cardiovascular disease in the losartan group versus 234 deaths in the atenolol group (risk ratio 0.89; $P = 0.026$), but nonfatal stroke was significantly reduced, with a risk ratio of 0.75 ($P = 0.001$). Furthermore, new-onset diabetes mellitus was less frequent with losartan therapy. Again, the implications for these observations with respect to development of heart failure are great. Nonetheless, before one turns to angiotensin-receptor blocking drugs in this patient population, more definitive information must be made available. Furthermore, questions regarding secondary outcomes of cardiovascular events have blurred conclusions that can be made from these studies. Cardiovascular events actually may have increased in these two trials. As mentioned, these findings make the CHARM trial particularly important.[16] CHARM specifically is designed to evaluate candesartan in combination with ACE inhibition as well as in ACE intolerant patients with heart failure. The morbidity/mortality endpoints of this large heart failure clinical trial (9000 patients) will likely answer these questions. But one must still remember that angiotensin-converting enzyme inhibitors still produce substantial benefit with respect to atherosclerotic cardiovascular endpoints generally. A recently published substudy from the Heart Outcomes Prevention Evaluation trial (HOPE) found that ramipril reduces the incidence of stroke in high-risk patients even if blood pressure is not significantly reduced.[8]

New Pharmacologic Agents for Heart Failure

Several new drugs have undergone evaluation in heart failure populations. Interestingly, despite beneficial observations in earlier studies, the angiotensin-converting enzyme and neutral endopeptidase inhibitor omapatrilat, was not superior to the ACE inhibitor enalapril in the Omapatrilat Versus Enalapril Randomized Trial of Utility in Reducing Events (OVERTURE) study.[21] It did appear that the two drugs were equivalent with respect to outcomes. This is a bit perplexing, as the dual mechanism of action of omapatrilat theoretically would produce substantive benefit. Perhaps if omapatrilat had been compared to placebo it would have shown a more clear benefit, but the drug probably needs to show a benefit over angiotensin-converting enzyme inhibitors in order to have a place in heart failure therapeutics. Details of the study show that OVERTURE included 5770 patients with NYHA class II–IV heart failure symptoms and left ventricular ejection fraction less than 30%. Patients were required to have been hospitalized for heart failure within 12 months of randomization. All were to receive optimal therapies for heart failure and 50% were on beta-blockers, 40% on spironolactone, and 60% on digoxin. They were then randomized to enalapril 10 mg b.i.d. or omapatrilat 50 mg q.d. The primary endpoint was all-cause mortality and congestive heart failure hospitalizations. There was a 6% reduction in this endpoint with omapatrilat, but this did not reach statistical significance. All of the predefined subgroup analyses showed similar results, with trends toward benefit with omapatrilat in all groups, but none that reached statistical significance. Adverse effects showed a lower rate of heart failure and impaired renal function with omapatrilat, but a higher rate of hypotension and dizziness. Angioedema, which has been an issue with omapatrilat in hypertensive patients, was slightly higher in the omapatrilat group, but it was not a meaningful or statistically significant observation. It is important to remember that omapatrilat is a potent antihypertensive drug. Possibly, in the heart failure patients, this turned out to be a detrimental effect. The observations in the OVERTURE trial should be put into the perspective of omapatrilat hypertension studies.[20,21] The Omapatrilat Cardiovascular Treatment Assessment Versus Enalapril (OCTAVE) trial showed that omapatrilat was associated with greater reductions in blood pressure than enalapril, which was seen across all types of patients and suggested that the agent was the most effective hypertensive agent yet developed and studied.[20] The major issue was whether or not angioneurotic edema would limit its utility. A total of 2.17% of patients with omapatrilat versus 0.68% of patients on enalapril developed angioneurotic edema over this 24-week hypertension trial. The risk of angioedema was higher in black patients than nonblacks and in smokers than nonsmokers

The Endothelin Antagonist Bosentan for Lowering Cardiac Events (ENABLE) trial studied the endothelin antagonist bosentan in patients with congestive heart failure.[17] Because endothelin is a powerful vasoconstricting agent thought to be important in detrimental remodeling of the pulmonary and peripheral vasculature (and the myocardium), blocking this agent's receptor site has appeal. Preliminary studies had suggested that bosentan produced seemingly beneficial hemodynamic changes in heart failure patients. In the ENABLE trial, however, there were nonsignificant trends to reduction in all-cause mortality and the composite of death and congestive heart failure hospitalization favoring bosentan. The fact that the ENABLE program did not demonstrate significant reduction in major heart failure morbidity and mortality was disappointing, given the fact that endothelin is such a potent vasoconstricting agent and an attractive target for therapeutics in heart failure. There was some suggestion that the dose of bosentan in the ENABLE trials was excessive. As with omapatrilat, perhaps overly aggressive blood pressure reduction created difficulties. Also important in the ENABLE study was that some patients on bosentan demonstrated excessive fluid retention, reflected by early and sustained increases in body weight, decreases in hemoglobin, and increases in peripheral edema. Indeed, the early fluid retention state was associated with a greater risk of adverse outcomes. Perhaps future studies can be performed at lower doses of bosentan. But the observations on bosentan in heart failure should be placed in the perspective of the Bosentan Randomized Trial of Endothelin Antagonist Therapy.[18] This study focused on pulmonary hypertension patients and did demonstrate that bosentan was beneficial in this group and well tolerated. Indeed, this trial has led to the approval of bosentan as an endothelin-receptor antagonist useful for primary pulmonary hypertension.

Eplerenone is an aldosterone antagonist similar to spironolactone, but devoid of some of the nuisance complications such as painful gynecomastia.[31] Results of one eplerenone study suggest that in patients with mild to moderate hypertension and left ventricular hypertrophy by echocardiography who were randomized to receive eplerenone (added onto a thiazide diuretic and/or amlodipine), the drug reduced left ventricular mass. This observation is quite interesting, though still a surrogate for adverse clinical outcome. If studies confirm these findings, perhaps eplerenone will be an agent to study further in heart failure. Indeed, an ongoing clinical trial, the Eplerenone Post-AMI Heart Failure Efficacy and Survival Study (EPHESUS), is now underway, with over 6400 patients enrolled.[31] This trial is investigating whether use of eplerenone will have a beneficial effect on survival and morbidity in patients with myocardial infarction and left ventricular systolic dysfunction over and above all other medications.

Levosimendan

Levosimendan is a newer myocyte calcium-sensitizing agent currently being developed for short-term treatment of decompensated congestive heart failure patients.[6,7] Experimental studies have indicated that levosimendan increases myocardial contractility, reduces filling pressure, and dilates both the peripheral and coronary blood vessels. The positive inotropic action of levosimendan is brought about by the calcium-dependent binding of the drug troponin, whilst its vasodilative mechanism of actions due to the opening of adenosine 5-triphosphate (ATP)-dependent K-channels in vascular smooth muscle. Although levosimendan acts preferentially as a calcium sensitizer, it also has demonstrated selective phosphodiesterase-3 inhibitory effects *in vitro* at high combinations. This selective inhibition does not contribute to the positive inotropic action at pharmacologically relevant concentrations. Previous studies have suggested that levosimendan is beneficial in decompensated congestive heart failure patients. Interestingly, in two clinical trials, the Levosimendan Infusion versus Dobutamine (LIDO) and RUSSLAN studies, acute exposure to the drug seemed to beneficially affect mortality at the 6-month follow-up point. Clinical trials are currently being designed to evaluate the potential for this drug to reduce morbidity and mortality in acutely hospitalized heart failure patients. One would hope that the detrimental effects in decompensated heart failure patients previously seen with parenteral inotropes will not be noted with this agent.

Nesiritide versus Milrinone in Acute Decompensated Heart Failure

Two important clinical trials of heart failure management strategies were recently reported.[19,31,32] Results of the Vasodilation in the Management of Acute Congestive Heart Failure (VMAC) trial demonstrated that intravenous nesiritide or B-type natriuretic peptide (BNP) improves hemodynamic functions and symptoms of heart failure better than nitroglycerine in patients with acute decompensated congestive heart failure necessitating hospital admission.[19] On the other hand, the Outcomes of a Prospective Trial of Intravenous Milrinone for Exacerbations of Chronic Heart Failure (OPTIME-CHF) study showed no benefit and some harm when routine milrinone was administered to hospitalized heart failure patients.[32,33] Milrinone seemingly caused more symptomatic hypotension and problematic arrhythmias than did placebo. The VMAC trial randomized 489 patients with decompensated congestive heart failure and dyspnea at rest to receive either intravenous nesiritide or intravenous nitroglycerine or a placebo.[19] The primary endpoints were change in pulmonary capillary wedge pressure (PCWP) among catheterized patients and patients' self-evaluation of dyspnea at three hours. Nesiritide was more effective than nitroglycerine or placebo in reducing PCWP and more effective than placebo in relief of dyspnea but not significantly different than nitroglycerine in this regard.

OPTIME-CHF was also a placebo-controlled trial that included 951 patients admitted to the hospital with an exacerbation of systolic heart failure.[32,33] Patients were randomized to a 48-h infusion of either milrinone or placebo in addition to standard therapy. Although milrinone is indicated for, and often used, to treat patients with decompensated heart failure, OPTIME-CHF patients were not in such severe heart failure that, in the opinion of the treating physician, inotropic or vasopressor agents were absolutely required. With respect to the primary endpoints, there was no difference in the number of days hospitalized for cardiovascular causes within 60 days after randomization, or in-hospital mortality, 60-day mortality, or the composite of death and readmission, between patients receiving milrinone or not. However, the incidence of sustained hypotension requiring intervention was significantly higher in the milrinone group, as was the incidence of new atrial arrhythmias.

B-Type Natriuretic Peptide as a Diagnostic Test

In addition to mechanical and pharmacologic agents emerging as important in the treatment of heart failure, new diagnostic tools are becoming available.[4,29,30] Implantable hemodynamic monitoring devices and techniques to assess transthoracic bio-impedance produce, perhaps, important information that might be helpful in managing heart failure patients. A simple, relatively inexpensive point-of-care test to quantify serum B-type natriuretic peptide levels has recently been developed and introduced into practice. Small and now larger-sized clinical trials have studied the utility of this measurement. The Breathing Not Properly (BNP) trial suggested that serum levels of brain natriuretic peptide could be helpful to differentiate symptomatic congestive heart failure from other difficulties causing dyspnea.[30] In a 1586-patient, prospective, blinded study evaluating rapid B-type natriuretic peptide level measurements in individuals presenting to the emergency room, those who ultimately proved to have significant congestive heart failure had significantly higher levels of B-type natriuretic peptide than those not having heart failure. Indeed, in patients with NYHA class 1 heart failure, the average BNP level was 150 pg/mL versus those who were in class II (250 pg/mL), versus those in class III (550 pg/mL), versus those in class IV (900 pg/mL). Overall, the sensitivity of the BNP cut-off of 100 pg/mL was 90% and the specificity for a congestive heart failure diagnosis was 74%. This cut-off point provided for an accurate diagnosis 81% of the time. By comparison, clinical judgment produced an ultimately accurate diagnosis in only 74% of the patients. In terms of clinician diagnostic certainty, physicians indicated they were unsure of the appropriate diagnosis in 43% of cases, with BNP levels clarifying the situation in most of these instances. This study emphasized the importance of utilizing BNP measurements for diagnosing significant congestive heart failure. Other studies have shown the utility of the measurement for prognostication in patients with known heart failure syndromes.

Emerging Surgical Approaches to Heart Failure

Apart from the utilization of ventricular assist devices, surgical approaches to heart failure are continuing to play a substantive role in treating patients with ventricular dysfunction.[23] Arguably the most important of these are coronary revascularization strategies. It has been long known and well recognized that ischemic and viable but hibernating myocardium responds to restoration of perfusion and improved blood supply. More aggressive intervention in patients with depressed left ventricular ejection fraction and viable myocardium is justified. Coupling revascularization procedures to surgical remodeling of the heart is proving an effective means to alleviate congestive heart failure symptoms. So-called infarct exclusion procedures, where scarred myocardium is removed and more normal-shaped ventricles crafted, have great promise. Often, these operations are coupled with repair of the mitral valve when significant mitral regurgitation is present.

In those with dilated cardiomyopathy and significant mitral or tricuspid regurgitation, elimination of this volume overload condition has also helped selected patients improve symptoms and increase exercise tolerance. Other forms of surgical remodeling utilize devices to contain cardiac enlargement and dilation (the Acorn cardiac support device) or physically reshape the heart (the MyoSplint). The Acorn device is a sock-like fabric mesh covering that is rolled up over and around the heart, whereas the MyoSplint is a skewer placed across the left ventricular cavity chamber to produce a left ventricle with a figure-of-eight shape. This latter device will cause a reduction in wall stress by changing the dilated and globular-shaped left ventricle into a bilobed configuration.

For the moment, cell transplantation for myocardial failure is quite early with respect to clinical trials and still relegated to surgical injection of cultured cells into infarcted zones of the heart. Procedures utilizing cell-transforming agents can produce myoblasts from skeletal muscle biopsies that are introduced into tissue culture media. These cells can then be injected into the heart, with the hope that a matrix will develop of new myocytes that will contract, relax, and electrically conduct in a reasonably normal fashion. Another tissue-engineering technique is to stimulate the endogenous bone marrow production of stem cells that can then be released to migrate to acutely injured myocardium. Also possible is to use bone-marrow transplant techniques to harvest and later reinject appropriate myocyte progenitor cells. All of these techniques are quite experimental at the moment. We do not know the feasibility of this approach, and the risks of proarrhythmia or tumor formation are unclear. Nonetheless, this is a promising avenue of research, as is gene transfer. Transfer of genes capable of inducing new blood vessel formation may also be an attractive strategy to benefit patients with heart failure due to significant coronary heart disease.

Summary

With the development of newer pharmaceutical agents for heart failure and understanding new uses of currently available drugs, patients with significant left ventricular dysfunction and heart failure stand to benefit in the future. Furthermore, new surgical and electrophysiologic procedures hold great promise as well. Finally, gaining further insight into the pathophysiology of heart failure and, particularly, the molecular biodynamics and pharmacogenomics of this difficulty will spur along other new and exciting developments.

References

1. Young JB, Mills RM. *Clinical Management of Heart Failure.* West Islip, NY: Professional Communications, 2001.
2. Mills RM, Young JB. *Practical Approaches to the Treatment of Heart Failure.* Baltimore: Williams & Wilkins, 1998.

3. Kirklin JK, Young JB, McGiffin DC. *Heart Transplantation.* Philadelphia: Churchill Livingstone, 2002.
4. Young JB. Heart failure. *Cardiol Clin* 2001;19:541–681.
5. American Heart Association and American College of Cardiology Task Force on Diagnosis and Management of Heart Failure. *Pocket Guideline for the Diagnosis and Management of Heart Failure.* Bethesda, MD: American Heart Association and American College of Cardiology, 2002.
6. Foloath F, Slawsky MT, Nieminen MS, et al. Dose ranging and safety with intravenous levosimendan and low output heart failure: experience in three pilot studies and outline of Levosimendan Infusion versus Dobutamine (LIDO) trial. *Am J Cardiol* 1999;83(12B):21–25.
7. Moiseyev V, Poder P, Andrejevs N, et al. RUSSLAN Study Investigators. Safety and efficacy of a novel calcium sensitizer, levosimendan, in patients with left ventricular failure due to an acute myocardial infarction. *Eur Heart J* 2002;23:1422–1432.
8. Sica DA, Bakris GL. Type 2 diabetes: RENAAL and IDNT—the emergence of new treatment options. *J Clin Hypertens* 2002;4:52–57.
9. Epstein M, Tobe S. What is the optimal strategy to intensify blood pressure control and prevent progression of renal failure? *Curr Hypertens Rep* 2002;3: 422–428.
10. Coats AJ. Angiotensin receptor blockers—finally the evidence is coming in: IDNT and RENAAL. *Int J Cardiol* 2002;79:99–102.
11. Cohn JN, Tognoni G. A randomized trial of the angiotensin-receptor blocker valsartan for chronic heart failure. *N Engl J Med* 2001;345:1667–1675.
12. Dahlof B, Devereux RV, Kjeldsen SE, et al. Cardiovascular morbidity and mortality in the losartan intervention for endpoint reduction in hypertension study (LIFE): a randomized trial against atenolol. *Lancet* 2002;359:995–1003.
13. Lindholm LH, Ibsen H, Dahlof B, et al. Cardiovascular morbidity and mortality in patients with diabetes in the losartan intervention for endpoint reduction in hypertension study (LIFE): a randomized trial against atenolol. *Lancet* 2002;359:1004–1010.
14. Bosch J, Yusuf S, Pogue J, et al. Use of ramipril in preventing stroke: A double blind randomized trial. *BMJ* 2002;324:699–702.
15. Zanella M, Ribieiro A. The role of angiotensin II antagonism in type II diabetes mellitus: a review of renoprotection studies. *Clin Ther* 2002;24: 1019–1034.
16. [Web site]. Candesartan cilexetil (candesartan) in heart failure: assessment of reduction in mortality and morbidity (CHARM) program (www.charmnet.net).
17. [Web site]. ENABLE: Non-significant trend to benefit, but investigation into bosentan for CHF may continue (www.theheart.org).
18. Ruben LJ, Badesch DB, Barst RJ, et al. Bosentan therapy for pulmonary arterial hypertension. *N Engl J Med* 2002;346:896–903.
19. [Anonymous.] Intravenous nesiritide vs. nitroglycerin for treatment of decompensated congestive heart failure: a randomized controlled trial. *JAMA* 2002;287:1531–1540.
20. [Web site]. OCTAVE—Omapatrilat in hypertension: 2.17% of angioedema (www.theheart.org).
21. [Web site]. OVERTURE—Omapatrilat: no better than enalapril in heart failure (www.theheart.org).
22. Lisman KA, Stetson SJ, Koerner MM, et al. Managing heart failure with immunomodulatory agents. *Cardiol Clin* 2001;19:617–626.

23. Kumpati GS, McCarthy PM, Hoercher KJ. Surgical treatments for heart failure. *Cardiol Clin* 2001;19:669–682.
24. Rose EA, Gelijns AC, Moskowitz AJ, et al. Long-term use of a left ventricular-assist device for end-stage heart failure (REMATCH). *N Engl J Med* 2001;345: 1435–1443.
25. Stevenson LW. End-stage heart failure patients already prescribed IV inotropic drugs benefit most from LVAD (www.theheart.org).
26. Young JB. ICD plus bi-ventricular pacer safe and effective in severe heart failure: InSync ICD (www.theheart.org).
27. Moss AJ, Zareba W, Hall WJ, et al. Prophylactic implantation of a defibrillator in patients with myocardial infarction and reduced ejection fraction (MADIT-II). *N Engl J Med* 2002;346:877–883.
28. Pavia SV, Wilkoff BL. Biventricular pacing for heart failure. *Cardiol Clin* 2001;19:637–652.
29. Maisel A. B-type natriuretic peptide and the diagnosis and management of congestive heart failure. *Cardiol Clin* 2001;19:557–572.
30. [Web site]. Breathing Not Properly trial (BNP) indicates B-type natriuretic peptides tests should be incorporated into ACC/AHA CHF guidelines (www.theheart.org).
31. [Web site]. 4E Trial: eplerenone/enalapril combo reduces blood pressure and left ventricular hypertrophy in essential hypertension (www.theheart.org).
32. Cuff MS, Califf RM, Adams KF Jr, et al. Short-term intravenous milrinone for acute exacerbation of chronic heart failure: a randomized controlled trial (OPTIME-CHF). *JAMA* 2002;287:1541–1547.
33. Poole-Wilson PA. Treatment of acute heart failure: out with the old, in with the new. *JAMA* 2002;287:1578–1580.

Index

Page numbers in *italics* refer to figures and those in **bold** to tables